AF794458

Polysaccharide Biomaterials in Cancer Research and Therapy

Scrivener Publishing
100 Cummings Center, Suite 541J
Beverly, MA 01915-6106

Publishers at Scrivener
Martin Scrivener (martin@scrivenerpublishing.com)
Phillip Carmical (pcarmical@scrivenerpublishing.com)

Polysaccharide Biomaterials in Cancer Research and Therapy

From Lab to Life

Edited by

Luqman Jameel Rather

College of Sericulture, Textile and Biomass Science, Southwest University, Chongqing, P.R. China

Showkat Ali Ganie

College of Sericulture, Textile and Biomass Science, Southwest University, Chongqing, P.R. China

and

Mohammed A. Assiri

Department of Chemistry, Faculty of Science, King Khalid University, Abha, Saudi Arabia

Scrivener Publishing

WILEY

This edition first published 2026 by John Wiley & Sons, Inc., 111 River Street, Hoboken, NJ 07030, USA and Scrivener Publishing LLC, 100 Cummings Center, Suite 541J, Beverly, MA 01915, USA
© 2026 Scrivener Publishing LLC
For more information about Scrivener publications please visit www.scrivenerpublishing.com.

All rights reserved. No part of this publication may be reproduced, stored in a retrieval system, or transmitted, in any form or by any means, electronic, mechanical, photocopying, recording, or otherwise, except as permitted by law. Advice on how to obtain permission to reuse material from this title is available at http://www.wiley.com/go/permissions.

Wiley Global Headquarters
111 River Street, Hoboken, NJ 07030, USA

For details of our global editorial offices, customer services, and more information about Wiley products visit us at www.wiley.com.

The manufacturer's authorized representative according to the EU General Product Safety Regulation is Wiley-VCH GmbH, Boschstr. 12, 69469 Weinheim, Germany, e-mail: Product_Safety@wiley.com.

Limit of Liability/Disclaimer of Warranty
While the publisher and authors have used their best efforts in preparing this work, they make no representations or warranties with respect to the accuracy or completeness of the contents of this work and specifically disclaim all warranties, including without limitation any implied warranties of merchantability or fitness for a particular purpose. No warranty may be created or extended by sales representatives, written sales materials, or promotional statements for this work. The fact that an organization, website, or product is referred to in this work as a citation and/or potential source of further information does not mean that the publisher and authors endorse the information or services the organization, website, or product may provide or recommendations it may make. This work is sold with the understanding that the publisher is not engaged in rendering professional services. The advice and strategies contained herein may not be suitable for your situation. You should consult with a specialist where appropriate. Neither the publisher nor authors shall be liable for any loss of profit or any other commercial damages, including but not limited to special, incidental, consequential, or other damages. Further, readers should be aware that websites listed in this work may have changed or disappeared between when this work was written and when it is read.

Library of Congress Cataloging-in-Publication Data

ISBN 978-1-394-34544-1

Cover image: Generated with AI using Adobe Firefly
Cover design by Russell Richardson

Set in size of 11pt and Minion Pro by Manila Typesetting Company, Makati, Philippines

Printed in the USA

10 9 8 7 6 5 4 3 2 1

Contents

Preface

Cancer remains one of the most formidable health challenges of our time, demanding the continual pursuit of novel therapeutic approaches. Among the many recent advancements in oncology, polysaccharide-based biomaterials have emerged as highly promising candidates for enhancing cancer treatment strategies. Their biocompatibility, biodegradability, and multifunctional properties make them ideal for applications such as drug delivery, immunomodulation, and targeted therapy.

This book presents a comprehensive overview of the latest progress in this dynamic field. It compiles pioneering research on the structural, biophysical, and functional characteristics of various polysaccharides, detailing their therapeutic roles in oncology. By examining key materials such as inulin, chitosan, cyclodextrins, hyaluronic acid, and beta-glucans, the book underscores the transformative potential of these biomaterials in modern cancer treatment.

The chapters are designed to serve researchers, clinicians, and industry professionals alike—bridging the gap between foundational research and clinical application. With a multidisciplinary approach, the book integrates insights from material science, nanotechnology, and biomedical engineering to foster innovative solutions in cancer therapy.

We hope this volume proves to be a valuable resource for scholars and practitioners seeking efficient, biocompatible approaches to cancer treatment. As science continues to evolve, we believe polysaccharide biomaterials will play a vital role in shaping the future of oncology, offering safer and more effective therapeutic options.

Luqman Jameel Rather
Showkat Ali Ganie
Mohammed A. Assiri
December 2025

Preface

Acknowledgment

The completion of this book would not have been possible without the contributions, guidance, and encouragement of many individuals and organizations.

First and foremost, we extend our heartfelt gratitude to all the authors who contributed their invaluable research and insights. Their dedication and expertise have enriched this volume, making it a significant reference in the field of cancer research.

We sincerely appreciate the support of our respective institutions and research teams, who provided an environment conducive to scholarly pursuits. Their encouragement and collaboration played a crucial role in shaping this book.

Our deepest thanks go to our families and friends, whose patience, understanding, and unwavering support sustained us throughout this journey.

We also extend our appreciation to Martin Scrivener and Scrivener Publishing for their professionalism and commitment to bringing this book to life. Their editorial and production teams have been instrumental in refining and presenting our work in the best possible manner.

Finally, we acknowledge all researchers, scientists, and medical professionals working tirelessly in the field of cancer treatment. Their dedication inspires us to continue exploring new frontiers in biomedical innovation.

Luqman Jameel Rather
Showkat Ali Ganie
Mohammed A. Assiri

Acknowledgments

1

Introduction to Polysaccharides in Cancer Therapy: Unveiling the Therapeutic Potential

Suvarna Yenduri* **and Naga Prashant K.**

Faculty of Pharmacy, Sri Adichunchanagiri College of Pharmacy, Adichunchanagiri University, Karnataka, India

Abstract

Significant contributions of polysaccharides to a number of biological processes, including cell–cell interaction, inflammation, immunological response, and metabolism, have been demonstrated during the last 10 years by growing data. The possible therapeutic advantages of these complex carbohydrates in pathophysiological diseases, like cancer, have been studied. This chapter describes many traditional polysaccharide-based cancer therapy strategies together with the fundamental working principles of each. We also discuss recent neo-therapeutic developments in immunotherapy, imino sugars, small compounds, pro-drugs, and vaccinations. Correlating these therapeutic approaches with particular targets—be they proteins, enzymes, malfunctioning cell organelles, or genes expressed during cancer development—needs an understanding of the basic phases of cancer. The shift in cancer treatment approaches toward precision medicine represents a significant departure in the prevailing paradigm, made possible by the special qualities of polysaccharides such as antiangiogenic properties, antioxidant effects, regulating mitochondrial activity, antagonizing cell cycle checkpoints, immunomodulation, and ease of chemical modifications, which is also covered in this chapter. Lastly, the challenges and opportunities for the utilization of polysaccharides in neo-chemotherapeutic fields are discussed.

Keywords: Polysaccharides, neo-chemotherapy, cell cycle checkpoints, immunomodulation, antioxidant effect

**Corresponding author*: Suvarna.ph52@gmail.com

Luqman Jameel Rather, Showkat Ali Ganie and Mohammed A. Assiri (eds.) Polysaccharide Biomaterials in Cancer Research and Therapy: From Lab to Life, (1–24) © 2026 Scrivener Publishing LLC

1.1 Introduction

Polysaccharides are naturally derived polymeric macromolecules that are typically constituted with more than 10 saccharin units that are connected with each [1]. Long chains of monosaccharides interconnected by glycosidic links are known as polysaccharides or polymeric carbohydrate molecules [2]. Simple sugar polymers are also referred to as polysaccharides or nano polysaccharides (monosaccharide) [3]. Brown algae, photosynthetic plants, fungus, and bacteria can all be the primary producers of polysaccharides. The structural polysaccharides on an organism's membrane or cell wall, or the stored polysaccharides in the cytoplasm, are portrayed by the polysaccharide derivatives at the cellular level. The manner in which the polysaccharides are collected and refined is affected directly by their chemistry and assembly [4]. Polysaccharides are one of the widely used natural compounds in various fields especially in drug-delivery systems and also for several therapeutic effects. Polysaccharides are one of the important natural compounds used in cancer therapy. Because of the multiple side effects shown by the synthetic compounds during chemotherapy, there is a need for natural compounds for treatments of cancer [5–7].

1.1.1 Overview of Polysaccharides

Polysaccharides include substances like chitin, starch, and cellulose. In accordance with the sugar molecules, they can be categorized as homopolysaccharides and heteropolysaccharides (Figure 1.1). Polysaccharides are composed of distinct saccharin units interconnected by either α or β glycosidic linkage in the main or side branch. There are four basic forms of polysaccharide chains: primary, secondary, tertiary, and quaternary. These chains contain various kinds of connections and binding groups [3].

Bioactive biopolymers are mostly found in polysaccharides or polysaccharide–protein complexes as glucans having different glycosidic linkages like (1→3)-α-glucans and (1→3), (1→6)-α-glucans. These polysaccharides possess an array of fascinating properties, notably immunomodulation and anticancer effects. *Lentinus edodes*, *Schizophyllum commune*, and *Coriolus versicolor* produce lentinan, Schizophyllan, and protein-bound polysaccharides, respectively, which show antitumor properties [8]. Polysaccharide applications can be divided into two major categories: the first involves their role as an excipient in pharmaceutical formulations.

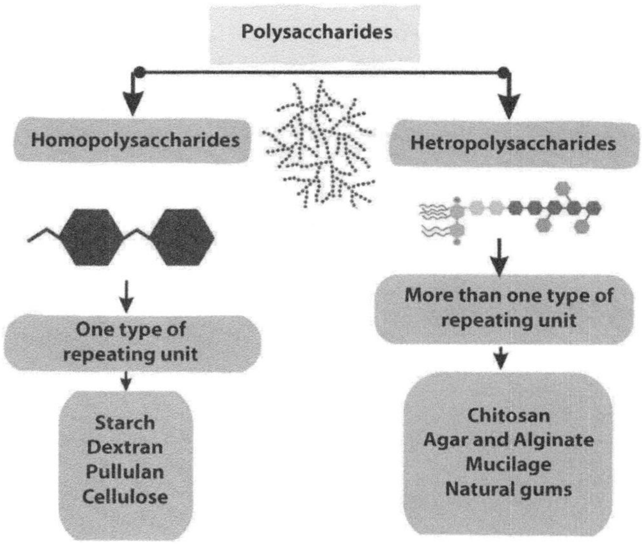

Figure 1.1 Classification of polysaccharides.

Polysaccharides may form gels, exert strong osmotic pressure, be viscous, and absorb water. Their unique physical and chemical properties make them appropriate for pharmaceutical substances, drug transporters, drug release agents, plasma replacements, etc. Plant, animal, seaweed, and fungal polysaccharides have attracted attention due to their wide spectrum of medicinal properties. All animals, microbes, algae, and plants contain polysaccharides in enormous amounts. Another use of polysaccharides is their biological activity, such as antitumor activity, antigenicity, and biological activity, related to preparing vaccines and new drugs (Figure 1.2) [1].

Polysaccharides, abundant in plants, are the source of biological energy. Seaweeds such agar, furcellaran, and alginates; seeds like tamarind gum, guar gum, and psyllium seed gum; extracts like pectin; and exudates like tragacanth, arabica, and karaya gums are the main sources of plant polysaccharides [9]. Plant polysaccharides are explored in food and medicine due to their many biological activities, safety, effectiveness, and low toxicity. Chemical structure determines plant polysaccharide biological activity. Immunoregulation, anti-oxidation, antiviral, hypoglycemic, anti-hepatic damage, and antineoplastic actions have been found [10].

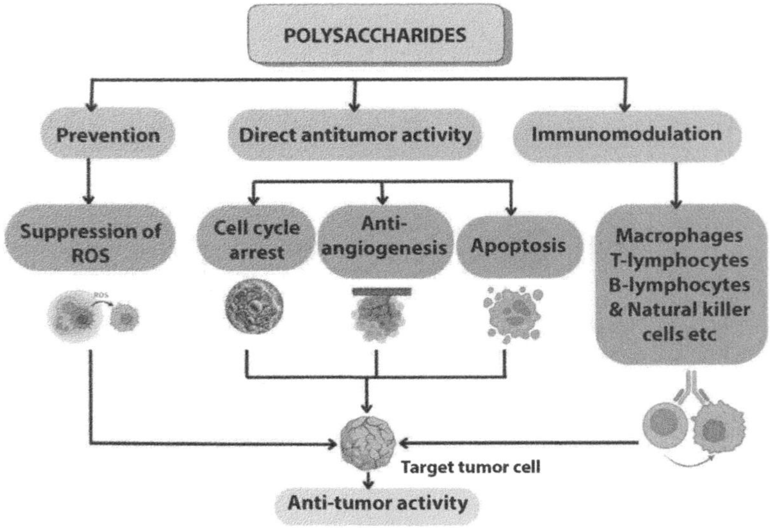

Figure 1.2 Various modes of action shown by polysaccharides for antitumor activity [1].

1.1.2 Historical Perspective in Medicine

Polysaccharides show a wide range of biological activities including immunoregulatory, anticancer, hypolipidemic, antioxidant, and hypoglycemic effects [11]. According to pharmacological research, polysaccharides offer several beneficial medical properties, including the ability to prevent cancer, increase plasma testosterone levels, reduce fatigue, inhibit fibrosis, provide hypoglycemic impact, and protect the kidneys from radiation [12]. Some of the polysaccharides and their therapeutic effects are listed in Table 1.1. Most of the polysaccharide's immunological activities are linked to bacterial lipopolysaccharides *via* lipid A. Despite lacking the lipid moiety, polysaccharides from plants, fungi, yeasts, and algae interact with humoral defense cells and molecules. Due to their immune system stimulatory effects, these interactions may increase innate and adaptive immune responses. These effects can be caused by interactions or complex reaction cascades. These polysaccharides may be employed as therapeutic agents due to their antibacterial, antiviral, antitussive, radioprotective, antiseptic shock, and antitumor immunological properties. Polysaccharides may interact with immune system components, causing cellular and molecular events that may stimulate the immune system. In reaction to polysaccharides, complement proteins attach to monocytes, macrophages, dendritic cells, neutrophils, and lymphocytes [19]. Molecular structure and weight

Table 1.1 Polysaccharides and their therapeutic effects.

S. no.	Polysaccharide source	Action	Therapeutic effect	Ref.
1	*Cyclocarya paliurus*	Anti-apoptotic protection, high insulin production, and moderate toxicity	Diabetes mellitus	[11]
2	Heparin	Blocking complement activation, deactivating chemokines, blocking neutrophil-derived elastase, and shielding vascular endothelial cells from harmful substances	Anti-inflammatory	[13]
3	*Salvia officinalis*	Anticancer, inhibited angiogenesis *via* VEGF, immunostimulatory effects on Sarcoma 180 tumor cells	Breast cancer	[14]
4	Astragalus polysaccharide (APS) and β-glucans from *Ganoderma lucidum*	Activates macrophages, monocytes, dendritic cells, Toll-like receptors (TLR) to produce cytokines, chemokines, and pro-inflammatory substances for robust immune response	Antitumor activity	[15, 16]
5	*Ganoderma atrum*	Activate spleen lymphocytes and peritoneal macrophages through chemoprotection	-	[17]
6	*D. indusiata's*	-	Immune-modulatory, antioxidant, and anticancer	[17]
7	*Cordyceps sinensis* mycelia	Stimulate dendritic and macrophage activities		[17]
8	*Lonicera japonica*	-	Anti-inflammatory, antiviral, anticoagulant, antioxidant, anticancer, and anti-atherosclerotic effects	[18]
9	Japanese ginseng (LJP-31)	Immunostimulant activity through the activation of MAPK and NF-kB signaling pathways mediated by TLR4	-	[18]

of dietary polysaccharides affect immune responses. Most marine algae rich in sulfated polysaccharides, which reduce inflammation and allergic responses, influence the innate immune system and complement system differently. Sulfated polysaccharides activate complement, promote nitric oxide synthase and cytokines, disrupt leukocyte migration, enhance primary antibody immune responses, bind to pattern recognition receptors, affect macrophage function, and alter cecum intestinal flora. They also boost lymphocyte, macrophage, and NK cell tumor cytotoxicity [20].

1.2 Role of Polysaccharides in Current Cancer Therapy

Because of their distinct biological characteristics and possible therapeutic advantages, polysaccharides are receiving a lot of interest as a cancer treatment. Their important roles in modern cancer therapies are immunomodulatory effects, cytotoxic effect, antagonistic effect on various cell cycle checkpoints, regulating mitochondrial functions, etc.

1.2.1 Immunomodulatory Effects of Polysaccharides

The primary mechanism underlying the immunostimulatory, antitumor, antibacterial, and other therapeutic effects of botanical polysaccharides seems to involve the regulation of the complement system and the stimulation of macrophages. Consequently, the modulation of innate immunity significantly influences the host's ability to respond rapidly and effectively to various infections [21]. TNF-α was reduced in RAW 264.7 cells by (1 → 3; 1 → 6)-β-D-polysaccharides from *P. linteus* and *P. igniarius*, indicating an immunosuppressive effect. Moreover, these polysaccharides strongly suppressed the transcription of IL-6 and elevated the IL-10 response [22]. Sulfated polysaccharides, which were either extracted from plants or synthesized artificially, found to possess superior biological characteristics compared with non-sulfated ones. Sulfated polysaccharides act as immunomodulators by controlling immune complement systems like T/B lymphocytes, natural killer cells (NK cells) and macrophages to preserve homeostasis. They stimulate the complement system, thereby inducing the production of antibodies and stimulating cytokine release. They also control the phagocytosis of macrophages and indirectly stimulate the release of nitric oxide (NO), interleukin (IL)-6, and other cytokines by macrophages. Immune function can also be enhanced by sulfate modification, which also has the potential to greatly increase the activities of both immunosuppressed and normal mice macrophages. This effect may be attributed to the control of immune cell signal transduction [23]. Porphyran, a sulfated polysaccharide obtained from red sea weeds (Porphyra), shows anticancer property through several pathways like immunomodulation, interfering in NF-kB pathway, inhibiting cell proliferation, inducing apoptosis, etc. [24].

Polysaccharides are a primary bioactive component present in mushrooms. In RAW264.7 macrophage cells, edible fungal polysaccharides regulate cytokines and other factors to execute immunomodulatory actions. Activated macrophages generate elevated levels of mediators such as TNF-α, ROS, NO, IL-1β, and IL-6. Macrophages play a vital role in the human immune system's defense against microbial infections. To attack pathogens such as viruses and bacteria, they emit various inflammatory mediators, cytokines, and engage in phagocytic activities. Activated macrophage host defense mechanisms are mediated by nitric oxide, a crucial intracellular signaling molecule. It also modulates the immune system by functioning as a cytotoxic agent. Pro-inflammatory factors TNF-α and IL-1β can increase the production of supplementary immunomodulatory molecules and enhance the immune response in macrophages. Besides controlling inflammation, phagocytosis, and antigen presentation, IL-6 provides T cells with the third signal that governs both humoral and cellular immunity [25].

Some of the polysaccharides obtained from mushrooms like Schizophyllan from *Schizophyllum commune*, Lentinan from *Lentinus edodes*, Grifolan from *Grifola frondose*, and polysaccharide protein complex and protein bound polysaccharides from *Trametes versicolor* were found to have potent anticancer properties by causing immunomodulatory effects with the activation of immunomodulatory cytokines [26]. Ginsenosides, or ginseng polysaccharides (GPs), activate and suppress the immune system. As an immunoadjuvant, they aid immunizations. Ginsenosides (GP) regulate several pathways, including MAPK. MAPKs are intracellular enzymes that stimulate cytokine production, which causes inflammation and GTPase stimulation to upstream protein kinases that are triggered by mitogens. Signaling enzymes monitor cellular mechanisms like activation, degranulation, and proliferation during this sequential activation pathway. These enzymes include p38, ERK, and JNK. After MPAK activation, serine/threonine kinases phosphorylate p38 MAPK. Inflammatory mediators are created by p38 MAPK-dependent transcription and post-transcriptional regulation. Mediators of inflammation and allergies are transcribed *via* the NF-κB pathway, activated by MAPKs and translocated into the nucleus. Innate immune cells like neutrophils and macrophages initiate the immune system's response. Invasive bacteria like lipopolysaccharide (LPS) or Th1 cytokines like IFNγ and TNF-α activate M1 macrophages, which are critical to inflammatory processes. They are also known for upregulating pro-inflammatory genes such COX-2, iNOS, TNF-α, IL-1β, and IL-6, which can lead to inflammatory disorders [27].

Ganoderma species are one of the major sources of polysaccharides and have been utilized as dietary supplements in Chinese medicine. These polysaccharides can exhibit antitumor, immunomodulatory, and anti-inflammatory effects. These polysaccharides contain β-(1 → 3)-D-glucan with (1 → 6)-β-D-glucosyl branches containing glucose, galactose, and mannose as saccharin units. Ganoderma polysaccharides (GLPs) show anticancer effect by activating different immune responses in host. Their unique immunomodulatory effects are because of binding to specific sites on monocytes, macrophages, neutrophils, NK cells, granulocytes, etc. [28]. Polysaccharide obtained from *Astragalus membranaceus* acts on various immune cells like lymphocytes, NK cells, macrophages, dendritic cells, chemokines, etc. to produce immunomodulatory effect and thus is useful for treating cancer, diabetes, asthma, auto-immune diseases, etc. It also acts on immune organs such as spleen, lymph nodes, thymus, bone marrow, etc. [29].

1.2.2 Selective Toxicity toward Cancer Cells

It has been shown that numerous types of polysaccharides exhibit cytotoxicity on different cancer cell lines without causing harm to healthy tissues. Polysaccharides that were extracted from various sources such as pomegranate fruit, edible fungus, shrimp shells, green tea leaves, and traditional Chinese herbs were found to have cytotoxic activity. The pomegranate-derived galactomannan (PSP001) showed anticancer efficacy by reducing the angiogenesis, invasion, migration, and colonization—four critical steps in the metastatic cascade [30]. Ulvan, a sulfated polysaccharide obtained from Ulva rigida, was found to have anticancer properties. When tested on cell lines, Ulvan showed significant cytotoxic effect on HCT-116. The study revealed the polysaccharide Ulvan as a potential anticancer agent for treating human colon cancer and also confirmed that no side effects were produced when it was tested on zebra fish [31].

1.2.3 Cell Cycle Checkpoint Antagonist

Cell cycle checkpoints are regulatory systems that ensure proper advancement of the eukaryotic cell cycle. Every checkpoint functions as a potential endpoint in the cell cycle, where the status of the cell is assessed, and only when favorable conditions are met does the cell proceed through its various phases. The cell cycle contains a number of checkpoints [32]. Although there are numerous checkpoints, the three primary ones are:

a) G1 checkpoint (Major checkpoint, Start checkpoint, or Restriction checkpoint)
b) G2/M checkpoint
c) Spindle check point (metaphase to anaphase transition check point) (Figure 1.3).

The cyclin-dependent kinases were activated by cyclins (regulatory protein subunits), which are synthesized in different forms at each phase of the cell cycle to control unique activities of that phase, and are mostly accountable for advancing through these checkpoints [33].

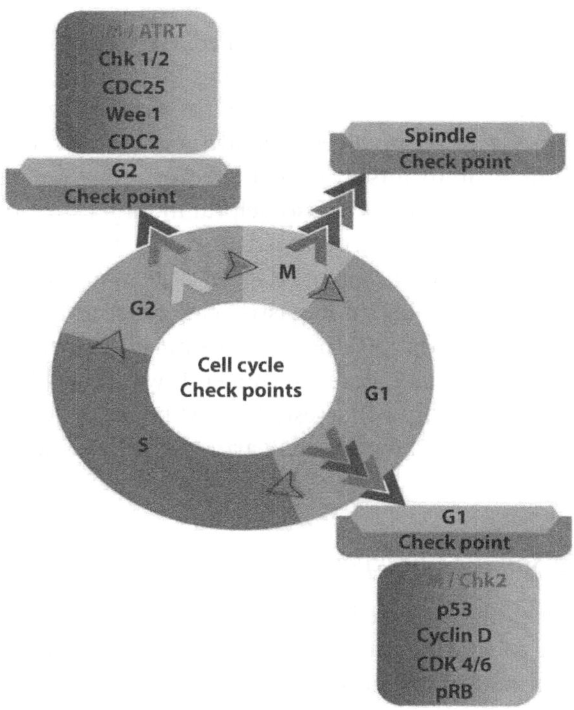

Figure 1.3 Cell cycle checkpoints.

1.2.3.1 G1 (Restriction) Checkpoint

At the G1 checkpoint, cell commits to the cell cycle. It is considered as restriction point mammalian cells; in case of yeast, it is the starting point. As the cell moves through G1, it can either delay G1, go through the restriction point, or enter a quiescent state called G0, depending on internal and external factors. The primary sign that a cell should "restrict" and avoid going through the cell cycle is DNA damage. The cell decides to enter the S phase and initiate cyclin-CDK-dependent transcription in order to initiate a new round of cell division. This checkpoint guarantees the subsequent steps [34]. A capsular polysaccharide obtained from marine G-ve bacteria *Kangiella japonica* was found to suppress T47D cell proliferation by arresting G0/G1 phase and inducing mitochondrial-dependent apoptosis. This sulfated polysaccharide was found to be efficient against human breast carcinoma cells (T-47D) [35].

1.2.3.2 G2 Checkpoint

A cell goes through a growth phase called G2. The production of the required mitotic proteins takes place during this period, and once again, regulatory process ensures cell readiness for mitotic proliferation. This transition from G2 to M involves several mechanistic checkpoints [36]. GPs were found as adjuvants in cancer therapy. They are also useful for promoting tumor immunity and also helpful in target therapy. Panax ginseng polysaccharide (PGP2a), obtained from the root of *Panax ginseng*, was found to inhibit proliferation of HGC-27 cells by arresting G2/M phase of the cell cycle and thus useful in gastric cancer treatment [37]. Ginseng berry polysaccharide extract (GBPE) and its purified portion (GBPP) was found to be potent against colorectal cancer. It was found that GBPE (300 μg/ml) and GBPP (600 μg/ml) arrested G2/M phase of cell cycle in HCT-116 cell lines, and in HT-29 cells, they arrested both G1 and G2/M phase [38].

1.2.3.3 The Spindle Checkpoint

At the M checkpoint, the cell checks if each sister chromatid is properly connected to spindle microtubules. The cycle will not resume until all chromosomes are stably connected to at least two spindle fibers from opposing cell poles because sister chromatid separation during anaphase is irreversible [39]. A wide range of cell cycle checkpoint inhibitors, including ATM/ATR/CHK1/CHK2/WEE1 inhibitors, has been developed in order to precisely disrupt the processes by which tumor cells react to agents that damage DNA. This is due to the fact that these checkpoints play a major role in the DNA damage response. Originally created to treat p53 mutated tumors due to their compromised G1/S checkpoint, this class of compounds has since been found to be applicable to p53 wild-type tumors as well [40].

Astragalus polysaccharides (APSs) obtained from the dried root of soyabean (*Astragalus*) were found to exhibit antitumor activity. APS is a mixture of macromolecules like glucans and heteropolysaccharides and shows a wide spectrum of pharmacological activities. There is increased research attention toward APS because of its high efficacy and low toxicity properties. An *in vitro* study on MG63 cells revealed that APS downregulated cyclin D1, which helps in the promotion of mitotic cell division from the G1 phase to S phase [41]. APS also showed activity against proliferation of HCC cells by arresting the G1 phase of human hepatoma HepG2 cells and also found to inhibit proliferation of SW620 cells (colon cancer) by arresting G2/M phase and thus showed antitumor activity [42].

Polysaccharide extract of fruits of *Rosa roxburghii* showed potential effects on DU145 prostate cancer cell proliferation and apoptosis. RTDP of dose 6 mg/ml showed significant cell cycle arrest of the G0/G1 phase and thus confirmed dose-dependent cell cycle arrest [43]. WSG, a water-soluble glucose enriched polysaccharide obtained from *Ganoderma lucidum*, was found to induce sub G1 and G2/M phase of cell cycle and reduces colony. [44]. *Gayralia brasiliensis* polysaccharide Gb1 may arrest cells in the G1 phase, therefore stopping DNA replication from starting. Moreover, the over-sulfurized derivative of Gb1, known as Gb1-OS, could cause cell arrest in S and G2 phases quite drastically [73]. The polysaccharide derived from *Salvia miltiorrhiza* (SMP) has anti-proliferative properties against cancer cells by halting the cell cycle at the S phase [74].

1.2.3.4 ATM (Ataxia-Telangiectasia Mutated Kinase) and ATR Inhibitors

KuDOS Pharmaceuticals, AstraZeneca produced KU-55933, the first potent ATM inhibitor. Hickinson and colleagues found that KU-55933 increases sensitivity to ionizing radiation and chemotherapeutics that produce DNA double-strand breaks (DSBs), such as topoisomerase II inhibitors (etoposide and doxorubicin in cancer cells) [45]. KU-55933 selects ATM above ATR, DNA-PK, and PI3K by more than 100 times. KU-55933 exposure made cells more susceptible to DNA-damaging chemotherapeutic medicines (etoposide, doxorubicin, and camptothecin) and IR cytotoxicity. This enhances the possibility of these chemicals affecting cells [46]. CP466722 may also inhibit. It was shown that this compound totally inhibited ATM kinase at 6 nmol/L or greater, like KU-60019. Cell culture is sensitive to IR. This molecule may be changed to boost potency and specificity, making it more effective in animal models, and sensitize cells in culture with minimal exposure. But none of these drugs were tested on animals in preclinical studies [47]. GLPs obtained from *Ganoderma lucidum* inhibit DNA-PK and ATM and thus interfere in DNA damage repair. This can be made by inhibiting PI3K/ATK signaling and thus preventing tumor cells in DNA damage repair [48].

1.2.3.5 CHK1/CHK2 Inhibitors

A family of cancer treatments known as CHK1/CHK2 inhibitors specifically target the CHK1 and CHK2 protein kinases. These inhibitors have demonstrated therapeutic effectiveness against a range of cancer types, such as ovarian cancer, triple-negative breast cancer, and solid tumors. Selective inhibitors targeting CHK1 and CHK2 kinases, such as V158411, have shown strong efficacy against cancer cell lines, particularly those with triple-negative breast cancer [49]. Dual CHK1/CHK2 inhibitors, like LY2606368, are being investigated in clinical trials for their potential to treat various types of cancer, including BRCA1/BRCA2-mutant breast and ovarian cancer. These inhibitors can sensitize cancer cells to DNA-damaging treatments, such as radiation therapy, by inhibiting the checkpoint kinases that repair DNA damage. Preclinical studies have shown that CHK1/CHK2 inhibitors can enhance the effectiveness of chemotherapy and radiation therapy in treating cancer. Clinical trials are ongoing to evaluate the safety and efficacy of CHK1/CHK2 inhibitors in combination with other cancer therapies. Overall, CHK1/CHK2 inhibitors hold promise as a new approach to cancer treatment, especially in combination with existing therapies [50].

1.2.3.6 WEE1 Inhibitors

WEE1 inhibitors have been created in large quantities with the goal of blocking cell cycle checkpoint signaling and increasing tumor cells' susceptibility to the harmful effects of various genotoxic substances. A class of cancer treatments known as WEE1 inhibitors specifically target the WEE1 kinase family, which is essential for regulating the cell cycle and identifying and repairing DNA damage in both non-malignant and malignant cells. Within non-cancerous cells, WEE1 functions as a suppressor of tumor growth by inhibiting the reproduction of cells with modified DNA. Nevertheless, in cancer cells, WEE1 functions as an oncogene, often having excessive expression in both solid and hematological tumors [40]. WEE1 inhibitors have shown single agent and chemosensitizer effects in various cancer models, making them a promising therapeutic target for hematological and solid tumors. Several pharmacological inhibitors have been designed and validated in different cancer models, including hematological malignancies such as acute lymphoblastic leukemia, multiple myeloma, and solid tumors like hepatocellular carcinoma, colon cancer, and non-small-cell lung cancer. By targeting WEE1, these inhibitors aim to exploit the oncogenic role of WEE1 in cancer cells, providing a new approach to cancer treatment [51]. The extract of polysaccharides of *Polygonatum cyrtonema* Hua were found to have activity against human cervical cancer cells (Hela). The chelating agent soluble solid fraction (CASS) of polysaccharide extract showed cell cycle block at the G2/M phase by lowering the expression of WEE1, CHK2, CDK1, etc. CASS activated caspase-3 through the cell death receptor and mitochondrial pathways [52].

1.2.4 Mitochondrial Function Regulations

Mitochondria perform various metabolic functions in cancer. In addition to generating ATP through OXPHOS, mitochondria are needed to metabolize lipids, amino acids, the TCA cycle, and nucleic acids [53]. Energy generation, cellular metabolism, apoptosis, calcium and redox balance, and mitochondrial function modulation are critical to cancer progression and development. Mitochondrial failure shifts cancer cells from aerobic respiration to aerobic glycolysis, increasing growth and proliferation [54]. Alterations in mitochondrial dynamics regulators impact mitochondrial fusion and fission, which affects cancer growth. These modifications promote cancer growth, emphasizing mitochondrial function control in cancer [55]. Cancer cells modify mitochondrial fusion and fission, affecting mitochondrial function and progression. In cancer cells, mitochondrial transcription factors change, affecting mitochondrial function and progression [56]. Mutations in mitochondrial DNA, which encodes electron transport and other mitochondrial proteins, cause cancer. Cellular dynamics, transcription, and mitochondrial function determine cancer development. Effective cancer therapies need understanding these pathways [57].

For the polysaccharides obtained from *Dendrobium officinale* (DOP), when studied for its mechanism on colon cancer therapy, it was found that DOP has inhibited the CT26 cell proliferation and increased autophagy level. DOP altered mitochondrial function by raising reactive oxygen species (ROS) and decreasing mitochondrial membrane potential (MMP), limiting ATP production and activating AMPK/mTOR autophagy signaling [58]. Polysaccharide from *Schisandra chinensis* (Turcz.) Baill (SCP) demonstrated strong cytotoxic potential in Caki-1 cells by generating apoptosis, which was associated to inhibiting ERK1/2 phosphorylation and subsequently causing apoptosis in the mitochondrial pathway. *Polygala tenuifolia* Willd. polysaccharide (PTP) treatment in OVCAR-3 cells can inhibit NF-κB expression, leading to cell death signals in the tumor cells' programmed external route [59].

1.2.5 Polysaccharides as Drug Carriers

Polysaccharides are long chains of sugar molecules that can be used as drug carriers due to their unique properties. They offer several advantages, including biodegradability, mucoadhesiveness, and modifiable molecular weight and particle size, making them a safe and effective option for drug delivery. Various types of polysaccharides, such as chitosan, alginate, starch, cellulose, and dextran, can be used as drug carriers. They have applications in oral, injectable, topical, and gene delivery and can be used to enhance drug absorption, provide sustained drug release, and deliver genetic material [60]. Polysaccharides are being studied for use as drug carriers due to their biodegradability, mucoadhesiveness, and ability to modify molecular weight and particle size [61]. Here are some ways polysaccharides are being used as drug carriers. Polysaccharides prevalent in marine environments have been discovered to possess pharmacological properties, including anticancer, immunomodulatory, antioxidant, and anti-inflammatory activity capabilities. The combination of these effects and the medications that are being utilized can have a synergistic therapeutic impact. Microsystems that have a high drug entrapment efficiency may be created in a relatively straightforward and low-cost manner because of their capabilities. Chitosan, alginate, fucoidan, carrageenan, and other polysaccharides are among the aforementioned polysaccharides that have been the focus of intensive investigation as drug carriers during the past several years [57].

Chitosan is a polysaccharide that has been found to have mucoadhesive properties, making it suitable for drug delivery. It has been used to deliver drugs such as vancomycin hydrochloride and betahistine.

Chitosan microparticles can enhance the skin's absorption of proteins, peptides, and low molecular weight polar drugs [62]. Alginate is a polysaccharide that has been found to possess mucoadhesive qualities, which makes it appropriate for the delivery of drugs. Insulin and acyclovir are two medications that have been administered with it [63]. Natural polymers called alginates are frequently used in pharmaceuticals as stabilizing, gel-forming, and viscosity-enhancing agents. Drug-delivery systems that are frequently utilized are membrane microstructures or alginate matrix. Alginate microparticles are used as non-toxic, biocompatible, and biodegradable drug carriers for encasing hydrophilic and hydrophobic active ingredients, such as cells and bioproducts. Natural water-soluble polysaccharides called alginates are taken out of the cell walls of different kinds of brown algae [64]. Fucoidan microparticles are a form of drug delivery that utilizes fucoidan, a sulfated polysaccharide found in brown seaweed. In order to achieve controlled and targeted drug release, fucoidan microparticles have been developed as oral and vaginal delivery systems for the sustained release of antibiotics and antifungal agents. Ofloxacin and posaconazole have been incorporated into fucospheres using a variety of preparation methods, including spray-drying, complexation, and precipitation techniques [65]. Microparticles based on fucoidan have been proposed as viable pulmonary drug-delivery systems for tuberculosis treatment. Doxorubicin-loaded fucoidan-coated microparticles are an additional illustration of the potential of these formulations as drug-delivery vehicles for cancer treatment [66]. It was also studied that anticancer agents along with polysaccharides have shown synergistic effect. In recent studies, irinotecan was combined with fucoidan-based nanoparticles and showed enhanced cytotoxic effect by the increase in their cellular reuptake, especially by colorectal cancer cells and thus showed synergistic effect [67]. Because of high drug-delivery efficacy, controlled drug release, and precise tumor target of polysaccharides, they were considered as the primary choice in formulating nanocarriers, especially in cancer therapy [68].

1.2.6 Polysaccharides in Precision Medicine

Polysaccharides were found to have a major role in precision medicine especially in cancer therapy because of their unique and wide characteristics. As chemotherapy causes toxicity to normal cells, this effect can be overcome by target-based therapy. This can be made possible by polysaccharide-based carriers that act as drug-delivery systems to deliver drug only to cancer cells. The stability and bioavailability of the polysaccharide carriers can be improved by chemical modification. Cyclodextrins, chitin, alginates, chitosan, pectin, cellulose, dextran, and hyaluronic acid are the most widely used polysaccharides in anticancer drug-delivery systems [69].

1.2.7 Role of Artificial Intelligence in Polysaccharide-Based Therapy

AI and ML are significantly altering cancer treatment research and development in modern oncology. Overcoming conventional drug development pipeline restrictions, these technologies enable scientists to create new anticancer treatments more quickly. To uncover new treatment targets, forecast patient reactions, and overcome cancer medicine resistance, artificial intelligence and machine learning can replicate human cognitive processes. The importance of artificial intelligence in identifying novel drug targets has increased [75].

Advancing this field are AI-powered tools such as the largest public cancer drug discovery knowledgebase, canSAR. Using several data sources, canSAR fuels AI-driven models, hence advancing drug discovery. By exposing how cancer-related proteins like tumor-cell signal transduction components and effectors interact with drugs and provide new therapeutic routes, AlphaFold has also improved protein structure prediction. Many issues persist even with these encouraging developments. Big datasets are required to teach these algorithms as data quality and biases might compromise AI model performance. Still, advances in data collecting and sharing will help AI-driven model performance flourish [76].

1.3 Challenges

As polysaccharides are complex macromolecules, there is difficulty in degradation, which results in poor bioavailability and less therapeutic effect [77]. Limited clinical data availability is another drawback to utilize polysaccharide in cancer treatment as the safety and efficacy of polysaccharides in humans are not validated. Gaining regulatory approvals for polysaccharide-based therapy is a lengthy process that delays its availability for treatment [78].

1.4 Future Directions and Potential Therapies

With continued research and development, polysaccharide cancer therapies have a bright future ahead of them. Targeted drug-delivery systems, immunotherapy, and cancer vaccines are being developed to capitalize on the potential of polysaccharides; gene therapy and personalized medicine approaches are also being investigated; polysaccharides are being investigated for their potential to target cancer stem cells, thereby preventing tumor recurrence and metastasis. As research advances, polysaccharide-based therapies are likely to become an essential component of cancer treatment, providing patients with new hope for improved outcomes and an enhanced quality of life [70]. Polysaccharide-based nanoparticles will be engineered to deliver drugs directly to tumors, stimulate antitumor immunity, and deliver genetic material to cancer cells. Personalized polysaccharide-based therapies will be tailored to individual patients' needs, and combination therapies will enhance efficacy [71, 72].

1.5 Conclusion

Polysaccharides have shown promise for cancer treatment because of their ability to target many pathways, offering a multimodal approach to therapy. The selective toxicity of these macromolecules against cancer cells may help to reduce the unpleasant side effects that are sometimes connected to conventional chemotherapy. Because they affect the immune system, polysaccharides can enhance the body's own defenses against the development of cancerous cells. More understanding of polysaccharide participation in cancer therapy will be made possible by the continuing of study into their structural and functional properties, which will pave the way for the creation of revolutionary drugs. This problem underlines the potential of polysaccharides as a cancer therapy. It demonstrates the unique characteristics of polysaccharides and the positive outlook for next studies and medical uses of these substances.

AI disclosure statement: The author acknowledges the use of AI-based tools for minor language editing or grammatical correction. However, all intellectual contributions, analyses, and conclusions presented in this chapter are entirely the author's own.

References

1. Yu, Y., Shen, M., Song, Q., Xie, J., Biological activities and pharmaceutical applications of polysaccharide from natural resources: A review. *Carbohydr. Polym.*, 183, 91–101, 2018, https://doi.org/10.1016/j.carbpol.2017.12.009.
2. Miao, T., Wang, J., Zeng, Y., Liu, G., Chen, X., Polysaccharide-Based Controlled Release Systems for Therapeutics Delivery and Tissue Engineering: From Bench to Bedside. *Adv. Sci.*, 5, 1700513, 2018, https://doi.org/10.1002/advs.201700513.
3. Chaudhary, S., Jain, V.P., Jaiswar, G., The composition of polysaccharides: monosaccharides and binding, group decorating, polysaccharides chains, in: *Innovation in Nano-Polysaccharides for Eco-sustainability*, pp. 83–118, Elsevier, 2022.
4. Leung, M.Y.K., Liu, C., Koon, J.C.M., Fung, K.P., Polysaccharide biological response modifiers. *Immunol. Lett.*, 105, 101–114, 2006, https://doi.org/10.1016/j.imlet.2006.01.009.
5. Manojmouli, C., Pasha, T., Nagaprashant, K., Ramesh, B., Ul, E., Purushotham, K., Flavonoid derivatives as anticancer moiety and its effect on cancer cell lines: An updated review. *J. Serb. Chem. Soc.*, 88, 937–957, 2023, https://doi.org/10.2298/JSC221228041M.
6. Pasha, T.Y., Manojmouli, C., Ramesh, B., Prashant, K.N., Purushotham, K.N., Eain, N.U., Shankar, M., Therapeutic Importance of Biological Half-Life of Antineoplastic Agents- A Review. *Adv. Pharmacol. Pharm.*, 10, 265–272, 2022, https://doi.org/10.13189/app.2022.100405.
7. Koppuravuri, N.P., Bharath, S., Pasha, Y., Car-T Cell Therapy for Cancer: A Review. *Adv. Biores.*, 14, 354–360, 2023, https://doi.org/10.15515/abr.0976-4585.14.4.354360.
8. Ooi, V.E.C. and Liu, F., A Review of Pharmacological Activities of Mushroom Polysaccharides. *Int. J. Med. Mushrooms*, 1, 195–206, 1999, https://doi.org/10.1615/IntJMedMushrooms.v1.i3.10.
9. Bisht, S., Kant, R., Kumar, V., α-d-Glucosidase inhibitory activity of polysaccharide isolated from Acacia tortilis gum exudate. *Int. J. Biol. Macromol.*, 59, 214–220, 2013, https://doi.org/10.1016/j.ijbiomac.2013.04.057.
10. Tan, X., Zhou, X., Chen, H.-G., Structure-activity relationship of plant polysaccharides. *Zhongguo Zhong Yao Za Zhi*, 42, 4104–4109, 2017, https://doi.org/10.19540/j.cnki.cjcmm.20170928.016.
11. Zhu, Z., Lin, W., Ma, J., Li, N., Wang, J., Li, J., The physiochemical characteristics of Cyclocarya paliurus polysaccharides and *in vitro* anti-diabetic effects of their different fractions. *Ind. Crops Prod.*, 211, 118188, 2024, https://doi.org/10.1016/j.indcrop.2024.118188.
12. Meng, L., Sun, S., Li, R., Shen, Z., Wang, P., Jiang, X., Antioxidant activity of polysaccharides produced by Hirsutella sp. and relation with their chemical characteristics. *Carbohydr. Polym.*, 117, 452–457, 2015, https://doi.org/10.1016/j.carbpol.2014.09.076.

13. Brito, A.S., Arimatéia, D.S., Souza, L.R., Lima, M.A., Santos, V.O., Medeiros, V.P., Ferreira, P.A., Silva, R.A., Ferreira, C.V., Justo, G.Z., Leite, E.L., Andrade, G.P.V., Oliveira, F.W., Nader, H.B., Chavante, S.F., Anti-inflammatory properties of a heparin-like glycosaminoglycan with reduced anti-coagulant activity isolated from a marine shrimp. *Bioorg. Med. Chem.*, 16, 9588–9595, 2008, https://doi.org/10.1016/j.bmc.2008.09.020.
14. Cai, Z., Li, W., Wang, H., Yan, W., Zhou, Y., Wang, G., Cui, J., Wang, F., Antitumor and immunomodulating activities of a polysaccharide from the root of Sanguisorba officinalis L. *Int. J. Biol. Macromol.*, 51, 484–488, 2012, https://doi.org/10.1016/j.ijbiomac.2012.05.029.
15. Cheng, B.-H., Chan, J.Y.-W., Chan, B.C.-L., Lin, H.-Q., Han, X.-Q., Zhou, X., Wan, D.C.-C., Wang, Y.-F., Leung, P.-C., Fung, K.-P., Lau, C.B.-S., Structural characterization and immunomodulatory effect of a polysaccharide HCP-2 from Houttuynia cordata. *Carbohydr. Polym.*, 103, 244–249, 2014, https://doi.org/10.1016/j.carbpol.2013.12.048.
16. Qiu, W.-L., Lo, H.-C., Lu, M.-K., Lin, T.-Y., Significance of culture period on the physiochemistry and anti-cancer potentials of polysaccharides from mycelia of Ganoderma lucidum. *Int. J. Biol. Macromol.*, 242, 125181, 2023, https://doi.org/10.1016/j.ijbiomac.2023.125181.
17. Deng, C., Shang, J., Fu, H., Chen, J., Liu, H., Chen, J., Mechanism of the immunostimulatory activity by a polysaccharide from Dictyophora indusiata. *Int. J. Biol. Macromol.*, 91, 752–759, 2016, https://doi.org/10.1016/j.ijbiomac.2016.06.024.
18. Fang, Q., Wang, J.-F., Zha, X.-Q., Cui, S.-H., Cao, L., Luo, J.-P., Immunomodulatory activity on macrophage of a purified polysaccharide extracted from Laminaria japonica. *Carbohydr. Polym.*, 134, 66–73, 2015, https://doi.org/10.1016/j.carbpol.2015.07.070.
19. Ferreira, S.S., Passos, C.P., Madureira, P., Vilanova, M., Coimbra, M.A., Structure–function relationships of immunostimulatory polysaccharides: A review. *Carbohydr. Polym.*, 132, 378–396, 2015, https://doi.org/10.1016/j.carbpol.2015.05.079.
20. Bhatia, S., Rathee, P., Sharma, K., Chaugule, B.B., Kar, N., Bera, T., Immuno-modulation effect of sulphated polysaccharide (porphyran) from Porphyra vietnamensis. *Int. J. Biol. Macromol.*, 57, 50–56, 2013, https://doi.org/10.1016/j.ijbiomac.2013.03.012.
21. Schepetkin, I.A. and Quinn, M.T., Botanical polysaccharides: Macrophage immunomodulation and therapeutic potential. *Int. Immunopharmacol.*, 6, 317–333, 2006, https://doi.org/10.1016/j.intimp.2005.10.005.
22. Suabjakyong, P., Nishimura, K., Toida, T., Griensven, V., L.J.L.D., Structural characterization and immunomodulatory effects of polysaccharides from Phellinus linteus and Phellinus igniarius on the IL-6/IL-10 cytokine balance of the mouse macrophage cell lines (RAW 264.7). *Food Funct.*, 6, 2834–2844, 2015, https://doi.org/10.1039/C5FO00491H.

23. Huang, L., Shen, M., Morris, G.A., Xie, J., Sulfated polysaccharides: Immunomodulation and signaling mechanisms. *Trends Food Sci. Technol.*, 92, 1–11, 2019, https://doi.org/10.1016/j.tifs.2019.08.008.
24. Pradhan, B., Rout, L., Ki, J.-S., Immunomodulatory and anti-inflammatory and anticancer activities of porphyran, a sulfated galactan. *Carbohydr. Polym.*, 301, 120326, 2023, https://doi.org/10.1016/j.carbpol.2022.120326.
25. Yin, Z., Liang, Z., Li, C., Wang, J., Ma, C., Kang, W., Immunomodulatory effects of polysaccharides from edible fungus: a review. *Food Sci. Hum. Wellness*, 10, 393–400, 2021, https://doi.org/10.1016/j.fshw.2021.04.001.
26. Krishnakumar, N.M., Ramesh, B.T., Ceasar, S.A., Medicinal mushrooms as potential sources of anticancer polysaccharides and polysaccharide–protein complexes, in: *Studies in Natural Products Chemistry*, pp. 113–148, 2023.
27. Balasubramaniam, M., Sapuan, S., Hashim, I.F., Ismail, N.I., Yaakop, A.S., Kamaruzaman, N.A., Ahmad Mokhtar, A.M., The properties and mechanism of action of plant immunomodulators in regulation of immune response – A narrative review focusing on Curcuma longa L., Panax ginseng C. A. Meyer and Moringa oleifera Lam. *Heliyon*, 10, e28261, 2024, https://doi.org/10.1016/j.heliyon.2024.e28261.
28. Ren, L., Zhang, J., Zhang, T., Immunomodulatory activities of polysaccharides from Ganoderma on immune effector cells. *Food Chem.*, 340, 127933, 2021, https://doi.org/10.1016/j.foodchem.2020.127933.
29. Li, C., Liu, Y., Zhang, Y., Li, J., Lai, J., Astragalus polysaccharide: a review of its immunomodulatory effect. *Arch. Pharm. Res.*, 45, 367–389, 2022, https://doi.org/10.1007/s12272-022-01393-3.
30. Khan, T., Date, A., Chawda, H., Patel, K., Polysaccharides as potential anticancer agents—A review of their progress. *Carbohydr. Polym.*, 210, 412–428, 2019, https://doi.org/10.1016/j.carbpol.2019.01.064.
31. García-Márquez, J., Moreira, B.R., Valverde-Guillén, P., Latorre-Redoli, S., Caneda-Santiago, C.T., Acién, G., Martínez-Manzanares, E., Marí-Beffa, M., Abdala-Díaz, R.T., *In Vitro* and *In Vivo* Effects of Ulvan Polysaccharides from Ulva rigida. *Pharmaceuticals*, 16, 660, 2023, https://doi.org/10.3390/ph16050660.
32. Hartwell, L.H. and Weinert, T.A., Checkpoints: Controls That Ensure the Order of Cell Cycle Events. *Science (1979)*, 246, 629–634, 1989, https://doi.org/10.1126/science.2683079.
33. Morgan, D.O., Cyclin-dependent Kinases: Engines, Clocks, and Microprocessors. *Annu. Rev. Cell Dev. Biol.*, 13, 261–291, 1997, https://doi.org/10.1146/annurev.cellbio.13.1.261.
34. Bertoli, C., Skotheim, J.M., de Bruin, R.A.M., Control of cell cycle transcription during G1 and S phases. *Nat. Rev. Mol. Cell Biol.*, 14, 518–528, 2013, https://doi.org/10.1038/nrm3629.
35. Kuzmich, A.S., Romanenko, L.A., Kokoulin, M.S., Cell-cycle arrest and mitochondria-dependent apoptosis induction in T-47D cells by the capsular polysaccharide from the marine bacterium Kangiella japonica KMM

3897. *Carbohydr. Polym.*, 320, 121237, 2023, https://doi.org/10.1016/j.carbpol.2023.121237.

36. Wang, Z., Regulation of Cell Cycle Progression by Growth Factor-Induced Cell Signaling. *Cells*, 10, 3327, 2021, https://doi.org/10.3390/cells10123327.
37. Li, C., Tian, Z.-N., Cai, J.-P., Chen, K.-X., Zhang, B., Feng, M.-Y., Shi, Q.-T., Li, R., Qin, Y., Geng, J.-S., Panax ginseng polysaccharide induces apoptosis by targeting Twist/AKR1C2/NF-1 pathway in human gastric cancer. *Carbohydr. Polym.*, 102, 103–109, 2014, https://doi.org/10.1016/j.carbpol.2013.11.016.
38. Wang, C.-Z., Hou, L., Wan, J.-Y., Yao, H., Yuan, J., Zeng, J., Park, C.W., Kim, S.H., Seo, D.B., Shin, K.-S., Zhang, C.-F., Chen, L., Zhang, Q.-H., Liu, Z., Sava-Segal, C., Yuan, C.-S., Ginseng berry polysaccharides on inflammation-associated colon cancer: inhibiting T-cell differentiation, promoting apoptosis, and enhancing the effects of 5-fluorouracil. *J. Ginseng Res.*, 44, 282–290, 2020, https://doi.org/10.1016/j.jgr.2018.12.010.
39. Darbary, H., Stoler, D.L., Anderson, G.R., Family Cancer Syndromes: Inherited Deficiencies in Systems for the Maintenance of Genomic Integrity. *Surg. Oncol. Clin. N. Am.*, 18, 1–17, 2009, https://doi.org/10.1016/j.soc.2008.08.001.
40. Ghelli Luserna di Rora, A., Iacobucci, I., Martinelli, G., The cell cycle checkpoint inhibitors in the treatment of leukemias. *J. Hematol. Oncol.*, 10, 77, 2017, https://doi.org/10.1186/s13045-017-0443-x.
41. Chu, Y., Fang, Y., Chi, J., Li, J., Zhang, D., Zou, Y., Wang, Z., Astragalus polysaccharides decrease proliferation, migration, and invasion but increase apoptosis of human osteosarcoma cells by up-regulation of microRNA-133a. *Braz. J. Med. Biol. Res.*, 51, 2018, https://doi.org/10.1590/1414-431x20187665.
42. Yang, Q., Meng, D., Zhang, Q., Wang, J., Advances in research on the antitumor mechanism of Astragalus polysaccharides. *Front. Oncol.*, 14, 2024, https://doi.org/10.3389/fonc.2024.1334915.
43. Yang, Z. and Chen, G., Inhibition of Proliferation and Induction of Apoptosis in Prostatic Carcinoma DU145 Cells by Polysaccharides from Yunnan Rosa roxburghii Tratt. *Molecules*, 29, 1575, 2024, https://doi.org/10.3390/molecules29071575.
44. Hsu, W.-H., Hua, W.-J., Qiu, W.-L., Tseng, A.-J., Cheng, H.-C., Lin, T.-Y., WSG, a glucose-enriched polysaccharide from Ganoderma lucidum, suppresses tongue cancer cells *via* inhibition of EGFR-mediated signaling and potentiates cisplatin-induced apoptosis. *Int. J. Biol. Macromol.*, 193, 1201–1208, 2021, https://doi.org/10.1016/j.ijbiomac.2021.10.146.
45. Hickson, I., Zhao, Y., Richardson, C.J., Green, S.J., Martin, N.M.B., Orr, A.I., Reaper, P.M., Jackson, S.P., Curtin, N.J., Smith, G.C.M., Identification and Characterization of a Novel and Specific Inhibitor of the Ataxia-Telangiectasia Mutated Kinase ATM. *Cancer Res.*, 64, 9152–9159, 2004, https://doi.org/10.1158/0008-5472.CAN-04-2727.

46. Lito, P., Solomon, M., Li, L.-S., Hansen, R., Rosen, N., Allele-specific inhibitors inactivate mutant KRAS G12C by a trapping mechanism. *Science (1979)*, 351, 604–608, 2016, https://doi.org/10.1126/science.aad6204.
47. Rainey, M.D., Charlton, M.E., Stanton, R.V., Kastan, M.B., Transient Inhibition of ATM Kinase Is Sufficient to Enhance Cellular Sensitivity to Ionizing Radiation. *Cancer Res.*, 68, 7466–7474, 2008, https://doi.org/10.1158/0008-5472.CAN-08-0763.
48. Wang, M. and Yu, F., Research Progress on the Anticancer Activities and Mechanisms of Polysaccharides From Ganoderma. *Front. Pharmacol.*, 13, 891171, 2022, https://doi.org/10.3389/fphar.2022.891171.
49. Sofianidi, A., Dumbrava, E.E., Syrigos, K.N., Nasrazadani, A., Triple-Negative Breast Cancer and Emerging Therapeutic Strategies: ATR and CHK1/2 as Promising Targets. *Cancers (Basel)*, 16, 1139, 2024, https://doi.org/10.3390/cancers16061139.
50. Gillespie, D.A., Targeting CHK1 for Cancer Therapy: Rationale, Progress and Prospects, in: *Targeting the DNA Damage Response for Anti-Cancer Therapy*, pp. 209–240, 2018.
51. Ghelli Luserna di Rorà, A., Cerchione, C., Martinelli, G., Simonetti, G., A WEE1 family business: regulation of mitosis, cancer progression, and therapeutic target. *J. Hematol. Oncol.*, 13, 126, 2020, https://doi.org/10.1186/s13045-020-00959-2.
52. Li, L., Thakur, K., Cao, Y.-Y., Liao, B.-Y., Zhang, J.-G., Wei, Z.-J., Anticancerous potential of polysaccharides sequentially extracted from Polygonatum cyrtonema Hua in Human cervical cancer Hela cells. *Int. J. Biol. Macromol.*, 148, 843–850, 2020, https://doi.org/10.1016/j.ijbiomac.2020.01.223.
53. Wallace, D.C., Mitochondria and cancer. *Nat. Rev. Cancer*, 12, 685–698, 2012, https://doi.org/10.1038/nrc3365.
54. Wang, S.-F., Tseng, L.-M., Lee, H.-C., Role of mitochondrial alterations in human cancer progression and cancer immunity. *J. Biomed. Sci.*, 30, 61, 2023, https://doi.org/10.1186/s12929-023-00956-w.
55. Kumar, S., Ashraf, R., C.K., A., Mitochondrial dynamics regulators: implications for therapeutic intervention in cancer. *Cell Biol. Toxicol.*, 38, 377–406, 2022, https://doi.org/10.1007/s10565-021-09662-5.
56. Lei, T., Rui, Y., Xiaoshuang, Z., Jinglan, Z., Jihong, Z., Mitochondria transcription and cancer. *Cell Death Discov.*, 10, 168, 2024, https://doi.org/10.1038/s41420-024-01926-3.
57. Wagner, A., Kosnacova, H., Chovanec, M., Jurkovicova, D., Mitochondrial Genetic and Epigenetic Regulations in Cancer: Therapeutic Potential. *Int. J. Mol. Sci.*, 23, 7897, 2022, https://doi.org/10.3390/ijms23147897.
58. Zhang, K., Zhou, X., Wang, J., Zhou, Y., Qi, W., Chen, H., Nie, S., Xie, M., Dendrobium officinale polysaccharide triggers mitochondrial disorder to induce colon cancer cell death *via* ROS-AMPK-autophagy pathway. *Carbohydr. Polym.*, 264, 118018, 2021, https://doi.org/10.1016/j.carbpol.2021.118018.

59. Gan, Q., Wang, J., Hu, J., Lou, G., Xiong, H., Peng, C., Huang, Q., Modulation of Apoptosis by Plant Polysaccharides for Exerting Anti-Cancer Effects: A Review. *Front. Pharmacol.*, 11, 792, 2020, https://doi.org/10.3389/fphar.2020.00792.
60. Kudłacik-Kramarczyk, S., Drabczyk, A., Krzan, M., Advanced Drug Carriers: A Review of Selected Protein, Polysaccharide, and Lipid Drug Delivery Platforms. *Int. J. Mol. Sci.*, 25, 786, 2024, https://doi.org/10.3390/ijms25020786.
61. BeMiller, J.N., Polysaccharides, in: *Encyclopedia of Life Sciences*, Wiley, 2001.
62. Di Filippo, L.D., Duarte, J.L., Roque-Borda, C.A., Pavan, F.R., Meneguin, A.B., Chorilli, M., Melero, A., Guillot, A.J., Spagnol, C.M., Correa, M.A., *In Vitro* Skin Co-Delivery and Antibacterial Properties of Chitosan-Based Microparticles Containing Ascorbic Acid and Nicotinamide. *Life*, 12, 1049, 2022, https://doi.org/10.3390/life12071049.
63. Lukova, P. and Katsarov, P., Contemporary Aspects of Designing Marine Polysaccharide Microparticles as Drug Carriers for Biomedical Application. *Pharmaceutics*, 15, 2126, 2023, https://doi.org/10.3390/pharmaceutics15082126.
64. Wang, L., Li, W., Qin, S., Three Polymers from the Sea: Unique Structures, Directional Modifications, and Medical Applications. *Polymers (Basel)*, 13, 2482, 2021, https://doi.org/10.3390/polym13152482.
65. Sezer, A.D. and Akbuğa, J., The design of biodegradable ofloxacin-based core-shell microspheres: Influence of the formulation parameters on *in vitro* characterization. *Pharm. Dev. Technol.*, 17, 118–124, 2012, https://doi.org/10.3109/10837450.2010.529145.
66. Wang, P., Kankala, R.K., Fan, J., Long, R., Liu, Y., Wang, S., Poly-L-ornithine/fucoidan-coated calcium carbonate microparticles by layer-by-layer self-assembly technique for cancer theranostics. *J. Mater. Sci. - Mater. Med.*, 29, 68, 2018, https://doi.org/10.1007/s10856-018-6075-z.
67. Pai, F.-T. and Lin, W.J., Synergistic cytotoxicity of irinotecan combined with polysaccharide-based nanoparticles for colorectal carcinoma. *Biomater. Adv.*, 153, 213577, 2023, https://doi.org/10.1016/j.bioadv.2023.213577.
68. Jiang, Y., Yan, C., Li, M., Chen, S., Chen, Z., Yang, L., Luo, K., Delivery of natural products *via* polysaccharide-based nanocarriers for cancer therapy: A review on recent advances and future challenges. *Int. J. Biol. Macromol.*, 278, 135072, 2024, https://doi.org/10.1016/j.ijbiomac.2024.135072.
69. Yadav, N., Francis, A.P., Priya, V.V., Patil, S., Mustaq, S., Khan, S.S., Alzahrani, K.J., Banjer, H.J., Mohan, S.K., Mony, U., Rajagopalan, R., Polysaccharide-Drug Conjugates: A Tool for Enhanced Cancer Therapy. *Polymers (Basel)*, 14, 950, 2022, https://doi.org/10.3390/polym14050950.
70. Guan, W.-L., He, Y., Xu, R.-H., Gastric cancer treatment: recent progress and future perspectives. *J. Hematol. Oncol.*, 16, 57, 2023, https://doi.org/10.1186/s13045-023-01451-3.

71. Peng, P., Yang, K., Tong, G., Ma, L., Polysaccharide Nanoparticles for Targeted Cancer Therapies. *Curr. Drug Metab.*, 19, 781–792, 2018, https://doi.org/10.2174/1389200219666180511153403.
72. Varghese, S., Joseph, M.M., Aravind, S.R., Unnikrishnan, B.S., Pillai, K.R., Sreelekha, T.T., Immunostimulatory plant polysaccharides impede cancer progression and metastasis by avoiding off-target effects. *Int. Immunopharmacol.*, 73, 280–292, 2019, https://doi.org/10.1016/j.intimp.2019.05.025.
73. Mazepa, E., Noseda, M.D., Ferreira, L.G., de Carvalho, M.M., Gonçalves, A.G., Ducatti, D.R.B., de L. Bellan, D., Gomes, R.P., da S. Trindade, E., Franco, C.R.C., Pellizzari, F.M., Winnischofer, S.M.B., Duarte, M.E.R., Chemical structure of native and modified sulfated heterorhamnans from the green seaweed Gayralia brasiliensis and their cytotoxic effect on U87MG human glioma cells. *Int. J. Biol. Macromol.*, 187, 710–721, 2021. https://doi.org/10.1016/j.ijbiomac.2021.07.145.
74. Wang, X., Gao, A., Jiao, Y., Zhao, Y., Yang, X., Antitumor effect and molecular mechanism of antioxidant polysaccharides from Salvia miltiorrhiza Bunge in human colorectal carcinoma LoVo cells. *Int. J. Biol. Macromol.*, 108, 625–634, 2018. https://doi.org/10.1016/j.ijbiomac.2017.12.006.
75. Shokrani, H., Shokrani, A., Seidi, F., Kucińska-Lipka, J., Makurat-Kasprolewicz, B., Saeb, M.R., Ramakrishna, S., Artificial intelligence for biomedical engineering of polysaccharides: A short overview. *Curr. Opin. Biomed. Eng.*, 27, 100463, 2023. https://doi.org/10.1016/j.cobme.2023.100463.
76. Adamopoulos, C., Papavassiliou, K.A., Papavassiliou, A.G.: Fusing Artificial Intelligence and Machine Learning for Anti-Cancer Drug Discovery. *Cancers (Basel)*, 16, 3522, 2024. https://doi.org/10.3390/cancers16203522.
77. Guo, R., Chen, M., Ding, Y., Yang, P., Wang, M., Zhang, H., He, Y., Ma, H.: Polysaccharides as Potential Anti-tumor Biomacromolecules —A Review. *Front. Nutr.*, 9, 2022. https://doi.org/10.3389/fnut.2022.838179.
78. Fan, J., Zhu, J., Zhu, H., Zhang, Y., Xu, H., Potential therapeutic target for polysaccharide inhibition of colon cancer progression. *Front. Med. (Lausanne)*, 10, 2024. https://doi.org/10.3389/fmed.2023.1325491.

2

Structural Insights and Biophysical Properties of Polysaccharide Biomaterials for Enhancing Cancer Therapy

Shahnawaz Ahamd Bhat[1], Zeenat Islam[2], Shazia Shaheen Mir[3*] and Luqman Jameel Rather[4]

[1]Department of Chemistry, Jamia Millia Islamia, New Delhi, India
[2]Advanced Research Laboratory, Department of Zoology, School of Life Sciences, University of Kashmir, Srinagar, Jammu & Kashmir, India
[3]Laboratory Medicine Department, Faculty of Applied Medical Sciences, Al Baha University, Al Baha, Saudi Arabia
[4]College of Sericulture, Textile and Biomass Science, Southwest University, Chongqing, PR China

Abstract

This chapter will discuss the role of polysaccharide biomaterials in new frontiers of cancer therapy, with an emphasis on their structural, biophysical, and functional properties, which turn them ideal for biomedical applications. Starting with a brief overview of the polysaccharides normally used in cancer treatment, such as chitosan, hyaluronic acid, and alginates, this chapter sets the contributions related to their compatibility, degradability, and versatility. Its chemical versatility and finally the form of hydrogels and nanoparticles preset great advantages in drug delivery, tissue engineering, and immunomodulation. In such a context, detailed studies of the structural and biophysical properties of natural polymers are discussed with an emphasis on how these directly influence the mode by which they interact with cancer cells and the tumor microenvironment. By modulating cellular uptake, targeting tumor-specific receptors, and enabling controlled release in response to environmental stimuli, polysaccharides enhance the precision and efficacy of therapeutic delivery. Furthermore, this chapter outlines challenges regarding clinical

**Corresponding author*: smir@bu.edu.sa

Luqman Jameel Rather, Showkat Ali Ganie and Mohammed A. Assiri (eds.) Polysaccharide Biomaterials in Cancer Research and Therapy: From Lab to Life, (25–56) © 2026 Scrivener Publishing LLC

translation on issues related to scalability, stability, and regulatory hurdles, while the futures are personalized medicine, integration with immunotherapy, and decision-making through artificial intelligence (AI) in system design. In a nutshell, polysaccharide-based delivery systems may likely offer a promising versatile approach in oncology. Thanks to continuous innovation and interdisciplinary collaboration, they will be able to reshape the concept of cancer treatment toward safer, more effective, and targeted therapeutic options.

Keywords: Polysaccharide-based biomaterials, cancer therapy, biophysical properties, drug delivery systems, tumor microenvironment, biocompatibility and biodegradability

2.1 Introduction

Cancer is among the major fatal diseases worldwide; the quest to develop effective therapies against this disease is still an uphill task [1]. The conventional therapeutic approaches for cancer are chemotherapy, radiation therapy, and surgery. These are associated with serious side effects and several other disadvantages, toxic effects among both healthy tissues, and a lack of targeting accuracy [2]. The approach toward cancer therapy from the very beginning has moved toward more selectivity with minimum invasiveness, mainly to reduce adverse events and improve therapeutic efficacy. Several important developments have been made in targeted drug delivery systems, immunotherapy approaches, and personalized medicine, with the intent of greater specificity coupled with higher effectiveness [3]. In this regard, biomaterials of natural origin polysaccharides have received considerable interest due to their versatility as vectors of cancer therapy. These biomaterials provide not only biological compatibility but also the ability to tailor at a molecular level to achieve heightened therapeutic specificity [4]. The prospects of polysaccharides acting as drug carriers, imaging agents, and structural scaffolds have heralded new directions in cancer therapy, whereby the biocompatibility, degradability, and ease of functionalization contribute in dual ways to therapeutic and diagnostic applications [5].

Biomaterials play a variety of roles in modern cancer therapies, especially as carriers in drug delivery systems. Biomaterials accomplish controlled release to the tumor site by providing a structured scaffold for anticancer agents, minimizing systemic toxicity [6]. Recent innovations in biomaterial design have resulted in the development of "smart" systems responding to the tumor microenvironment (TME), such as pH-responsive, enzyme-responsive, and redox-responsive systems that enhance the targeting efficiency as well as the release kinetics of the encapsulated drugs [7]. Among all biomaterials, polysaccharides have become preferred candidates for such applications due to their natural abundance, structural diversity, and ease of functionalization. These materials can be engineered to optimize the pharmacokinetics and pharmacodynamics of therapeutic agents, which permits higher efficiency in drug absorption and prolongs circulation times. Their capability for interaction with biological macromolecules opens wider perspectives for targeting receptors on cancer cells regarding improvement in therapeutic efficacy [8].

Polysaccharides are one of the important biomaterials that possess physicochemical properties suitable for various biomedical applications [9]. Their molecular structures include repeating units of sugar that can easily be modified to provide functional groups, thus enhancing interaction with therapeutic agents for purposeful delivery to cancer cells. Such flexibility means immense possibilities in modifying polysaccharides for specific therapeutic needs ranging from increasing solubility to the attainment of sustained drug release. For example, polysaccharides possess inherent biocompatibility and are normally degraded to non-toxic by-products inside the body, which minimizes adverse immune responses and guarantees safety within the body [10]. Recently, polysaccharide nanoparticles, hydrogels, and film substrates have been demonstrated to carry anticancer drugs, genes, and imaging agents effectively to the tumor sites. For instance, one recent 2023 study demonstrated that the nanoparticles based on hyaluronic acid (HA) effectively delivered a common chemotherapy drug, doxorubicin, into breast cancer cells by taking advantage of CD44 receptor overexpression within the cancer microenvironment. This form of targeted delivery not only enhances the therapeutic effect but also diminishes the chances of drug resistance and off-target effects. Besides drug delivery, this biomaterial class of polysaccharides has also shown immense promise as active immunomodulatory agents [11]. Certain polysaccharides, such as β-glucans, for instance, are known to activate immune cells like macrophages and T-cells, hence facilitating an anti-tumor immune response. This dual functionality of serving both as a delivery vector and an immune enhancer places polysaccharide biomaterials as poised tools in combination therapies, synergizing with other modes of treatment to enhance their overall effectiveness [12, 13].

2.2 Structural Aspects of Polysaccharides

2.2.1 Chemical Structure and Composition

Polysaccharides are complex macromolecules composed of long chains of monosaccharide units linked by glycosidic bonds. The structures of these carbohydrate polymers show a diversity ranging from a linear to a highly branched form depending on the type of glycosidic linkages and the nature of the monosaccharides joining them [14]. Common monosaccharides in polysaccharides include glucose, mannose, galactose, and glucuronic acid, among others. These units happen in many ways, and different bonds among these units, such as linking α- or β-glycosidic, will confer special structural properties on each polysaccharide; it is such structural characteristics that determine the functions of the polysaccharides in biomedical applications [15]. The use of the term primary structure in polysaccharides reflects the sequence of the monosaccharide unit and their types of linkages. For instance, chitosan is a cationic polysaccharide that highly consists of D-glucosamine and N-acetyl-D-glucosamine units connected by β (1→4) glycosidic bonds (Figure 2.1) [16], whereas alginate is a linear copolymer containing homogeneous blocks of mannuronic acid and guluronic acid residues (Figure 2.2) [17]. This sequential and linked pattern defines its basic properties, including solubility, biodegradability, and reactivity—all very important features in biomedical applications, with special reference to cancer therapy [18]. Due to the existence of these functional groups at the molecular level, such as hydroxyls, amines, and carboxylic acids, they provide potential sites for various kinds of chemical modification. Thus, therapeutic agents, imaging molecules, or targeting ligands can be attached. For instance, chitosan contains amino groups that should render it a good candidate for conjugation with negatively charged drugs or targeting ligands, whereas HA has carboxyl groups that enable it to form hydrogels or bind to cationic molecules. These various modifications allow polysaccharides to become very versatile

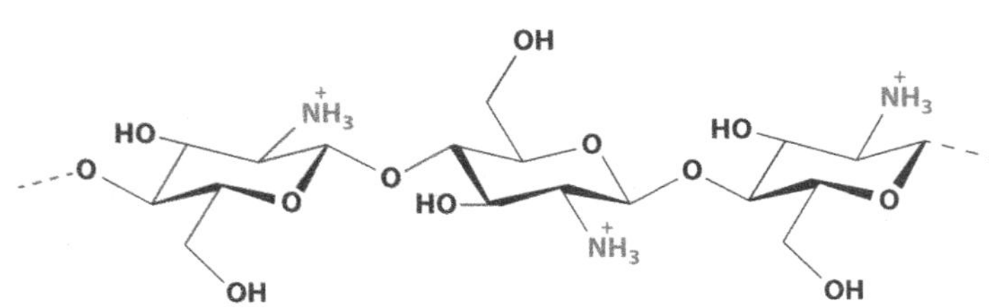

Figure 2.1 Structure of chitosan [16].

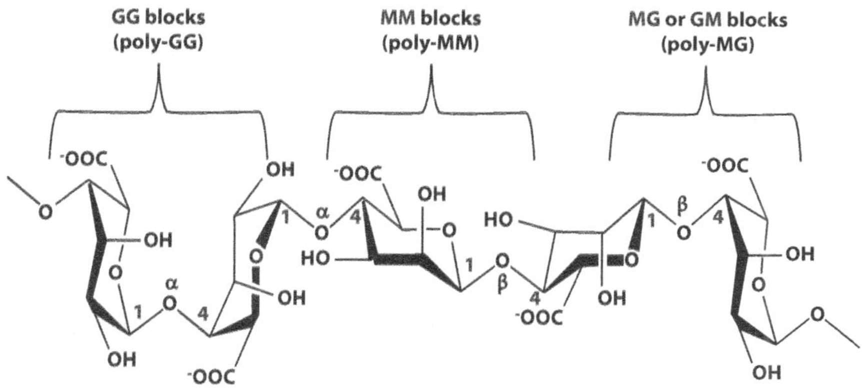

Figure 2.2 Structure of alginate (GG: guluronic acid and MM: mannuronic acid) [17].

carriers in drug delivery systems, thus being able to load protect and control the release of therapeutic agents [19].

2.2.2 Structural Variability among Polysaccharides

The variability in the structure of polysaccharides emanates from a difference in composition, linkage types, chain length, and, importantly, the degree of branching. This leads to a wide range of physical and chemical properties, allowing the polysaccharides to be tailored toward specific biomedical applications [20]. For example, the linear morphology of alginate, composed of repeating units of mannuronic and guluronic acid, enables the polysaccharide to form hydrogels upon its interaction with divalent cations such as calcium. This gelling property is very useful in fabricating drug delivery matrices for localized cancer therapy [21]. On the other hand, polysaccharides like dextran and HA have a branched or semi-branched structure that dictates their solubility and thereby their interactions with biological tissues [22]. The branch patterns affect the polysaccharide molecular weight and its spatial arrangement of the functional groups, both important parameters to determine its biocompatibility and bioavailability. For example, the branched structure of dextran allows it to function as a substitute for blood plasma and also as a drug carrier due to its excellent water solubility and nontoxic nature [23]. The semi-branched structure of HA and high molecular weight successor endow viscoelastic properties for targeted drug delivery in TMEs [24]. The degree of polymerization of a polysaccharide chain, referring to the number of monosaccharide units, then extensively influences its physical properties. Generally speaking, low-molecular-weight polysaccharides have better solubility and faster degradation rates, while most high-molecular-weight ones are stable with slower degradation [20]. This property is very important for the design of cancer therapy systems, where stability and the drug carrier release profile must be tailored according to the therapeutic requirement. For instance, high-molecular-weight chitosan is preferred in systems for prolonged drug release [25], while low-molecular-weight chitosan offers advantages in those formulations that require rapid degradation and clearance [26].

2.2.3 Impact of Structural Modifications on Biological Activity

Further modification of the inherent properties of polysaccharides could be done through structural modifications that enable them to function even better in cancer therapy. Common chemical modifications of polysaccharides, such as phosphorylation, sulfation, acetylation, and carboxymethylation, generally alter the charge, solubility, and binding of polysaccharides. Such modification makes the polysaccharide interact more effectively with either the cancerous cells or results in controlled drug delivery [27]. For example, carboxymethylated chitosan is more soluble in neutral and basic media and, therefore, best suited for drug delivery at physiological conditions. Phosphorylation of polysaccharides might achieve the appropriate insertion of negatively charged phosphate groups, which may ensure interaction between the latter and a positively charged drug or biomolecule. Sulfated polysaccharides like fucoidan have been reported with anti-tumor and anti-metastatic activities by inhibiting tumor cell adhesion, migration, and invasion [28]. In return, this structural modification of polysaccharides increases targeting toward cancer cells and hence greatly enhances their therapeutic efficacy. The nano-formulation represents another method of the structural modification with an aim for drug delivery. Therefore, nanoparticles made from polysaccharides, like chitosan and HA, enable the encapsulation of hydrophobic drugs and protection of sensible therapeutic agents against degradation [29].

Nanoparticles have the advantage of an enhanced permeability and retention (EPR) effect by means of which they selectively accumulate in tumor tissues. More recently, there have been reports that HA-modified nanoparticles target CD44 receptors, which are highly expressed in many types of cancer cells, resulting in an increase in cellular uptake and therapeutic effect [30]. Modulation in structure can also enhance immunomodulatory properties of the polysaccharide. Carbohydrates, such as β-glucans, can modulate the immune responses and will enhance the body's reaction against tumor cells. Different structural modifications, like acetylation and sulfation, have been reported to enhance the binding of β-glucans to the immune receptors such as Dectin-1 and CR3, which could further increase macrophage activation along with tumoricidal effects. By carrying out these immunomodulating effects, the modified polysaccharides also position themselves for combination therapies: to act both as drug carriers and immune stimulants in synergy with other cancer treatments [31].

2.3 Biophysical Properties Relevant to Cancer Therapy

The biophysical properties of polysaccharide-based biomaterials play a crucial role in determining their effectiveness as carriers and scaffolds in cancer therapy. Key properties, including mechanical strength, hydration and swelling behavior, and thermal stability, dictate how well these materials can perform under physiological conditions, respond to environmental triggers, and release therapeutic agents in a controlled manner [32]. Tailoring these biophysical characteristics can significantly enhance the functionality of polysaccharide biomaterials, making them more effective for cancer treatment applications [15].

2.3.1 Mechanical Properties and Strength

The mechanical strength and elasticity of polysaccharide biomaterials are essential factors in their application as drug delivery vehicles and tissue engineering scaffolds. In cancer therapy, materials with suitable mechanical properties can serve as implantable carriers or protective coatings for drug-loaded particles, providing structural integrity while minimizing the risk of premature degradation or release. Mechanical properties are influenced by the molecular weight of the polysaccharide, the degree of polymerization, and the presence of cross-linking agents that reinforce the structure [32]. For example, chitosan-based hydrogels, commonly used for localized drug delivery, are often modified to improve their mechanical strength through physical or chemical cross-linking. By cross-linking chitosan with biocompatible agents like genipin or tripolyphosphate, the resultant hydrogel exhibits enhanced strength and elasticity, allowing it to withstand physiological stresses and provide a prolonged drug release profile [33]. Similarly, alginate can form ionically cross-linked hydrogels with divalent cations (e.g., calcium), creating a mechanically stable gel network that can encapsulate and protect cancer drugs [34]. Mechanical properties are also crucial in designing injectable hydrogels or microparticles that must navigate complex tumor environments. Injectable formulations require an optimal balance of stiffness and flexibility to ensure they can be administered through a syringe yet retain their integrity once within the body [35]. For instance, HA-based hydrogels with adjustable stiffness have been explored for their ability to selectively target tumor sites, with recent studies showing that stiffer hydrogels may inhibit tumor growth by altering cell signaling pathways and limiting cellular proliferation [36]. Thus, controlling the mechanical properties of polysaccharide biomaterials is essential for achieving specific therapeutic outcomes in cancer therapy [37].

2.3.2 Hydration and Swelling Behavior

Hydration and swelling properties of polysaccharides are vital for their performance as drug delivery systems. Many polysaccharides, such as HA and alginate, are highly hydrophilic and can absorb large amounts of water, resulting in swelling. This property is particularly advantageous in cancer therapy, as it allows polysaccharide-based hydrogels to expand upon contact with physiological fluids, creating a hydrogel matrix that can encapsulate and protect drugs while providing a sustained release. The swelling behavior of polysaccharides is influenced by factors such as molecular weight, cross-linking density, and the ionic environment [37]. For instance, alginate hydrogels swell differently in the presence of various cations, with calcium ions forming a more compact and less swellable gel compared to sodium ions. This ion-dependent swelling behavior can be exploited to design drug delivery systems that respond to changes in the TME [38], which often has altered pH and ionic concentrations compared to normal tissues [39]. By adjusting the cross-linking density and ionic composition of polysaccharide-based hydrogels, researchers can create systems that swell and release drugs specifically in response to the acidic and ionic conditions found within tumors. Swelling behavior also impacts the release kinetics of encapsulated drugs. More swelling typically results in faster drug diffusion, which may be beneficial for immediate therapeutic effects. However, for sustained release applications, a controlled swelling rate is necessary to prevent premature drug depletion. Recent studies have explored dual-cross-linked hydrogels, combining ionic and covalent cross-links, to achieve more stable and tunable swelling profiles in polysaccharide matrices. For example, a dual-cross-linked chitosan hydrogel demonstrated prolonged and controlled release of doxorubicin, an anticancer drug, in breast cancer models by maintaining an optimal swelling profile. Such advancements highlight the importance of tailoring swelling behavior to achieve desired drug release profiles for specific cancer therapies [40].

2.3.3 Thermal Stability and Biostability

Thermal stability and biostability are important factors for the practical application of polysaccharide biomaterials, especially in cancer therapy, where materials may be subjected to temperature fluctuations or need to remain stable over extended periods. Thermal stability refers to the ability of a material to retain its structural integrity at different temperatures, while biostability indicates the resistance of the material to enzymatic degradation in biological environments [41]. Polysaccharides like chitosan and alginate are relatively stable at physiological temperatures, making them suitable for *in vivo* applications. However, modifications are often necessary to enhance their thermal stability for specific applications. For instance, the introduction of cross-linking agents can improve thermal stability by restricting molecular mobility, thereby enhancing the structural robustness of the material. This property is beneficial for polysaccharide-based nanoparticles, which may need to withstand high temperatures during sterilization processes without degrading or losing properties [42].

Biostability is equally crucial, as polysaccharides must be able to resist degradation until they reach the target site, after which controlled degradation can facilitate drug release. Enzymatic degradation of polysaccharides, such as the breakdown of HA by hyaluronidase or chitosan by lysozyme, can be leveraged to create responsive drug delivery systems. In the TME, where enzymes like hyaluronidase are often overexpressed, polysaccharides like HA can degrade selectively, releasing encapsulated drugs in a controlled manner at the cancer site [43]. Recent studies have focused on chemically modifying polysaccharides to enhance their biostability while maintaining biodegradability in specific environments. For instance, sulfation and phosphorylation of polysaccharides can reduce their susceptibility to enzymatic degradation, thus prolonging their circulation time and enhancing drug delivery efficacy. Sulfated polysaccharides, such as carrageenan, have shown promise in cancer therapy due to their stability and ability to inhibit tumor growth by interacting with cellular receptors. By balancing stability with degradability, researchers can optimize polysaccharide-based carriers for targeted, prolonged release, ultimately improving the therapeutic efficacy of cancer treatments [44].

2.4 Interaction Mechanisms with Cancer Cells and the TME

The interaction of polysaccharide-based biomaterials with cancer cells and the TME is fundamental to their effectiveness as drug delivery systems in cancer therapy. The TME, which is composed of cancer cells, immune cells, fibroblasts, blood vessels, and extracellular matrix (ECM) components, plays a significant role in tumor progression and resistance to therapies. Polysaccharides can be engineered to exploit the unique characteristics of the TME, such as its acidic pH, overexpressed receptors, and hypoxic conditions, to improve targeting specificity and therapeutic outcomes [45].

2.4.1 Cellular Uptake Mechanisms

The cellular uptake of polysaccharide-based nanoparticles and drug carriers is crucial for the efficient delivery of therapeutic agents directly into cancer cells [45]. Various endocytic pathways, such as clathrin-mediated endocytosis, caveolae-mediated endocytosis, and macropinocytosis, facilitate the internalization of polysaccharide-based materials. The choice of cellular uptake pathway depends on the size, surface charge, and structural characteristics of the polysaccharide carrier [46]. For instance, polysaccharides like HA can target cancer cells by binding to the CD44 receptor, which is often overexpressed on the surface of many tumor cells. HA–CD44 interactions trigger receptor-mediated endocytosis, allowing HA-based nanoparticles or hydrogels to enter cancer cells and release their therapeutic payloads intracellularly [47]. A recent study demonstrated that HA-conjugated nanoparticles effectively delivered doxorubicin to CD44-overexpressing breast cancer cells, resulting in enhanced cytotoxicity compared to non-targeted delivery systems [48]. Similarly, chitosan-based nanoparticles can enter cells through electrostatic interactions between the positively charged chitosan and the negatively charged cell membrane. This interaction facilitates cellular uptake *via* endocytosis, making chitosan a popular choice for delivering anticancer drugs and genes. By manipulating the surface charge and size of chitosan-based nanoparticles, researchers can enhance cellular uptake and improve drug delivery efficiency. Additionally, polysaccharide carriers can be modified with targeting ligands, such as folic acid or peptides, to improve specificity for certain cancer cell types, further enhancing cellular internalization and therapeutic efficacy [49].

2.4.2 Modulation of the TME

Polysaccharide-based biomaterials could modulate the TME, which can improve the efficacy of cancer therapies by overcoming certain barriers that hinder treatment. The TME is characterized by a high degree of acidity, elevated levels of specific enzymes, and abnormal vasculature, all of which can be targeted by smart polysaccharide systems. One of the key features of the TME is its acidic pH, resulting from the high metabolic rate of cancer cells and the production of lactic acid through anaerobic glycolysis (the Warburg effect). This acidity can be exploited by pH-sensitive polysaccharide-based drug carriers, which are engineered to release their therapeutic payloads selectively in the acidic environment of tumors [50]. For example, polysaccharides like alginate and chitosan can be modified to form pH-responsive nanoparticles that swell and release drugs under acidic conditions, improving localized drug delivery to the tumor site. Such pH-responsive systems minimize off-target effects by ensuring that drugs are released primarily in the acidic TME rather than in normal, neutral pH tissues [45].

Enzymatically responsive polysaccharide systems are another approach to modulating the TME. Enzymes such as matrix metalloproteinases (MMPs) and hyaluronidase are often overexpressed in the TME, facilitating cancer cell invasion and metastasis [51]. Polysaccharides such as HA can be used to develop enzyme-sensitive drug carriers that degrade in response to elevated hyaluronidase levels, resulting in localized drug release within the TME. This approach has been shown to improve the penetration of anticancer agents into tumor tissue, as well as to enhance drug uptake by cancer cells [52]. A recent study on HA-based nanoparticles demonstrated that these carriers could effectively release paclitaxel, a chemotherapy drug, in the presence of hyaluronidase, enhancing drug accumulation in the tumor tissue and suppressing tumor growth [53]. The TME also promotes immune evasion, where cancer cells avoid detection and elimination by the immune system. Certain polysaccharides, such as β-glucans, exhibit immunomodulatory properties that can help stimulate the body's immune response against tumors. β-Glucans bind to receptors on immune cells, such as Dectin-1 on macrophages and neutrophils, activating an immune response that targets cancer cells. This immunomodulatory action can be leveraged in combination therapies, where β-glucan-based carriers are used to deliver chemotherapy drugs while simultaneously boosting the immune response. By enhancing immune cell infiltration and activation within the TME, polysaccharide-based materials contribute to a more favorable environment for cancer therapy [31].

2.4.3 Targeted Delivery and Controlled Release of Therapeutics

One of the most critical functions of polysaccharide-based biomaterials in cancer therapy is their ability to deliver therapeutic agents in a targeted and controlled manner. Targeted delivery minimizes damage to healthy tissues and enhances drug accumulation at the tumor site, improving therapeutic outcomes. Polysaccharides can be functionalized with targeting ligands or antibodies that recognize specific receptors overexpressed on cancer cells, such as HER2, folate receptor, or integrins, to achieve targeted delivery [54]. For example, chitosan nanoparticles functionalized with folic acid have been widely explored for targeting folate receptor-positive cancers, such as ovarian and breast cancers. The folic acid-modified nanoparticles specifically bind to folate receptors on cancer cells, allowing the nanoparticles to be internalized and release their drug payload within the target cells. This receptor-mediated targeting enhances the selectivity and efficacy of the treatment while reducing side effects associated with conventional chemotherapy [55]. Controlled release is another crucial aspect, as it enables a sustained therapeutic effect and reduces the frequency of drug administration. Polysaccharides like alginate, when cross-linked with divalent cations like calcium, form hydrogel networks that can encapsulate drugs and release them gradually over time. This slow release can be further modulated by adjusting the cross-linking density, molecular weight, or degree of modification of the polysaccharide [56].

In cancer therapy, such sustained release systems are particularly beneficial for maintaining therapeutic drug concentrations within the TME, minimizing fluctuations that could lead to drug resistance. Responsive release mechanisms are also being developed to enhance the specificity and efficiency of drug delivery. These mechanisms take advantage of the unique characteristics of the TME, such as low pH, high enzyme levels, or redox gradients, to trigger drug release in response to environmental changes [43]. For instance, redox-responsive polysaccharide nanoparticles containing disulfide bonds release their payload in the presence of high intracellular glutathione levels, which are often elevated in cancer cells. This redox-sensitive release provides another layer of specificity, ensuring that drugs are released primarily within cancer cells, minimizing off-target toxicity [76]. In addition to chemical targeting and controlled release, polysaccharide-based carriers can be modified to penetrate the dense ECM within tumors. The ECM often acts as a barrier to drug delivery, limiting the penetration of therapeutic agents into the deeper regions of solid tumors [57]. Polysaccharides like HA, which naturally interacts with

ECM components, can enhance tissue penetration and improve drug distribution within the tumor. Moreover, enzymatically degradable polysaccharides that break down ECM components further facilitate drug delivery by reducing physical barriers within the TME [58].

2.5 Polysaccharide-Based Delivery Systems for Cancer Therapy

Polysaccharide-based delivery systems have emerged as promising tools in cancer therapy due to their biocompatibility, biodegradability, and ability to carry therapeutic agents in a controlled manner [52]. These systems are engineered to overcome various barriers in cancer treatment, including drug solubility, stability, targeted delivery, and controlled release. Polysaccharides such as chitosan, HA, alginate, and dextran offer unique structural properties that can be tailored for specific drug delivery applications, providing versatility in designing delivery systems with nano- and micro-structures, conjugated therapeutic agents, and stimuli-responsive mechanisms [15].

2.5.1 Nano- and Micro-Structured Delivery Systems

Nanoparticles and microparticles made from polysaccharides provide effective platforms for delivering anticancer drugs due to their ability to encapsulate therapeutic agents, protect them from premature degradation, and enhance cellular uptake. Nano- and micro-sized delivery systems offer a range of advantages in cancer therapy, including increased surface area, improved biodistribution, and EPR effect, which allows particles to accumulate in tumor tissues selectively [59].

a. **Nanoparticles**: Polysaccharide-based nanoparticles, typically in the size range of 10 to 200 nm, can penetrate tumor tissues more effectively due to their small size and ability to evade the immune system. Nanoparticles made from chitosan, for example, have been widely studied for their capability to encapsulate hydrophobic drugs, genes, and proteins (Figure 2.3). The cationic nature of chitosan facilitates interactions with the negatively charged cell membrane, enhancing cellular uptake and promoting the release

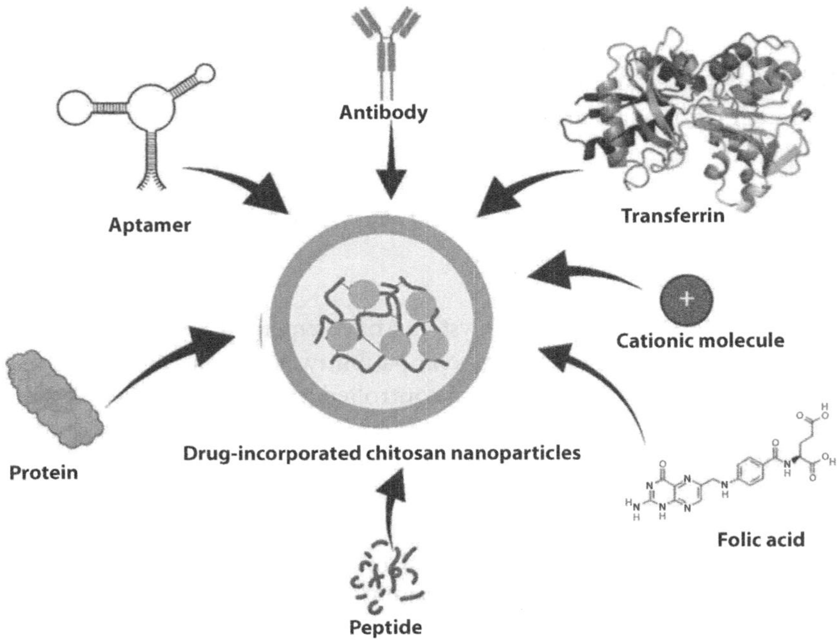

Figure 2.3 Graphical representation of different ligands affixed to the surface of chitosan nanoparticles to enhance tumor targeting efficacy [61].

of encapsulated drugs within the cell. Additionally, chitosan nanoparticles can be functionalized with targeting ligands like folic acid or antibodies to increase selectivity for specific cancer cell types [60].

HA nanoparticles represent another example, particularly in targeting tumors with overexpressed CD44 receptors. HA–CD44 interaction facilitates receptor-mediated endocytosis, allowing HA-based nanoparticles to deliver drugs directly to cancer cells while minimizing off-target effects [48, 61, 62]. Recent studies have shown that HA nanoparticles loaded with chemotherapeutic drugs like doxorubicin exhibit enhanced cytotoxicity in CD44-positive breast cancer cells, demonstrating the potential of HA-based nanoparticles in targeted cancer therapy (Figure 2.4) [63].

b. **Microparticles**: Polysaccharide microparticles, usually in the range of 1 to 100 μM, offer a different set of advantages for cancer therapy. Due to their larger size, microparticles are less likely to be cleared by the kidneys, allowing for

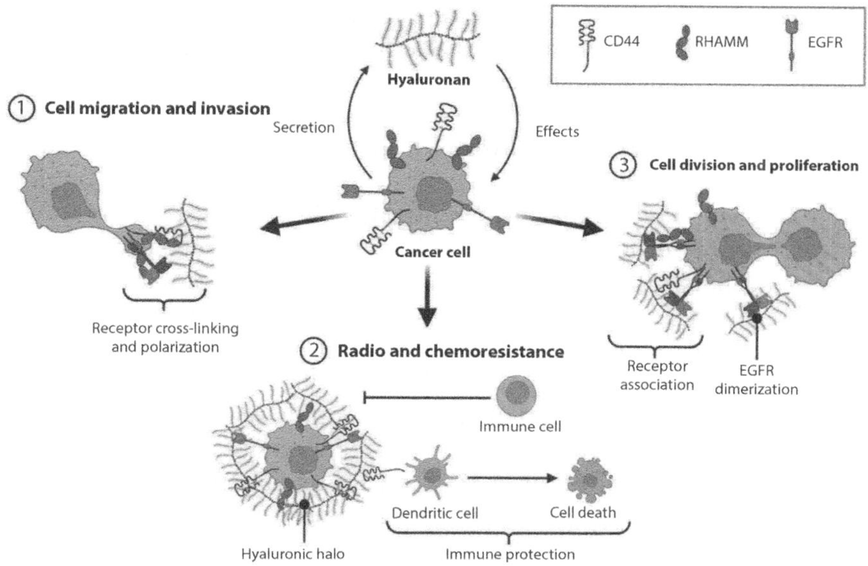

Figure 2.4 Hyaluronan impacts cancer cells by interacting with its receptors, CD44 and RHAMM [62].

prolonged circulation times. Alginate microparticles, for instance, have been used to encapsulate and deliver chemotherapeutic agents, providing sustained drug release and protection from enzymatic degradation. The gel-forming ability of alginate, especially in the presence of divalent cations, enables the formation of stable microparticles that can be injected directly into tumor sites, offering localized and controlled drug release [64].

Microparticles are also beneficial for cancer vaccines, where they serve as carriers for antigens and adjuvants, enhancing immune response against tumors. Chitosan and β-glucan microparticles, for example, have been explored for cancer immunotherapy, as they can activate immune cells such as macrophages and dendritic cells, promoting an anti-tumor immune response [65].

2.5.2 Conjugation with Therapeutic Agents

Polysaccharides can be chemically modified to conjugate therapeutic agents, providing a stable linkage that allows for precise control over drug release. Conjugation can improve the pharmacokinetic properties of drugs, increase their half-life in circulation, and enable targeted delivery to tumor sites. Conjugation strategies typically involve attaching drugs, imaging agents, or targeting moieties to functional groups present in the polysaccharide backbone, such as hydroxyl, amino, or carboxyl groups [66].

a. **Drug–Polysaccharide Conjugates**: By conjugating anticancer drugs directly to polysaccharides, researchers can enhance drug solubility, stability, and release profiles. For instance, doxorubicin, a commonly used chemotherapeutic drug, has been conjugated to HA to target CD44 receptors on cancer cells. The HA–doxorubicin conjugate ensures that the drug accumulates at the tumor site, allowing for a higher therapeutic index and reduced systemic toxicity. Additionally, the drug is gradually released in the acidic tumor environment, where the conjugate bond is cleaved, providing a controlled release mechanism [67]. Another example is the conjugation of methotrexate to chitosan. This conjugation improves methotrexate's solubility and bioavailability, while chitosan's positive charge facilitates interaction with the negatively charged cell membrane, enhancing drug uptake by cancer cells. These drug–polysaccharide conjugates have shown promising results in preclinical studies, providing targeted delivery with minimal side effects [68].
b. **Targeting Ligands and Imaging Agents**: Polysaccharides can also be modified with targeting ligands or imaging agents to enhance the selectivity and functionality of delivery systems. Targeting ligands such as peptides, antibodies, and folic acid can be conjugated to polysaccharides like chitosan and HA to direct the delivery system to specific receptors on cancer cells. For instance, the conjugation of folic acid to chitosan nanoparticles enables targeted delivery to folate receptor-positive cancer cells, commonly found in ovarian and breast cancers [69]. In addition, imaging agents like fluorescent dyes or contrast agents for magnetic resonance imaging can be attached to polysaccharides, allowing for real-time tracking of drug distribution and accumulation within the tumor. These theranostic systems (therapeutic + diagnostic) provide dual functions of both treatment and monitoring of drug delivery [70].

2.5.3 Responsive and Stimuli-Activated Delivery Systems

Responsive or stimuli-activated delivery systems are designed to release drugs in response to specific triggers within the TME, such as pH, enzymes, and redox potential. These systems improve drug targeting and minimize off-target effects by ensuring that drugs are released only in the presence of specific stimuli found predominantly in tumor tissues [71].

a. **pH-Responsive Systems**: Tumors are typically characterized by a more acidic microenvironment than normal tissues due to high metabolic activity and poor vascularization. Polysaccharides like chitosan and alginate can be modified to form pH-sensitive delivery systems that release drugs selectively in the acidic TME [72]. Chitosan, for example, becomes soluble in acidic conditions, allowing it to release encapsulated drugs when it encounters the low pH of tumors. This pH responsiveness has been utilized in chitosan-based nanoparticles to deliver doxorubicin selectively to acidic tumor sites, minimizing systemic exposure and reducing side effects [73].
b. **Enzyme-Responsive Systems**: The TME contains elevated levels of specific enzymes, such as MMPs and hyaluronidase, which facilitate cancer invasion and metastasis [74]. Polysaccharides like HA can be used to design enzyme-responsive delivery systems that degrade in the presence of these enzymes, releasing drugs directly at the tumor site. For instance, HA nanoparticles loaded with paclitaxel were shown to degrade in the presence of hyaluronidase, resulting in targeted drug release and improved therapeutic outcomes in animal models of cancer [29].
c. **Redox-Responsive Systems**: Cancer cells often exhibit a higher concentration of intracellular glutathione (GSH) than normal cells, creating a reducing environment that can trigger drug release from redox-responsive delivery systems [75]. Polysaccharide-based nanoparticles with disulfide linkages have been developed to take advantage of this redox gradient. When these nanoparticles enter cancer cells, the high levels of GSH reduce the disulfide bonds, triggering drug release within the cell. For example, redox-sensitive HA nanoparticles containing disulfide bonds have been used to

deliver chemotherapeutic agents selectively to cancer cells, improving intracellular drug accumulation and reducing systemic toxicity [76].

Responsive polysaccharide-based therapeutic systems provide a sophisticated approach to cancer treatment, allowing for the precise release of drugs in response to the unique characteristics of the TME. By exploiting these stimuli, researchers can enhance the selectivity, efficacy, and safety of cancer treatments, opening new possibilities for personalized and targeted therapies.

2.6 Challenges and Future Perspectives

Polysaccharide-based delivery systems have shown great potential for enhancing cancer therapy due to their biocompatibility, biodegradability, and versatility in drug delivery applications. However, despite these advantages, several challenges remain that hinder their clinical translation and widespread adoption in oncology. Addressing these challenges requires a combination of advanced research, technological innovation, and regulatory adaptation. Here, we outline the major challenges faced by polysaccharide-based systems in cancer therapy and discuss potential future directions to overcome these obstacles and realize the full therapeutic potential of these biomaterials [77].

2.6.1 Challenges

a. **Scalability and Production Costs:** One of the primary challenges in developing polysaccharide-based delivery systems is scaling up production for clinical use. Many polysaccharides are derived from natural sources, such as plants, algae, and microbial cultures, which may vary in yield, purity, and quality based on environmental conditions. This variability can lead to inconsistencies in the properties of polysaccharide-based materials, complicating large-scale production. Additionally, the extraction, purification, and functionalization processes are often labor-intensive and costly, which can make the final product prohibitively expensive for widespread clinical use. Furthermore, producing polysaccharide-based nanoparticles, hydrogels, or conjugates with precise structural and functional attributes requires specialized equipment and expertise, adding another layer of complexity to scaling up [78]. To address these issues, future research could focus on optimizing the extraction and synthesis processes for key polysaccharides, developing synthetic analogs or bioengineered versions with improved consistency, and establishing cost-effective production methods to ensure affordability and accessibility of polysaccharide-based therapies.

b. **Stability and Storage:** The stability of polysaccharide-based delivery systems is crucial for their effectiveness in drug delivery applications. Many polysaccharides are sensitive to environmental conditions such as temperature, humidity, and light, which can lead to degradation and loss of functionality over time [79]. For instance, chitosan is susceptible to hydrolysis in acidic or alkaline conditions, while HA can degrade in the presence of enzymes like hyaluronidase [45]. This sensitivity poses challenges for the storage and transport of polysaccharide-based products, especially if they require specific temperature and humidity controls to maintain their stability. Addressing stability issues may involve modifying the polysaccharide structure to enhance resistance to degradation or developing new formulations that incorporate stabilizing agents. Future research could focus on identifying optimal storage conditions, enhancing the thermal stability of polysaccharides through chemical modifications, and exploring protective packaging or encapsulation techniques that prolong the shelf life of these biomaterials.

c. **Targeting Efficacy and Drug Release Control:** Although polysaccharides offer advantages in targeted drug delivery, achieving precise targeting and controlled release remains a significant challenge. The heterogeneity of tumor tissues, including variations in receptor expression and microenvironmental conditions, can limit the targeting efficiency of polysaccharide-based systems [80]. For instance, while HA-based systems target CD44 receptors, not all cancer types or patients overexpress CD44, which can reduce the efficacy of HA-based targeting in certain cases. Additionally, ensuring that the drug release occurs at the optimal time and location within the tumor tissue remains a challenge, as premature release can lead to off-target effects and reduced therapeutic efficacy. Future directions in this area include the development of multi-targeting systems that incorporate multiple ligands or stimuli-responsive mechanisms to increase specificity and adaptability to various tumor types. Advancements in nanotechnology and molecular engineering could enable more precise tuning of release profiles, allowing for on-demand drug release in response to environmental cues. For example, combining pH- and enzyme-responsive mechanisms within a single delivery system could provide dual control, releasing drugs selectively in the acidic and enzyme-rich TME while remaining stable in normal tissues.

d. **Biocompatibility and Immunogenicity:** Although polysaccharides are generally considered biocompatible and non-toxic, some may elicit an immune response or cause adverse reactions in certain individuals [81]. For example, chitosan can cause mild irritation or an inflammatory response due to its cationic nature, while some sulfated polysaccharides have been shown to interact with immune receptors, leading to unintended immune activation. Additionally, polysaccharides that are derived from non-human sources, such as alginate from algae or fucoidan from seaweed, may introduce immunogenicity concerns when used in humans [82]. To mitigate these risks, future research could focus on engineering polysaccharides with improved biocompatibility profiles, such as by removing reactive functional groups or shielding them with inert materials. Additionally, exploring human-derived or synthetic polysaccharide analogs that mimic the structure and function of natural polysaccharides could reduce the risk of immune responses. Advanced testing and preclinical evaluation will be essential to understand the immunogenicity profiles of new polysaccharide-based materials before they proceed to clinical trials.

e. **Regulatory and Clinical Hurdles:** The regulatory landscape for polysaccharide-based delivery systems is complex and evolving, as these systems often fall into the category of advanced therapeutic products that combine elements of drugs, biologics, and medical devices. Obtaining regulatory approval for polysaccharide-based systems can be challenging due to the need for rigorous safety, efficacy, and quality evaluations [83]. Furthermore, variations in regulatory requirements between regions (e.g., FDA in the United States, EMA in Europe) add another layer of complexity for companies seeking to bring polysaccharide-based therapies to the global market [84]. To overcome regulatory hurdles, collaboration between researchers, industry stakeholders, and regulatory agencies is essential. Establishing clear guidelines for the development, testing, and approval of polysaccharide-based therapies could streamline the regulatory process. Additionally, conducting comprehensive preclinical studies that address potential safety and efficacy concerns will be crucial for facilitating the transition of these materials from the laboratory to the clinic.

2.6.2 Future Perspectives

a. **Advanced Functionalization and Smart Drug Delivery Systems:** Future developments in polysaccharide-based systems are likely to focus on creating "smart" delivery systems that respond to multiple stimuli, enabling more precise control over drug release in response to complex tumor environments. For instance, combining pH-sensitive, enzyme-sensitive, and redox-sensitive elements within a single delivery system could create a multifunctional platform capable of adapting to various tumor characteristics, ensuring that the drug is released only under specific conditions found in the TME [85]. Advances in synthetic chemistry and molecular engineering could also allow for more sophisticated functionalization of polysaccharides, enabling the incorporation of targeting ligands, imaging agents, or theranostic capabilities. The development of multi-functional polysaccharide-based nanoparticles with real-time imaging capabilities would enable clinicians to monitor drug delivery and therapeutic efficacy, paving the way for personalized cancer treatment.
b. **Integration with Immunotherapy:** The combination of polysaccharide-based delivery systems with immunotherapy is a promising area of research, as polysaccharides such as β-glucans possess inherent immunomodulatory properties [86]. Future research may focus on designing polysaccharide-based systems that can deliver immune-stimulating agents, such as cytokines, checkpoint inhibitors, or tumor

antigens, directly to the tumor site. These systems could stimulate an anti-tumor immune response, working synergistically with conventional chemotherapy or immunotherapy to enhance overall efficacy. By combining drug delivery with immunomodulation, polysaccharide-based systems could play a key role in the development of next-generation cancer immunotherapies, helping to overcome immune resistance and promote long-lasting anti-tumor immunity.

c. **Personalized and Precision Medicine Approaches:** Personalized medicine, which involves tailoring treatments to individual patient profiles, is a growing trend in cancer therapy [87]. In the future, polysaccharide-based systems could be customized to meet the specific needs of each patient based on their tumor type, genetic profile, and TME characteristics. For instance, using bioinformatics and machine learning (ML), researchers could design polysaccharide-based systems that deliver optimal drug combinations and doses based on predictive models of patient response. Personalized polysaccharide-based therapies could also incorporate patient-specific targeting ligands or unique biomarkers, ensuring that the delivery system is tailored precisely to the individual's tumor characteristics. Such precision approaches hold the potential to improve treatment efficacy and reduce adverse effects, ultimately leading to more effective and patient-centric cancer therapies.

d. **AI and ML for System Design:** The integration of AI and ML in the design and optimization of polysaccharide-based delivery systems represents an exciting future direction. AI and ML can analyze vast datasets to predict how specific structural modifications in polysaccharides influence drug release, targeting, and biocompatibility [88]. By leveraging computational modelling, researchers can efficiently screen and identify the most promising polysaccharide structures and functionalization, accelerating the development process and reducing experimental costs. AI-driven approaches can also assist in optimizing formulations, identifying optimal dosing regimens, and predicting patient responses, paving the way for more robust and effective polysaccharide-based cancer therapies.

2.7 Conclusion

Polysaccharide-based delivery systems have emerged as promising tools in the fight against cancer, offering biocompatibility, biodegradability, and versatility in designing drug carriers that address some of the most pressing challenges in cancer therapy. With the capacity to be modified for targeted delivery, controlled release, and responsiveness to the TME, polysaccharide-based biomaterials provide unique advantages over traditional drug delivery systems. Their ability to be functionalized with therapeutic agents, imaging compounds, and targeting ligands enables precise control over drug distribution, potentially reducing side effects and enhancing therapeutic outcomes. Despite their potential, challenges such as scalability, stability, targeting specificity, and regulatory hurdles continue to limit the clinical translation of polysaccharide-based systems. However, ongoing advancements in molecular engineering, synthetic chemistry, and nanotechnology are paving the way to overcome these obstacles. Future directions, including the integration of stimuli-responsive mechanisms, combination with immunotherapy, and incorporation of AI in design optimization, offer exciting possibilities for enhancing the effectiveness and precision of these delivery systems.

As research progresses, polysaccharide-based biomaterials are likely to play an increasingly important role in personalized and precision medicine, allowing for treatments tailored to individual patient profiles and tumor characteristics. The synergy of polysaccharide-based systems with current cancer therapies has the potential to improve patient outcomes, making them a valuable component in the arsenal against cancer. With continued innovation and collaboration across research, industry, and regulatory sectors, polysaccharide-based delivery systems hold the promise to revolutionize cancer treatment, transforming it into a more targeted, effective, and patient-centered approach.

AI disclosure statement: The author acknowledges the use of AI-based tools for minor language editing or grammatical correction. However, all intellectual contributions, analyses, and conclusions presented in this chapter are entirely the author's own.

References

1. Zugazagoitia, J., Guedes, C., Ponce, S., Ferrer, I., Molina-Pinelo, S., Paz-Ares, L., Current Challenges in Cancer Treatment. *Clin. Ther.*, 38, 1551–66, 2016, https://doi.org/10.1016/J.CLINTHERA.2016.03.026.
2. Kaur, R., Bhardwaj, A., Gupta, S., Cancer treatment therapies: traditional to modern approaches to combat cancers. *Mol. Biol. Rep.*, 50, 9663–76, 2023, https://doi.org/10.1007/S11033-023-08809-3.
3. Deivayanai, V.C., Thamarai, P., Karishma, S., Saravanan, A., Yaashikaa, P.R., Vickram, A.S., *et al.*, A comprehensive review on advances in nanoparticle-mediated cancer therapeutics: Current research and future perspectives. *Cancer Pathog. Ther.*, 2024, https://doi.org/10.1016/J.CPT.2024.11.002.
4. Prateeksha, Sharma, V.K., Liu, X., Oyarzún, D.A., Abdel-Azeem, A.M., Atanasov, A.G., *et al.*, Microbial polysaccharides: An emerging family of natural biomaterials for cancer therapy and diagnostics. *Semin. Cancer Biol.*, 86, 706–31, 2022, https://doi.org/10.1016/J.SEMCANCER.2021.05.021.
5. Alshangiti, D.M., El-Damhougy, T.K., Zaher, A., Madani, M., Mohamady ghobashy, M., Revolutionizing biomedicine: advancements, applications, and prospects of nanocomposite macromolecular carbohydrate-based hydrogel biomaterials: a review. *RSC Adv.*, 13, 35251–91, 2023, https://doi.org/10.1039/D3RA07391B.
6. Wang, Q.H., Cheng, S., Han, C.Y., Yang, S., Gao, S.R., Yin, W.Z., *et al.*, Tailoring cell-inspired biomaterials to fuel cancer therapy. *Mater. Today Bio*, 300, 101381, 2025, https://doi.org/10.1016/J.MTBIO.2024.101381.
7. Mazidi, Z., Javanmardi, S., Naghib, S.M., Mohammadpour, Z., Smart stimuli-responsive implantable drug delivery systems for programmed and on-demand cancer treatment: An overview on the emerging materials. *Chem. Eng. J.*, 433, 1, 134569, 2022, https://doi.org/10.1016/J.CEJ.2022.134569.
8. Tiwana, G., Cock, I.E., Cheesman, M.J., Phytochemical Analysis and Antimicrobial Activity of *Terminalia bellirica* (Gaertn.) Roxb. and *Terminalia chebula* Retz. Fruit Extracts Against Gastrointestinal Pathogens: Enhancing Antibiotic Efficacy. *Microorg*, 12, 2664, 2024, https://doi.org/10.3390/MICROORGANISMS12122664.
9. Han, X., Alu, A., Liu, H., Shi, Y., Wei, X., Cai, L., *et al.*, Biomaterial-assisted biotherapy: A brief review of biomaterials used in drug delivery, vaccine development, gene therapy, and stem cell therapy. *Bioact. Mater.*, 17, 29–48, 2022, https://doi.org/10.1016/J.BIOACTMAT.2022.01.011.
10. Sood, A., Gupta, A., Agrawal, G., Recent advances in polysaccharides based biomaterials for drug delivery and tissue engineering applications. *Carbohydr. Polym. Technol. Appl.*, 2, 100067, 2021, https://doi.org/10.1016/J.CARPTA.2021.100067.
11. Gómez-Pastor, S., Maugard, A., Walker, H.R., Elies, J., Borsum, K., Grimaldi, G., *et al.*, CD-44 targeted nanoparticles for combination therapy in an *in vitro* model of triple-negative breast cancer: Targeting the tumour inside out.

Colloids Surf. B Biointerfaces, 249, 114504, 2025, https://doi.org/10.1016/J.COLSURFB.2025.114504.

12. Wani, S.M., Gani, A., Mir, S.A., Masoodi, F.A., Khanday, F.A., β-Glucan: A dual regulator of apoptosis and cell proliferation. *Int. J. Biol. Macromol.*, 182, 1229–37, 2021, https://doi.org/10.1016/J.IJBIOMAC.2021.05.065.
13. De Marco Castro, E., Calder, P.C., Roche, H.M., β-1,3/1,6-Glucans and Immunity: State of the Art and Future Directions. *Mol. Nutr. Food Res.*, 65, 1901071, 2021, https://doi.org/10.1002/MNFR.201901071.
14. Chaudhary, S., Jain, V.P., Jaiswar, G., The composition of polysaccharides: monosaccharides and binding, group decorating, polysaccharides chains, in: *Innov Nano-Polysaccharides Eco-Sustainability From Sci to Ind Appl*, pp. 83–118, 2022, https://doi.org/10.1016/B978-0-12-823439-6.00005-2.
15. Rumon, M.M.H., Akib, A.A., Sarkar, S.D., Khan, M.A.R., Uddin, M.M., Nasrin, D., *et al.*, Polysaccharide-Based Hydrogels for Advanced Biomedical Engineering Applications. *ACS Polym. Au*, 4, 463–86, 2024, https://doi.org/10.1021/ACSPOLYMERSAU.4C00028/ASSET/IMAGES/LARGE/LG4C00028_0009.JPEG.
16. Guarnieri, A., Triunfo, M., Scieuzo, C., Ianniciello, D., Tafi, E., Hahn, T., *et al.*, Antimicrobial properties of chitosan from different developmental stages of the bioconverter insect Hermetia illucens. *Sci. Rep.*, 12, 1, 1–12, 2022, https://doi.org/10.1038/s41598-022-12150-3.
17. Abka-khajouei, R., Tounsi, L., Shahabi, N., Patel, A.K., Abdelkafi, S., Michaud, P., Structures, Properties and Applications of Alginates. *Mar. Drugs*, 20, 364, 2022, https://doi.org/10.3390/MD20060364.
18. Quiñones, J.P., Peniche, H., Peniche, C., Chitosan Based Self-Assembled Nanoparticles in Drug Delivery. *Polymers (Basel)*, 10, 235, 2018, https://doi.org/10.3390/POLYM10030235.
19. Adhikari, H.S. and Yadav, P.N., Anticancer Activity of Chitosan, Chitosan Derivatives, and Their Mechanism of Action. *Int. J. Biomater.*, 2018, 2952085, 2018, https://doi.org/10.1155/2018/2952085.
20. Chen, Y., Zhang, N., Chen, X., Structurally Modified Polysaccharides: Physicochemical Properties, Biological Activities, Structure-Activity Relationship, and Applications. *J. Agric. Food Chem.*, 72, 3259–76, 2024, https://doi.org/10.1021/ACS.JAFC.3C06433/ASSET/IMAGES/MEDIUM/JF3C06433_0004.GIF.
21. Urbanova, M., Pavelkova, M., Czernek, J., Kubova, K., Vyslouzil, J., Pechova, A., *et al.*, Interaction Pathways and Structure-Chemical Transformations of Alginate Gels in Physiological Environments. *Biomacromolecules*, 20, 4158–70, 2019, https://doi.org/10.1021/ACS.BIOMAC.9B01052/ASSET/IMAGES/LARGE/BM9B01052_0014.JPEG.
22. Carvalho, T., Bártolo, R., Pedro, S.N., Valente, B.F.A., Pinto, R.J.B., Vilela, C., *et al.*, Injectable Nanocomposite Hydrogels of Gelatin-Hyaluronic Acid Reinforced with Hybrid Lysozyme Nanofibrils-Gold Nanoparticles for the Regeneration of Damaged Myocardium. *ACS Appl. Mater. Interfaces*,

15, 25860–72, 2023, https://doi.org/10.1021/ACSAMI.3C03874/ASSET/IMAGES/LARGE/AM3C03874_0009.JPEG.
23. Narayan, R., Arcovito, A., Dahiya, D., Singh Nigam, P., Dextran of Diverse Molecular-Configurations Used as a Blood-Plasma Substitute, Drug-Delivery Vehicle and Food Additive Biosynthesized by Leuconostoc, Lactobacillus and Weissella. *Appl. Sci.*, 13, 12526, 2023, https://doi.org/10.3390/APP132212526.
24. Carvalho, E.M., Ding, E.A., Saha, A., Weldy, A., Zushin, P.-J.H., Stahl, A., *et al.*, Viscoelastic high-molecular-weight hyaluronic acid hydrogels support rapid glioblastoma cell invasion with leader-follower dynamics. *Adv. Mater.*, 36, 50, 2404885, 2024, https://doi.org/10.1101/2024.04.04.588167.
25. Morales-Quintana, L., Salagean, A.-A., Moldovan, C-A-D, Slevin, M., Mures, T., Utilisation of High Molecular Weight and Ultra-High Molecular Weight Hyaluronan in Management of Glioblastoma. *Gels*, 11, 50, 2025, https://doi.org/10.3390/GELS11010050.
26. de Farias, B.S., Grundmann, D.D.R., Rizzi, F.Z., Martins, N.S.S., Sant'Anna Cadaval Junior, T.R., de Almeida Pinto, L.A., Production of low molecular weight chitosan by acid and oxidative pathways: Effect on physicochemical properties. *Food Res. Int.*, 123, 88–94, 2019, https://doi.org/10.1016/J.FOODRES.2019.04.051.
27. Udaipuria, N. and Bhattacharya, S., Novel Carbohydrate Polymer-Based Systems for Precise Drug Delivery in Colon Cancer: Improving Treatment Effectiveness With Intelligent Biodegradable Materials. *Biopolymers*, 116, e23632, 2025, https://doi.org/10.1002/BIP.23632.
28. Abu, R., Jiang, Z., Ueno, M., Isaka, S., Nakazono, S., Okimura, T., *et al.*, Anti-metastatic effects of the sulfated polysaccharide ascophyllan isolated from Ascophyllum nodosum on B16 melanoma. *Biochem. Biophys. Res. Commun.*, 458, 727–32, 2015, https://doi.org/10.1016/J.BBRC.2015.01.061.
29. Alsaikhan, F. and Farhood, B., Recent advances on chitosan/hyaluronic acid-based stimuli-responsive hydrogels and composites for cancer treatment: A comprehensive review. *Int. J. Biol. Macromol.*, 280, 135893, 2024, https://doi.org/10.1016/J.IJBIOMAC.2024.135893.
30. Hussain, Z., Akbari, A.H., Barbuor, S.H., Dawood Alshetiwi, D.S., Ahmed, I.S., Rawas-Qalaji, M., Hyaluronic acid based functionalization of nanodelivery systems: A promising strategy for CD44-receptors-mediated targeted therapy of lung cancer. *J. Drug Deliv. Sci. Technol.*, 101, 106183, 2024, https://doi.org/10.1016/J.JDDST.2024.106183.
31. Iwai, A., Involvement of β-glucan receptors on the antitumor activity of β-glucans. *Clin. Immunol. Commun.*, 7, 1–17, 2025, https://doi.org/10.1016/J.CLICOM.2024.12.002.
32. Farasati Far, B., Taromi, P., Jamshidi, E., Deheshjoo, M., Physicochemical and Mechanical Properties of Green Biomaterials, in: *Green Biomaterials in Tissue Engineering*, pp. 55–88, 2025, https://doi.org/10.1021/BK-2025-1497.CH002.

33. Xu, Z., Zhang, H., Huang, Y., Zhong, H., Qin, P., Cheng, S., *et al.*, Tough and Biocompatible Hydrogel Tissue Adhesives Entirely Based on Naturally Derived Ingredients. *ACS Appl. Polym. Mater.*, 6, 1141–51, 2024, https://doi.org/10.1021/ACSAPM.3C01926/SUPPL_FILE/AP3C01926_SI_001.PDF.
34. Wang, Y., Shen, Z., Wang, H., Song, Z., Yu, D., Li, G., *et al.*, Progress in Research on Metal Ion Crosslinking Alginate-Based Gels. *Gels*, 11, 16, 2025, https://doi.org/10.3390/GELS11010016.
35. Vernerey, F.J., Lalitha Sridhar, S., Muralidharan, A., Bryant, S.J., Mechanics of 3D Cell-Hydrogel Interactions: Experiments, Models, and Mechanisms. *Chem. Rev.*, 121, 11085–148, 2021, https://doi.org/10.1021/ACS.CHEMREV.1C00046/ASSET/IMAGES/MEDIUM/CR1C00046_0031.GIF.
36. Han, X., Li, G., You, S., Shen, M., Xu, Y., Yang, H., *et al.*, Injectable bio-multifunctional hyaluronic acid-based hydrogels loaded with poly ADP-ribose polymerase inhibitors for ovarian cancer therapy. *Int. J. Biol. Macromol.*, 270, 132275, 2024, https://doi.org/10.1016/J.IJBIOMAC.2024.132275.
37. Yang, X., Wang, B., Peng, D., Nie, X., Wang, J., Yu, C.Y., *et al.*, Hyaluronic Acid-Based Injectable Hydrogels for Wound Dressing and Localized Tumor Therapy: A Review. *Adv. NanoBiomed Res.*, 2, 2200124, 2022, https://doi.org/10.1002/ANBR.202200124.
38. Murdan, S., Electro-responsive drug delivery from hydrogels. *J. Control. Release*, 92, 1–17, 2003, https://doi.org/10.1016/S0168-3659(03)00303-1.
39. Zhou, J., Wang, H., Chen, H., Ling, Y., Xi, Z., Lv, M., *et al.*, pH-responsive nanocomposite hydrogel for simultaneous prevention of postoperative adhesion and tumor recurrence. *Acta Biomater.*, 158, 228–38, 2023, https://doi.org/10.1016/J.ACTBIO.2022.12.025.
40. Taghikhani, A., Babazadeh, M., Davaran, S., Ghasemi, E., Facile preparation of a pH-sensitive biocompatible nanocarrier based on magnetic layered double hydroxides/Cu MOFs-chitosan crosslinked κ-carrageenan for controlled doxorubicin delivery to breast cancer cells. *Colloids Surf. B Biointerfaces*, 243, 114122, 2024, https://doi.org/10.1016/J.COLSURFB.2024.114122.
41. Cheroni, S., Gatti, B., Margheritis, G., Formantici, C., Perrone, L., Galante, Y.M., Enzyme resistance and biostability of hydroxyalkylated cellulose and galactomannan as thickeners in waterborne paints. *Int. Biodeterior. Biodegrad.*, 69, 106–12, 2012, https://doi.org/10.1016/J.IBIOD.2011.06.009.
42. Zhang, J.T., Huang, S.W., Zhuo, R.X., Temperature-Sensitive Polyamidoamine Dendrimer/Poly(N-isopropylacrylamide) Hydrogels with Improved Responsive Properties. *Macromol. Biosci.*, 4, 575–8, 2004, https://doi.org/10.1002/MABI.200400003.
43. Gagneja, S., Capalash, N., Sharma, P., Hyaluronic acid as a tumor progression agent and a potential chemotherapeutic biomolecule against cancer: A review on its dual role. *Int. J. Biol. Macromol.*, 275, 133744, 2024, https://doi.org/10.1016/J.IJBIOMAC.2024.133744.

44. Cunha, L. and Grenha, A., Sulfated Seaweed Polysaccharides as Multi-functional Materials in Drug Delivery Applications. *Mar. Drugs*, 14, 42, 2016, https://doi.org/10.3390/MD14030042.
45. Wu, Q., Hu, Y., Yu, B., Hu, H., Xu, F.J., Polysaccharide-based tumor micro-environment-responsive drug delivery systems for cancer therapy. *J. Control. Release*, 362, 19–43, 2023, https://doi.org/10.1016/J.JCONREL.2023.08.019.
46. Sousa De Almeida, M., Susnik, E., Drasler, B., Taladriz-Blanco, P., Petri-Fink, A., Rothen-Rutishauser, B., Understanding nanoparticle endocytosis to improve targeting strategies in nanomedicine. *Chem. Soc. Rev.*, 50, 5397–434, 2021, https://doi.org/10.1039/D0CS01127D.
47. Qhattal, H.S.S. and Liu, X., Characterization of CD44-mediated cancer cell uptake and intracellular distribution of hyaluronan-grafted liposomes. *Mol. Pharm.*, 8, 1233–46, 2011, https://doi.org/10.1021/MP2000428/SUPPL_FILE/MP2000428_SI_001.PDF.
48. Wickens, J.M., Alsaab, H.O., Kesharwani, P., Bhise, K., Amin, M.C.I.M., Tekade, R.K., *et al.*, Recent advances in hyaluronic acid-decorated nanocarriers for targeted cancer therapy. *Drug Discov. Today*, 22, 665, 2016, https://doi.org/10.1016/J.DRUDIS.2016.12.009.
49. Heidari, R., Khosravian, P., Mirzaei, S.A., Elahian, F., siRNA delivery using intelligent chitosan-capped mesoporous silica nanoparticles for overcoming multidrug resistance in malignant carcinoma cells. *Sci. Rep.*, 11, 1, 1–14, 2021, https://doi.org/10.1038/s41598-021-00085-0.
50. Jiang, B., Aerobic glycolysis and high level of lactate in cancer metabolism and microenvironment. *Genes Dis.*, 4, 25–7, 2017, https://doi.org/10.1016/J.GENDIS.2017.02.003.
51. Winkler, J., Abisoye-Ogunniyan, A., Metcalf, K.J., Werb, Z., Concepts of extracellular matrix remodelling in tumour progression and metastasis. *Nat. Commun.*, 11, 1, 1–19, 2020, https://doi.org/10.1038/s41467-020-18794-x.
52. Miao, T., Wang, J., Zeng, Y., Liu, G., Chen, X., Polysaccharide-Based Controlled Release Systems for Therapeutics Delivery and Tissue Engineering: From Bench to Bedside. *Adv. Sci.*, 5, 1700513, 2018, https://doi.org/10.1002/ADVS.201700513.
53. Luo, K., Yin, S., Zhang, R., Yu, H., Wang, G., Li, J., Multifunctional composite nanoparticles based on hyaluronic acid-paclitaxel conjugates for enhanced cancer therapy. *Int. J. Pharm.*, 589, 119870, 2020, https://doi.org/10.1016/J.IJPHARM.2020.119870.
54. Ahmadi, M., Ritter, C.A., von Woedtke, T., Bekeschus, S., Wende, K., Package delivered: folate receptor-mediated transporters in cancer therapy and diagnosis. *Chem. Sci.*, 15, 1966–2006, 2024, https://doi.org/10.1039/D3SC05539F.
55. Angelopoulou, A., Kolokithas-Ntoukas, A., Fytas, C., Avgoustakis, K., Folic Acid-Functionalized, Condensed Magnetic Nanoparticles for Targeted Delivery of Doxorubicin to Tumor Cancer Cells Overexpressing the Folate Receptor. *ACS Omega*, 4, 22214–27, 2019, https://doi.org/10.1021/

ACSOMEGA.9B03594/ASSET/IMAGES/MEDIUM/AO9B03594_M002.GIF.

56. Donati, I. and Christensen, B.E., Alginate-metal cation interactions: Macromolecular approach. *Carbohydr. Polym.*, 321, 121280, 2023, https://doi.org/10.1016/J.CARBPOL.2023.121280.
57. Abyaneh, H.S., Regenold, M., McKee, T.D., Allen, C., Gauthier, M.A., Towards extracellular matrix normalization for improved treatment of solid tumors. *Theranostics*, 10, 1960, 2020, https://doi.org/10.7150/THNO.39995.
58. Luo, Z., Dai, Y., Gao, H., Development and application of hyaluronic acid in tumor targeting drug delivery. *Acta Pharm. Sin. B*, 9, 1099–112, 2019, https://doi.org/10.1016/J.APSB.2019.06.004.
59. Li, N., Chen, Y., Zhang, Y.M., Yang, Y., Su, Y., Chen, J.T., *et al.*, Polysaccharide-Gold Nanocluster Supramolecular Conjugates as a Versatile Platform for the Targeted Delivery of Anticancer Drugs. *Sci. Rep.*, 4, 1, 1–7, 2014, https://doi.org/10.1038/srep04164.
60. Liu, Y., Sun, M., Wang, T., Chen, X., Wang, H., Chitosan-based self-assembled nanomaterials: Their application in drug delivery. *View*, 2, 20200069, 2021, https://doi.org/10.1002/VIW.20200069.
61. Kesharwani, P., Halwai, K., Jha, S.K., Al Mughram, M.H., Almujri, S.S., Almalki, W.H., *et al.*, Folate-engineered chitosan nanoparticles: next-generation anticancer nanocarriers. *Mol. Cancer*, 23, 1, 1–51, 2024, https://doi.org/10.1186/S12943-024-02163-Z.
62. Cirillo, N., The Hyaluronan/CD44 Axis: A Double-Edged Sword in Cancer. *Int. J. Mol. Sci.*, 24, 21, 15812, 2023, https://doi.org/10.3390/IJMS242115812.
63. Zhong, Y., Zhang, J., Cheng, R., Deng, C., Meng, F., Xie, F., *et al.*, Reversibly crosslinked hyaluronic acid nanoparticles for active targeting and intelligent delivery of doxorubicin to drug resistant CD44 + human breast tumor xenografts. *J. Control. Release*, 205, 144–54, 2015, https://doi.org/10.1016/J.JCONREL.2015.01.012.
64. Lai, J., Azad, A.K., Sulaiman, W.M.A.W., Kumarasamy, V., Subramaniyan, V., Alshehade, S.A., Alginate-Based Encapsulation Fabrication Technique for Drug Delivery: An Updated Review of Particle Type, Formulation Technique, Pharmaceutical Ingredient, and Targeted Delivery System. *Pharm.*, 16, 370, 2024, https://doi.org/10.3390/PHARMACEUTICS16030370.
65. Melief, C.J.M., Cancer Immunotherapy by Dendritic Cells. *Immunity*, 29, 372–83, 2008, https://doi.org/10.1016/J.IMMUNI.2008.08.004.
66. Nichifor, M. and Mocanu, G., Polysaccharide-drug conjugates as controlled drug delivery systems. *ACS Symp. Ser.*, 934, 289–303, 2006, https://doi.org/10.1021/BK-2006-0934.CH015.
67. Liu, Y., Hinnant, B., Chen, S., Tao, H., Huang, Z., Qian, M., *et al.*, Hyaluronic acid-modified extracellular vesicles for targeted doxorubicin delivery in hepatocellular carcinoma. *Exp. Cell. Res.*, 443, 114332, 2024, https://doi.org/10.1016/J.YEXCR.2024.114332.

68. Soozanipour, A., Ejeian, F., Razmjou, A., Asadnia, M., Nasr-Esfahani, M.H., Taheri-Kafrani, A., Efficient PEGylated Dendrimer Nanoplatform for Codelivery of Hyaluronidase and Methotrexate: A New Frontier in Chemotherapeutic Efficacy and Tumor Penetration. *ACS Appl. Nano Mater.*, 7, 17262–77, 2024, https://doi.org/10.1021/ACSANM.4C01406/SUPPL_FILE/AN4C01406_SI_001.PDF.
69. Geethakumari, D., Bhaskaran Sathyabhama, A., Raji Sathyan, K., Mohandas, D., Somasekharan, J.V., Thavarool Puthiyedathu, S., Folate functionalized chitosan nanoparticles as targeted delivery systems for improved anticancer efficiency of cytarabine in MCF-7 human breast cancer cell lines. *Int. J. Biol. Macromol.*, 199, 150–61, 2022, https://doi.org/10.1016/J.IJBIOMAC.2021.12.070.
70. Ju, J., Xu, D., Mo, X., Miao, J., Xu, L., Ge, G., *et al.*, Multifunctional polysaccharide nanoprobes for biological imaging. *Carbohydr. Polym.*, 317, 121048, 2023, https://doi.org/10.1016/J.CARBPOL.2023.121048.
71. Majumder, J. and Minko, T., Multifunctional and stimuli-responsive nanocarriers for targeted therapeutic delivery. *Expert Opin. Drug Deliv.*, 18, 205–27, 2021, https://doi.org/10.1080/17425247.2021.1828339.
72. Feng, W., Nie, W., He, C., Zhou, X., Chen, L., Qiu, K., *et al.*, Effect of pH-responsive alginate/chitosan multilayers coating on delivery efficiency, cellular uptake and biodistribution of mesoporous silica nanoparticles based nanocarriers. *ACS Appl. Mater. Interfaces*, 6, 8447–60, 2014, https://doi.org/10.1021/AM501337S/SUPPL_FILE/AM501337S_SI_001.PDF.
73. Antoniraj, M.G., Jeeva Kumari, H.L., Shanmugarathinam, A., Kandasamy, R., pH-responsive chitosan copolymer synthesized *via* click chemistry for design of polymeric nanoparticles for targeted drug delivery. *Carbohydr. Res.*, 542, 109200, 2024, https://doi.org/10.1016/J.CARRES.2024.109200.
74. Yousefiasl, S., Zare, I., Ghovvati, M., Ghomi, M., Enzyme-Responsive Materials: Properties, Design, and Applications. *ACS Symp. Ser.*, 1436, 203–29, 2023, https://doi.org/10.1021/BK-2023-1436.CH009.
75. Guo, X., Cheng, Y., Zhao, X., Luo, Y., Chen, J., Yuan, W.E., Advances in redox-responsive drug delivery systems of tumor microenvironment. *J. Nanobiotechnol.*, 16, 1–10, 2018, https://doi.org/10.1186/S12951-018-0398-2/FIGURES/6.
76. Ma, W., Wang, X., Zhang, D., Mu, X., Research Progress of Disulfide Bond Based Tumor Microenvironment Targeted Drug Delivery System. *Int. J. Nanomed.*, 19, 7547–66, 2024, https://doi.org/10.2147/IJN.S471734.
77. Patra, P., Upadhyay, T.K., Alshammari, N., Saeed, M., Kesari, K.K., Alginate-Chitosan Biodegradable and Biocompatible Based Hydrogel for Breast Cancer Immunotherapy and Diagnosis: A Comprehensive Review. *ACS Appl. Bio Mater.*, 7, 3515–34, 2024, https://doi.org/10.1021/ACSABM.3C00984/ASSET/IMAGES/LARGE/MT3C00984_0003.JPEG.
78. Ravichandran, V., Kothandaraman, G.P., Bories, C., Loiseau, P.M., Jayakrishnan, A., Synthetic Polysaccharides as Drug Carriers: Synthesis of

Polyglucose-Amphotericin B Conjugates and *In Vitro* Evaluation of Their Anti-Fungal and Anti-Leishmanial Activities. *J. Nanosci. Nanotechnol.*, 18, 2405–14, 2018, https://doi.org/10.1166/JNN.2018.14296.

79. Hsu, C.Y., Allela, O.Q.B., Hussein, A.M., Mustafa, M.A., Kaur, M., Alaraj, M., *et al.*, Recent advances in polysaccharide-based drug delivery systems for cancer therapy: a comprehensive review. *Artif. Cells Nanomed. Biotechnol.*, 52, 564–86, 2024, https://doi.org/10.1080/21691401.2024.2436350.
80. Ezike, T.C., Okpala, U.S., Onoja, U.L., Nwike, C.P., Ezeako, E.C., Okpara, O.J., *et al.*, Advances in drug delivery systems, challenges and future directions. *Heliyon*, 9, e17488, 2023, https://doi.org/10.1016/J.HELIYON.2023.E17488.
81. Elieh Ali Komi, D., Sharma, L., Dela Cruz, C.S., Chitin and Its Effects on Inflammatory and Immune Responses. *Clin. Rev. Allergy Immunol.*, 54, 213, 2018, https://doi.org/10.1007/S12016-017-8600-0.
82. Ghattas, M., Dwivedi, G., Chevrier, A., Horn-Bourque, D., Alameh, M.G., Lavertu, M., Chitosan immunomodulation: insights into mechanisms of action on immune cells and signaling pathways. *RSC Adv.*, 15, 896–909, 2025, https://doi.org/10.1039/D4RA08406C.
83. How to Find and Effectively Use Predicate Devices, FDA, https://www.fda.gov/medical-devices/premarket-notification-510k/how-find-and-effectively-use-predicate-devices (accessed January 20, 2025).
84. Regulatory Controls, FDA, https://www.fda.gov/medical-devices/overview-device-regulation/regulatory-controls (accessed January 20, 2025).
85. Guo, J., Qiu, Y., Zhang, J., Xue, C., Zhu, J., A review on polysaccharide-based delivery systems for edible bioactives: pH responsive, controlled release, and emerging applications. *Int. J. Biol. Macromol.*, 291, 139178, 2025, https://doi.org/10.1016/J.IJBIOMAC.2024.139178.
86. Li, Q., Liu, X., Yan, C., Zhao, B., Zhao, Y., Yang, L., *et al.*, Polysaccharide-Based Stimulus-Responsive Nanomedicines for Combination Cancer Immunotherapy. *Small*, 19, 2206211, 2023, https://doi.org/10.1002/SMLL.202206211.
87. Toroghi, M.K., Cluett, W.R., Mahadevan, R., A Personalized Multiscale Modeling Framework for Dose Selection in Precision Medicine. *Ind. Eng. Chem. Res.*, 59, 9819–29, 2020, https://doi.org/10.1021/ACS.IECR.0C01070/SUPPL_FILE/IE0C01070_SI_001.PDF.
88. Hassanzadeh, P., Atyabi, F., Dinarvand, R., The significance of artificial intelligence in drug delivery system design. *Adv. Drug Deliv. Rev.*, 151–152, 169–90, 2019, https://doi.org/10.1016/J.ADDR.2019.05.001.

3

Inulin-Based Nanoparticles: Advancing Cancer Therapeutics through Biopolymer Innovations

Tariq Ahmad Mir[1], S. Wazed Ali[1] and Showkat Ali Ganie[2]*

[1]*Department of Textile and Fibre Engineering, Indian Institute of Technology Delhi, Delhi, India*
[2]*Department of Chemistry and Earth Sciences, College of Arts and Sciences, Qatar University, Doha, Qatar*

Abstract

Inulin-based nanoparticles have gained attention as a promising tool in cancer therapy due to their biocompatibility, biodegradability, and ability to respond to tumor-specific conditions. Derived from plant sources, inulin offers a unique structural foundation for the development of nanoparticles capable of targeted drug delivery and controlled release. Recent advancements include the creation of pH-responsive and redox-sensitive systems that exploit tumor microenvironment characteristics for precise therapeutic action. Inulin nanoparticles have demonstrated efficacy in encapsulating hydrophobic drugs, co-delivering multiple therapeutic agents, and inducing reactive oxygen species to promote apoptosis in cancer cells. Challenges such as optimizing drug loading and improving large-scale production remain, but emerging technologies, including hybrid systems and 3D printing, offer innovative solutions. Inulin nanoparticles hold immense potential for advancing personalized medicine, representing a significant leap forward in non-toxic, targeted cancer therapies.

Keywords: Inulin nanoparticles, biocompatible drug delivery, reactive oxygen species (ROS), pH-responsive nanocarriers, cancer nanomedicine, tumor microenvironment targeting

**Corresponding author*: alishowkat443@gmail.com

Luqman Jameel Rather, Showkat Ali Ganie and Mohammed A. Assiri (eds.) Polysaccharide Biomaterials in Cancer Research and Therapy: From Lab to Life, (57–86) © 2026 Scrivener Publishing LLC

3.1 Introduction

Cancer remains one of the most challenging diseases to treat, despite significant advancements in medicine [1]. Conventional therapies, such as chemotherapy and radiotherapy, often suffer from severe side effects, lack of specificity, and drug resistance [2]. Nanotechnology, particularly the development of nanoparticles as drug delivery systems, has revolutionized cancer therapeutics by offering targeted, controlled, and efficient delivery mechanisms [3]. Among the various nanocarriers, polysaccharide-based nanoparticles have shown immense potential due to their natural abundance, biocompatibility, and ability to be chemically tailored for specific applications [4]. In this context, **inulin**, a naturally occurring polysaccharide, has emerged as a highly promising material for nanoparticle synthesis aimed at enhancing cancer treatment outcomes [5]. Inulin is a plant-derived polysaccharide consisting of fructose units linked by β-(2→1) glycosidic bonds, with a terminal glucose molecule [6]. It is abundant in dietary sources such as chicory roots and Jerusalem artichokes [7]. Unlike many other biopolymers, inulin is resistant to enzymatic digestion in the human gastrointestinal tract, making it particularly useful for targeted drug delivery to the colon [8]. Additionally, its natural biodegradability and nontoxic profile make it ideal for biomedical applications [9]. These attributes have positioned inulin-based nanoparticles as a cutting-edge solution in modern nanomedicine, particularly for addressing the limitations of traditional cancer treatments [10]. The unique properties of inulin allow it to serve as a versatile platform for nanoparticle development [11]. Its chemical structure provides multiple functional groups that can be modified to enhance solubility, stability, and drug encapsulation efficiency. For example, functionalizing inulin with hydrophobic moieties enables the loading of poorly water-soluble chemotherapeutic agents such as camptothecin and paclitaxel [12]. Furthermore, inulin-based nanoparticles have been tailored to respond to specific stimuli in the tumor microenvironment, such as acidic pH or the presence of reactive oxygen species (ROS) [13]. These stimulus-responsive systems ensure that drugs are released precisely at the tumor site, thereby minimizing damage to healthy tissues [14].

In recent years, inulin nanoparticles have been explored for their ability to modulate biological pathways that are critical in cancer progression [15]. Studies have demonstrated that inulin-based nanocarriers can enhance ROS production in cancer cells, leading to oxidative stress, mitochondrial dysfunction, and apoptosis [16]. This mechanism has been particularly effective in targeting drug-resistant tumors [17].

Moreover, inulin nanoparticles have shown promise in delivering multiple therapeutic agents simultaneously [18]. Co-delivery systems that encapsulate chemotherapeutic drugs along with immune-modulating agents or genetic material, such as siRNA, have been developed to achieve synergistic therapeutic effects [19]. These systems not only enhance the efficacy of the primary drug but also target secondary pathways that contribute to tumor growth and metastasis [20]. One of the most promising applications of inulin nanoparticles is their use in colon-specific drug delivery [21]. The selective degradation of inulin by colonic microflora makes it an ideal carrier for treating colorectal cancer [8]. By encapsulating drugs in inulin nanoparticles, researchers have achieved improved drug stability and bioavailability in the gastrointestinal [22] tract. Additionally, inulin's ability to modulate the gut microbiome has opened new avenues for integrating microbiome-targeted therapies with conventional cancer treatments [23]. For instance, inulin nanoparticles have been combined with probiotics to create formulations that not only treat cancer but also restore the balance of gut flora, which is often disrupted by chemotherapy [24].

Despite their potential, the development of inulin nanoparticles faces certain challenges. Scalability in manufacturing, optimization of drug loading efficiency, and the need for clinical validation are critical areas that require further research. However, advancements in nanotechnology, including 3D printing and microfluidics, offer exciting possibilities for overcoming these hurdles. By integrating artificial intelligence (AI)-guided design and machine-learning algorithms, researchers can now optimize nanoparticle formulations more efficiently, paving the way for their clinical translation. In conclusion, inulin-based nanoparticles represent a transformative approach to cancer therapeutics. Their ability to enhance drug delivery, target tumor-specific environments, and modulate biological pathways makes them a valuable addition to the arsenal against cancer. As research progresses, the integration of inulin nanoparticles with advanced technologies and personalized medicine strategies is expected to further expand their therapeutic potential, offering hope for more effective and less invasive cancer treatments.

3.2 Chemistry and Structure of Inulin

Inulin is a natural polysaccharide that has garnered significant attention in biomedical applications due to its unique chemical structure, functional versatility, and inherent biocompatibility [11]. This section explores the chemical composition and structural features of inulin, its functionalization and modifications for enhanced properties, and its biocompatibility and biodegradability that make it ideal for nanoparticle-based cancer therapeutics. Inulin is primarily composed of linear chains of **β-(2→1)-linked fructose units** terminated by a glucose molecule (Figure 3.1) [15, 25]. This structural arrangement gives it a unique combination of hydrophilic and hydrophobic properties. Inulin molecules can have varying degrees of polymerization (DPs), typically ranging from 2 to 60 fructose units. Short-chain inulin is more soluble, whereas long-chain inulin provides higher stability in nanoparticle formulations [26].The water solubility ends on the polymer chain length and temperature, with higher solubility observed for shorter chains at room temperature [27]. Inulin exhibits excellent thermal stability, making it suitable for nanoparticle synthesis processes that involve high temperatures [28]. These properties allow inulin to serve as a stable and adaptable base material for the development of nanoparticles in cancer therapy. Its ability to withstand harsh gastrointestinal conditions while selectively degrading in the colon further enhances its utility in targeted drug delivery [5, 29]. The functional versatility of inulin lies in its hydroxyl groups, which can be chemically modified to enhance its properties for specific biomedical applications [11].

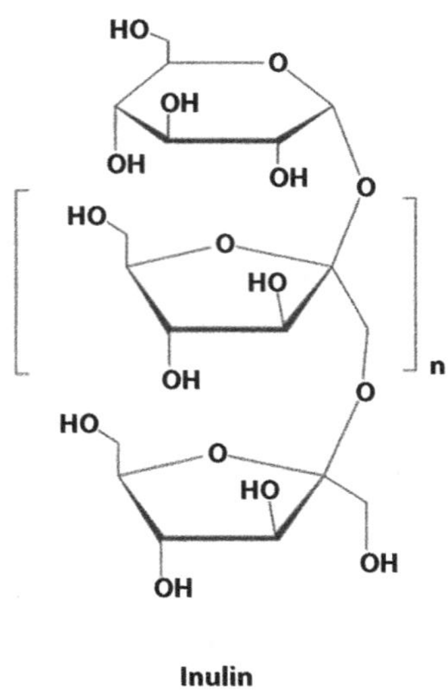

Figure 3.1 Structure of inulin.

Some common functionalization approaches include:

- **Hydrophobization**: Attaching hydrophobic moieties such as fatty acids or cholesterol enhances the encapsulation of hydrophobic drugs like paclitaxel and camptothecin [30].
- **Stimuli-Responsive Modifications**: Incorporating pH-sensitive or redox-sensitive functional groups allows inulin nanoparticles to release their payload specifically in acidic tumor microenvironments or under oxidative stress [31].
- **Targeting Ligands**: Conjugating targeting molecules, such as antibodies or peptides, enables specific binding to cancer cells, improving the therapeutic index [32].

Recent studies have shown that inulin modified with hydrophobic cholesterol derivatives forms self-assembling micelles capable of encapsulating hydrophobic drugs, significantly improving drug stability and bioavailability with pH-responsive properties, which have demonstrated controlled drug release in tumor sites, minimizing off-target effects and improving efficacy [33].

3.3 Biodegradability: Advantages for Biomedical Applications

Inulin's natural origin and biochemical properties make it inherently biocompatible and biodegradable, which are crucial for biomedical applications [34]. Inulin is recognized as Generally Regarded as Safe by the FDA, ensuring minimal risk of adverse reactions when used in pharmaceutical formulations [35]. The selective degradability resists enzymatic digestion in the upper gastrointestinal tract but is efficiently broken down by colonic microflora, making it highly suitable for colon-targeted drug delivery systems [36]. Immunomodulatory effect of inulin has been shown to positively influence the gut microbiome, enhancing host immunity and complementing cancer therapy by restoring microbial balance disrupted by chemotherapy [37]. These attributes allow inulin-based nanoparticles to deliver drugs effectively while minimizing systemic toxicity [38]. Their ability to degrade into non-toxic by-products ensures safe elimination from the body, a critical factor for clinical translation [39].

3.4 Synthesis and Fabrication of Inulin-Based Nanoparticles

3.4.1 Methods of Nanoparticle Formulations

The synthesis and fabrication of inulin-based nanoparticles have become a cornerstone in leveraging inulin's potential for cancer therapeutics [10]. By employing advanced techniques, researchers can create nanoparticles with enhanced stability, efficient drug encapsulation, and controlled release [40]. This section provides an in-depth exploration of the methodologies used for nanoparticle preparation, the roles of stabilizing agents and cross-linkers, and innovations in green synthesis techniques [41].

3.4.1.1 Ionic Gelation

Ionic gelation is a simple and cost-effective method for fabricating inulin nanoparticles [38]. This technique involves the interaction between the negatively charged inulin molecules and multivalent cations, such as calcium ions, to form nanoparticles. Key highlights are as follows:

- **Procedure**: Inulin is dissolved in aqueous solutions and mixed with ionic crosslinkers to initiate nanoparticle formation [42].
- **Advantages**: This method is efficient for encapsulating hydrophilic drugs and maintaining their bioactivity [43].
- **Applications**: Ionic gelation has been widely used to produce inulin nanoparticles for colon-targeted drug delivery, leveraging the selective degradability of inulin by colonic enzymes [44].

3.4.1.2 Self-Assembling Techniques

Self-assembling nanoparticles are formed by modifying inulin molecules with hydrophobic moieties, such as fatty acids or cholesterol derivatives [13]. These modifications enable the spontaneous formation of micelle-like structures in aqueous environments:

- **Mechanism**: Hydrophobic interactions drive the self-assembly of amphiphilic inulin derivatives into nanoscale structures [45].

- **Advantages**: These nanoparticles are particularly effective for encapsulating poorly water-soluble chemotherapeutics, such as paclitaxel and camptothecin [46].
- **Applications**: Self-assembling inulin nanoparticles are used in multidrug delivery systems and for targeted release in acidic tumor microenvironments [47].

3.4.1.3 Microfluidics and Spray Drying

These advanced fabrication techniques allow precise control over the size, shape, and drug loading efficiency of nanoparticles:

- ➢ **Microfluidics**: A continuous flow of inulin and drug solutions through microfluidic channels results in the formation of uniform nanoparticles [48].
  - **Benefits**: Microfluidics ensures reproducibility, scalability, and minimal solvent use [49].
  - **Applications**: Used for fabricating nanoparticles with targeted delivery capabilities and responsive release [50].
- ➢ **Spray Drying**: This method involves the atomization of inulin solutions into a hot chamber, where rapid solvent evaporation creates dry nanoparticles.
  - **Advantages**: Spray drying is ideal for large-scale production and provides good control over particle morphology [51].

3.4.2 Role of Stabilizing Agents and Crosslinkers

Stabilizing agents and crosslinkers are essential in enhancing the stability and functionality of inulin-based nanoparticles [52]. Materials like polyethylene glycol and polysorbates are often used to improve the dispersity and biocompatibility of nanoparticles [53]. They reduce aggregation, increase circulation time in the bloodstream, and improve cellular uptake [54]. Chemical agents such as glutaraldehyde or natural substances like genipin are employed to strengthen the nanoparticle matrix [55]. Crosslinking improves mechanical strength, drug retention, and resistance to premature degradation in physiological conditions [56].

3.4.3 Advances in Green Synthesis Techniques

Green synthesis methods emphasize the use of eco-friendly and sustainable approaches for nanoparticle fabrication [57]. Key innovations include the following: (a) natural extracts (e.g., phenolic compounds) are used to reduce inulin derivatives, eliminating the need for toxic chemical agents; (b) techniques such as ionic gelation and self-assembly avoid the use of organic solvents, ensuring safer formulations; and (c) natural crosslinkers like genipin offer enhanced biocompatibility compared to synthetic alternatives [58]. These green approaches not only reduce environmental impact but also ensure compatibility with clinical applications, where nontoxic and sustainable practices are paramount [59].

3.5 Applications in Cancer Therapy

Inulin-based nanoparticles have demonstrated exceptional potential in addressing the challenges of cancer therapy, such as drug resistance, systemic toxicity, and lack of tumor specificity [38]. These nanoparticles offer versatile platforms for delivering chemotherapeutic agents, targeting tumor microenvironments, and combining therapies for synergistic effects, thereby improving therapeutic outcomes. One of the most significant applications of inulin-based nanoparticles is their role as drug delivery platforms [60]. The unique chemical properties of inulin enable the design of nanoparticles that are pH-responsive, allowing drug release to be triggered specifically in the acidic microenvironment of tumors [61]. By incorporating functional groups sensitive to pH, inulin nanoparticles ensure that the therapeutic payload remains stable in the bloodstream but is released at the tumor site [23]. For instance, doxorubicin-loaded inulin nanoparticles have been shown to achieve selective release under acidic conditions, significantly reducing systemic toxicity while enhancing the drug's efficacy against cancer cells [22]. Furthermore, the crosslinking of inulin molecules or hydrophobic modifications can create nanoparticles capable of sustaining drug release over an extended period, maintaining therapeutic drug concentrations and improving treatment outcomes [62].

The tumor microenvironment plays a critical role in cancer progression, and inulin nanoparticles are well suited for targeting specific features of this environment [63]. Colon-specific drug delivery is one such application, leveraging the selective degradability of inulin by colonic microflora. This property enables inulin nanoparticles to protect drugs from degradation in the stomach and small intestine, ensuring that they are released only in the colon [44, 64]. This targeted approach is particularly effective for treating colorectal cancer, as it increases the concentration of the drug at the tumor site while minimizing adverse effects [65]. Additionally, functionalizing inulin nanoparticles with ligands such as folic acid or RGD peptides facilitates receptor-mediated targeting of tumors [11]. This strategy enhances the selective uptake of nanoparticles by cancer cells that overexpress specific receptors, such as folate or integrin receptors, further improving the specificity and efficacy of the treatment [66]. In addition to delivering single drugs, inulin-based nanoparticles are increasingly being used for the co-delivery of multiple therapeutic agents [52]. This approach allows for the simultaneous targeting of multiple pathways involved in cancer progression, leading to synergistic therapeutic effects [67]. For example, inulin nanoparticles have been developed to encapsulate both cisplatin and doxorubicin, two chemotherapeutic agents with complementary mechanisms of action [15]. This co-delivery system not only enhances the apoptotic effects on cancer cells but also reduces the likelihood of drug resistance [68]. Similarly, combining chemotherapeutics with gene therapies, such as siRNA, in inulin nanoparticles has shown promise in targeting genetic mutations while inducing cytotoxic effects, offering a powerful strategy for treating drug-resistant cancers [69].

The versatility of inulin-based nanoparticles extends beyond drug delivery to include modulation of the immune response and improved interaction with the tumor microenvironment [13]. By enhancing ROS production within cancer cells, inulin nanoparticles can induce oxidative stress, mitochondrial dysfunction, and apoptosis, effectively reducing tumor growth [70]. Moreover, the ability of inulin nanoparticles to restore the balance of the gut microbiome disrupted by chemotherapy highlights their potential for integrating microbiome-targeted therapies with conventional treatments, particularly for gastrointestinalcancers [71]. In conclusion, inulin-based nanoparticles represent a transformative approach to cancer therapy, combining precise targeting, controlled release, and multidrug delivery capabilities. Their ability to adapt to the complexities of the tumor microenvironment, coupled with their biocompatibility and biodegradability, positions them as a cornerstone in the advancement of nanomedicine. As research progresses, further optimization and clinical validation of these systems are expected to pave the way for more effective and personalized cancer treatments.

3.6 Mechanisms of Action in Cancer Cells

The therapeutic efficacy of inulin-based nanoparticles in cancer therapy lies in their ability to engage multiple cellular and molecular mechanisms to suppress tumor growth and enhance cancer cell death [72]. These nanoparticles operate through a variety of pathways, including the generation of ROS, induction of apoptosis, mitochondrial dysfunction, cell cycle arrest, and immunomodulation [73]. By targeting these pathways, inulin-based nanoparticles not only exert cytotoxic effects on cancer cells but also enhance the overall therapeutic impact of the encapsulated drugs [22]. One of the primary mechanisms by which inulin-based nanoparticles combat cancer is through the generation of ROS within cancer cells. Cancer cells often exhibit higher baseline ROS levels due to their rapid proliferation and metabolic activity [74]. Inulin-based nanoparticles, especially those modified with redox-sensitive functional groups, can further elevate intracellular ROS levels upon drug release, pushing the cells into oxidative stress. This oxidative stress damages critical cellular components such as DNA, lipids, and proteins, ultimately triggering apoptosis [75]. Studies have shown that the ROS-mediated mechanism of inulin nanoparticles amplifies the efficacy of encapsulated chemotherapeutic agents, such as doxorubicin, by enhancing their cytotoxicity while minimizing systemic side effects [16].

Mitochondrial dysfunction is another critical pathway targeted by inulin-based nanoparticles. The release of therapeutic agents from these nanoparticles can disrupt mitochondrial membrane potential, leading to the activation of intrinsic apoptotic pathways. This involves the release of cytochrome c from the mitochondria into the cytoplasm, which activates caspase-9 and downstream effector caspases, culminating in programmed cell death [76]. Additionally, the oxidative damage induced by ROS disrupts mitochondrial integrity, further amplifying apoptosis. Inulin nanoparticles have also been observed to arrest the cell cycle at critical checkpoints, such as the G2/M phase, by interfering with cell cycle regulatory proteins. This prevents cancer cells from proliferating and enhances their susceptibility to apoptosis [77].

Beyond direct cytotoxic effects, inulin-based nanoparticles also exhibit immunomodulatory properties that contribute to their anticancer activity. By interacting with the immune microenvironment, these nanoparticles can stimulate antitumor immune responses. For example, inulin nanoparticles have been shown to enhance dendritic cell activation and T-cell responses, improving the recognition and destruction of cancer cells [78].

Additionally, their ability to modulate the gut microbiota can indirectly influence systemic immunity, particularly in gastrointestinal cancers. Restoring a healthy microbiota composition can reduce inflammation and enhance the efficacy of immune checkpoint inhibitors or other immunotherapies when used in combination with inulin-based nanoparticles [79]. In summary, the mechanisms of action of inulin-based nanoparticles are multifaceted, targeting cancer cells through oxidative stress, mitochondrial dysfunction, cell cycle arrest, and immune modulation. These pathways not only directly kill cancer cells but also create an unfavorable environment for tumor growth and survival. The combination of these mechanisms, along with the ability of inulin nanoparticles to deliver therapeutic agents with high precision, underscores their potential as a powerful tool in modern oncology. Further exploration of these mechanisms in preclinical and clinical studies will help unlock the full potential of inulin-based nanoparticles in personalized cancer therapy.

3.7 Case Studies and Examples

Inulin-based selenium nanoparticle was designed and fabricated to overcome the inherent limitations of selenium nanoparticles of low bioavailability and low stability, extending the application of these nanoparticles in cancer treatment. 3-(4,5-dimethylthiazol-2-yl)-2,5-diphenyltetrazolium bromide (MTT) assay was used to examine the *in vitro* antitumor activity of inulin selenium nanoparticles on HepG2, HeLa, and A549 cells. Inulin selenium nanoparticles showed exceptional antitumor efficacy in Hela cells by boosting the formation of ROS. These nanoparticles could inhibit the proliferation of cancer cells by promoting apoptosis. The *in vivo* antitumor activity of inulin selenium nanoparticles was studied by using a zebrafish xenograft model, which showed that the anticancer activity of these nanoparticles might prevent the neovascularization of transgenic zebrafish and limit the proliferation and migration of tumors in the zebrafish xenograft [80, 81]. Selenium nanoparticles capped with inulin were prepared using sodium selenite through a redox reaction with ascorbic acid and were studied for their antitumor activity against a mouse forestomach carcinoma cell line. The nanoparticles had a substantial *in vitro* antiproliferative effect on mouse forestomach cancer cells, with a high inhibition rate, and the rate of late apoptosis in MFC cells increases with increasing nanoparticle concentration [82]. Inulin was used to stabilize selenium nanoparticles and were studied for the antihepatoma activities and intended to explore the potential applications in liver cancer by

Western blotting. The nanoparticles significantly increased the cleavage of poly ADP-ribose polymerase in a dose-dependent manner, validating the activation of apoptosis. These prevented the release of Bcl-2 as well, demonstrating that these nanoparticles led to mitochondrial dysfunction and, ultimately, cell death. Cleaved caspase-9 and cleaved caspase-3 protein expression levels decreased significantly as the concentration of these nanoparticles increased, whereas poly ADP-ribose polymerase and Bcl-2 protein expression levels increased significantly. This suggests that these nanoparticles can prevent 293T cells from going into apoptosis [83].

A biodegradable inulin-cholesterol derivative capable of generating core-shell nanostructures with micelle-like architecture, appropriate for the delivery of extremely hydrophobic anticancer drug 7-ethyl-10-hydroxy-camptothecin, was prepared. These nano-sized micelles were prepared by partially functionalizing inulin with thiocholesterol moieties *via* disulfide redox-sensitive bridges. The anticancer efficiency of these nano micelles was evaluated on human colorectal cancer cells, human breast cancer cells, and normal human bronchial epithelial cells by MTS assays. These micelles are capable of entering cancer cells and releasing their payload, particularly inside cell nuclei, where 7-ethyl-10-hydroxy-camptothecin can act and provide the greatest inhibition of its molecular target. The drug 7-ethyl-10-hydroxy-camptothecin is localized throughout the cell's cytoplasm, lysosomes, and nuclei where it acts as a topoisomerase inhibitor providing the main anticancer activity. The increased cytotoxicity reported in cancer cells may be attributed to the redox sensitivity of the disulfide bonds found in cancer cells, where the cytoplasmatic concentration of reduced glutathione is around tenfold higher than in normal cells. This means that the hydrophobic moieties linked by disulfide bridges inside lysosomes degrade quickly, resulting in rapid diffusion of 7-ethyl-10-hydroxy-camptothecin, which induces fast and unreversible cell damages [84] (Figure 3.2a). The nanoparticles were created with a core unit of lecithin sodium acetate ionic complex and a shell of quaternized inulin and were studied *in vitro* for their anticancer activity against breast cancer cell line by using MTT assay. Inulin was chemically modified by using glycidyl trimethyl ammonium chloride, which acts as a positively charged shell component and encapsulates the negatively charged surface of lecithin sodium acetate. Paclitaxel and curcumin are encapsulated in a new nano/micro drug delivery system with a lecithin-acetate core and an outer shell of quaternized inulin. This nano/micro drug delivery system's cytotoxicity is owing to effective cell internalization and drug release within the cell *via* enzymatic processes [85] (Figure 3.2b).

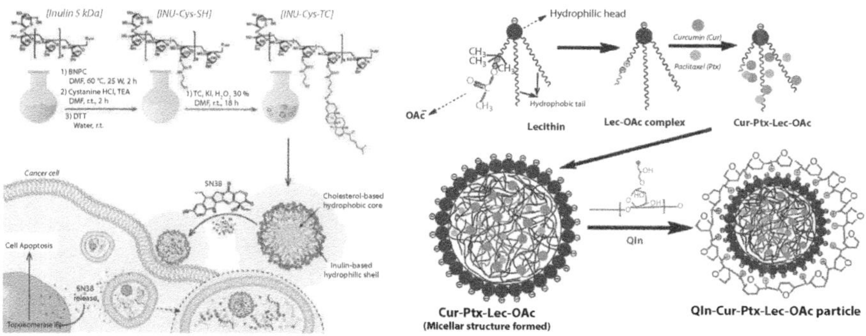

(a) (b)

Figure 3.2 (a) Cholesterol inulin conjugates. (b) Quaternized inulin-coated nanoparticles.

Inulin–stearic acid conjugate was used to create the self-assembling spherical nanoparticles, which were then tested for their ability to deliver genistein to targeted sites for the treatment of colon cancer. Hydrophobic genistein was enclosed within the hydrophobic stearic acid matrix of the nanoparticles by utilizing a solvent evaporation method. The hydrophobic chain of the inulin stearic acid conjugate aids in the production of drug-loaded, spontaneously assembling nanoparticles with fructose shell formation. The presence of inulin in the nanoparticles can prevent genistein from premature release in an acidic stomach environment while allowing the release in lower intestine-specific pH environments. The cytotoxicity profiles of the nanoparticles against human colorectal cancer cells were screened by MTT assay. Antiproliferation and apoptosis studies on the nanoparticles revealed potential cytotoxicity against human colorectal cancer cells. Due to the nanoparticles' strong cellular internalization, the observed half maximal inhibitory concentration value of the nanoparticles was much lower [86]. To increase the biocompatibility of the nanoformulation, boron-doped amine-functionalized carbon dots were coupled with a redesigned derivative of inulin using carbodiimide coupling reaction. The carbon dots were prepared using the solvothermal method in a single step. *In vitro* and *in vivo* tests on inulin-tethered boron-doped amine-functionalized carbon dots have shown that they are not harmful to the cell cultures. These inulin-based carbon dots exhibit no significant negative effects on mice at the levels evaluated according to tests on mice's survival, pathology, blood biochemical index, and biodistribution after inhalation exposure. With cell survival reaching 80% even at fairly high concentrations of these carbon dots, the biocompatibility MTT test on A549 cancer

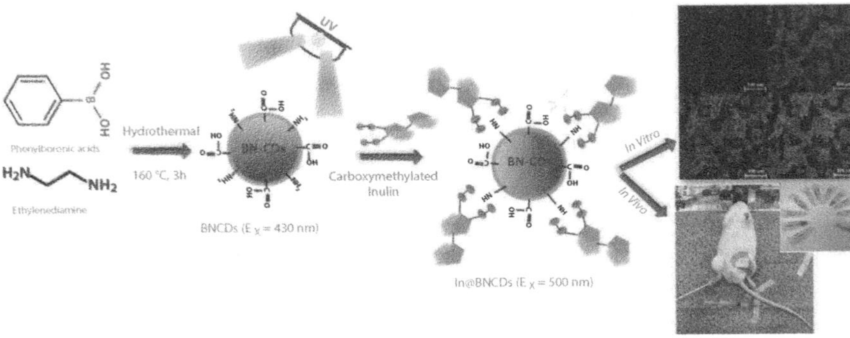

Figure 3.3 Inulin tethered boron-doped amine functionalized carbon dots.

cells demonstrated that these carbon dots did not clearly cause cytotoxicity [87] (Figure 3.3).

Inulin was used for coating the arginine stabilized manganese oxide nanocuboids for oral delivery of shRNA to the gut and was orally delivered to adenomatous polyposis coli knockout colon cancer mice models to evaluate the therapeutic possibility and effectiveness of this multimodal biodrug. The colon cancer cell line HCT-116 and a control cell line HEK293 were both subjected to an MTT experiment to determine the toxic effect of inulin-coated shRNA coupled arginine surface modified manganese oxide nanocuboids on their target (i.e., intestines). The Ephb4 gene was knocked down because of site-targeted administration of inulin-coated shRNA linked with surface modified manganese oxide nanocuboids, which enhanced survival without any known off-target effects. The inulin encapsulation prevents the breakdown of the nanoparticle shRNA complex and thus protecting it from the hostile stomach environment [88] (Figure 3.4a). The micellar aggregates up to 100 nm in size were created in aqueous solution above a critical concentration by using octenyl succinic anhydride inulin to solubilize doxorubicin. The CCK-8 method was used to determine the cytotoxicity of micelles toward MCF-7 cells, and BALB/c nude mice were used for the animal imaging tests. The octenyl succinic anhydride inulin micelles were suitable as delivery systems for doxorubicin with increased *in vitro* therapeutic efficacy because they had low cytotoxicity toward MCF-7 cells. This might be as a result of the polymer's size conforming to the increased permeability and retention impact, which improves the cells' ability to absorb doxorubicin loaded micelles. These also impeded macrophage identification in the reticuloendothelial system *via* the enhanced permeability and retention effect, resulting in extended blood circulation and increased tumor accumulation [89].

The paclitaxel-loaded oral colon double-targeted nanoparticles were synthesized by employing polylactic acid–polyethyleneimine and hyaluronic acid–inulin as an efficient delivery strategy that particularly targets the colon. Inulin can facilitate the secure distribution of nanoparticles to the colon because it is enzyme-sensitive and barely digested in the upper digestive tract. The nanoparticles were employed for proliferation inhibition research and *in vitro* anticancer studies, such as fluorescence labeling and flow cytometry. According to the investigation, the nanoparticles were more effectively absorbed by cancer cells and had a higher capacity to cause apoptosis and higher cytotoxicity. *In vivo* experiments demonstrated that the nanoparticles could stay for 24 hours and aggregate at the tumor site with significant therapeutic effect on tumor growth inhibition due to paclitaxel accumulation in tumors and excellent cancer cell uptake [15] (Figure 3.4b).

A human colon cancer cell line, human hepatic cancer cell line, and a human dermal fibroblast cell line were used in *in vitro* cell survival experiments on inulin-coated quercetin nanoparticles that were synthesized by using the spray dryer method. The nanoparticles facilitated the absorption of quercetin into Caco-2 cells, leading to an increase in its antiproliferative effects. The addition of inulin to the nanoparticles did not affect cell integrity, making the formulations biocompatible. The antiproliferative activity of quercetin was significantly enhanced by the nanoparticles, leading to a stronger inhibitory effect on HeLa cells. Overall, the nanoparticles show significant cytotoxicity against Caco-2 and HepG2 cells, while

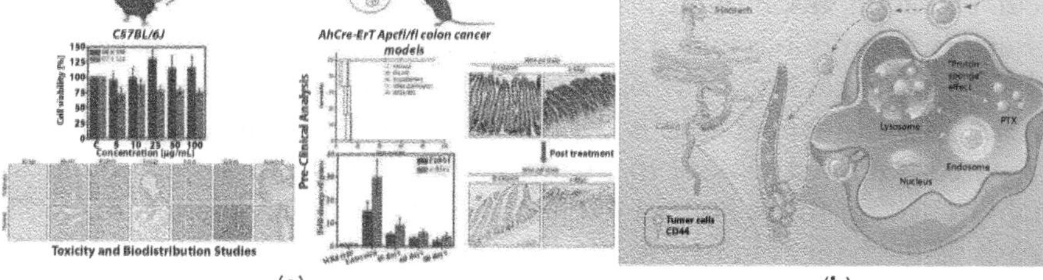

Figure 3.4 (a) Inulin-coated Mn_3O_4 nano cuboids and (b) paclitaxel-loaded composite nanoparticle delivery system.

having minimal effects on normal HDFa cells [90]. The ionotropic gelation method was used to synthesize inulin nanoparticles that were very stable and non-aggregatory. Calcium chloride was employed as the crosslinker, whereas natural honey served as the stabilizing agent. Several factors were found to influence the synthesis of inulin nanoparticles like concentration of inulin, honey, selection of counterions, $CaCl_2$, and stirring duration. An amorphous phase of the hydrophilic drug irinotecan hydrochloride trihydrate was encapsulated by the synthesized nanoparticles. The results of the colloidal stability investigations indicated that the inulin nanoparticles loaded with irinotecan hydrochloride trihydrate were more stable at room temperature, which could be attributed to the honey. The regulated release of irinotecan hydrochloride trihydrate from the nanoparticles was seen to be pH-dependent, suggesting that the nanoparticles were effective in targeting and releasing the drug specifically to the colon.

The MTT test was utilized on HCT 116 cells to study the *in vitro* evaluation of the anticancer activity of the nanoparticles. The control cells had a significant percentage of cell viability, suggesting a substantial quantity of viable cells. Conversely, cells that were exposed to the pure irinotecan hydrochloride trihydrate and nanoparticles exhibited a significant reduction in the percentage of cell viability. The proportion of viable cells in the cells treated with nanoparticles exhibited a notable decrease in comparison to the drug, suggesting a more pronounced anticancer impact of the nanoparticles on HCT 116 cells in contrast to the free irinotecan hydrochloride trihydrate. The inhibitory effects of the nanoparticles and free drug on HCT 116 cell colony formation were observed from colony formation assay. The nanoparticles exhibited a larger percentage of colony inhibition ability in comparison to the free drug. It was noted that nanoparticles greatly improved the suppression of colony formation in comparison to free drug, indicating that nanoparticles have a greater antiproliferative effect than free drug [91]. The successful synthesis of a novel bioconjugate was achieved by combining inulin, pluronic F68, and a lipid stearic acid. Due to its amphiphilic properties, the bioconjugate can undergo self-assembly into double-folded micelles. These micelles have the capacity to retain a significant quantity of hydrophobic resveratrol and subsequently release it in a manner that is dependent on pH. The micelles that were prepared exhibited a size at the nanoscale, a high level of physicochemical stability for up to 48 hours in colloidal form, and degradation that was sensitive to changes in pH. In the context of *in vitro* anticancer studies, it was observed that nomicelles exhibited superior efficacy in regulating the proliferation of human colorectal cancer cells compared to pure resveratrol. This was achieved through the induction of increased apoptosis and enhanced drug delivery *via* improved cellular uptake. Subsequently, the nomicelles were administered orally to animals in order to assess the pharmacokinetic parameter. The results indicated that the oral bioavailability of resveratrol was enhanced by the administration of these nomicelles. Therefore, the application of nanostructures based on inulin in the pH-responsive transportation of hydrophobic compounds in the gastrointestinal system exhibits promise and practicality [92].

3.8 Challenges and Limitations

Despite the promising potential of inulin-based nanoparticles in cancer therapy, several challenges and limitations must be addressed to ensure their successful translation from research to clinical applications. These obstacles include issues related to stability and scalability in production, optimization of drug loading efficiency, and overcoming multidrug resistance (MDR) in tumors [93]. One of the primary challenges in utilizing inulin-based nanoparticles is ensuring their stability and scalability for large-scale production. Nanoparticles often face issues such as aggregation, sedimentation, or premature degradation during storage and transportation, which can significantly impact their efficacy and shelf life [38]. Inulin-based nanoparticles, while inherently biocompatible and biodegradable, require additional stabilizing agents or surface modifications to enhance their colloidal stability over extended periods [94]. Furthermore, scaling up the production of these nanoparticles while maintaining their uniformity, size distribution, and encapsulation efficiency poses a significant technological and economic challenge. Techniques like spray drying and microfluidics offer potential solutions but require further optimization and cost-effective implementation for industrial-scale manufacturing [95].

Another critical limitation lies in optimizing the drug loading efficiency of inulin-based nanoparticles. Although inulin's chemical structure allows for functional modifications and drug encapsulation, achieving high drug loading capacity without compromising the structural integrity of the nanoparticles remains challenging [5]. Many chemotherapeutic agents, particularly hydrophobic drugs, exhibit limited solubility and compatibility with hydrophilic inulin matrices, necessitating the development of amphiphilic derivatives or specialized formulations [96]. Additionally, ensuring the controlled and sustained release of drugs from these nanoparticles requires precise crosslinking or encapsulation strategies, which can complicate the fabrication process and reduce production yields. MDR in tumors is another major obstacle to the efficacy of inulin-based nanoparticles [97].

Cancer cells often develop resistance to chemotherapeutic agents through various mechanisms, such as overexpression of efflux pumps (e.g., P-glycoprotein), alterations in drug targets, and enhanced DNA repair pathways [98]. While inulin-based nanoparticles can improve drug bioavailability and cellular uptake, overcoming MDR requires advanced strategies, such as co-delivery systems. These systems encapsulate multiple agents, such as chemotherapeutics and MDR inhibitors, within a single nanoparticle to simultaneously target multiple resistance pathways [16]. For instance, inulin nanoparticles co-loaded with siRNA and chemotherapeutic agents have shown potential in silencing resistance genes while delivering cytotoxic drugs. However, achieving effective co-delivery and ensuring the stability of such formulations remain significant hurdles [99]. In conclusion, while inulin-based nanoparticles hold immense potential in cancer therapy, addressing these challenges is critical for their clinical success. Advancements in fabrication techniques, incorporation of stabilizing agents, and the development of innovative drug delivery strategies can help overcome these limitations. Collaborative efforts between researchers, clinicians, and industry stakeholders are essential to optimize these systems and unlock their full potential in combating cancer.

3.9 Emerging Trends and Future Perspectives

Inulin-based nanoparticles are at the forefront of innovations in cancer therapeutics, and their potential continues to expand with the integration of advanced technologies and novel design strategies [5]. Emerging trends are shaping their development to address clinical challenges more effectively, paving the way for their transition from experimental models to widespread clinical application. Key advancements include the integration of cutting-edge technologies such as 3D printing and AI-guided design, the combination of inulin with other biopolymers, and efforts to bridge the gap between bench research and bedside applications. The integration of **3D printing technologies** is revolutionizing the development of personalized cancer therapies [100]. By using 3D printing, inulin-based nanoparticles can be incorporated into custom-designed drug delivery systems, such as implants, scaffolds, or microneedles, tailored to the unique anatomical and pathological features of individual patients. This level of customization ensures precise drug delivery to tumor sites, enhancing therapeutic efficacy while minimizing systemic side effects. Furthermore, 3D printing allows for the production of complex hybrid systems combining inulin nanoparticles with other therapeutic materials, such as hydrogels or bioresorbable polymers, enabling multifunctional platforms for cancer treatment [101, 102]. **AI-guided nanoparticle design** is another transformative trend that is streamlining the development of inulin-based nanoparticles. AI and machine-learning algorithms are being used to optimize nanoparticle formulations by predicting their physicochemical properties, drug loading capacities, and therapeutic outcomes [103]. These computational tools can analyze vast datasets to identify the most effective combinations of functional groups, drug payloads, and fabrication methods, significantly reducing the time and cost associated with experimental trials [104]. Moreover, AI can aid in the design of nanoparticles with enhanced targeting and release profiles, ensuring better interaction with tumor microenvironments and improving therapeutic precision [105].

Combining **inulin with other biopolymers** to create hybrid nanoparticle systems is another promising approach. Hybrid systems leverage the complementary properties of multiple materials to achieve enhanced performance [102]. For example, combining inulin with alginate or hyaluronic acid can improve the mechanical stability, drug encapsulation efficiency, and biological interactions of nanoparticles. These hybrid systems can also be engineered for dual stimuli responsiveness, such as pH and temperature, providing more sophisticated control over drug release in complex tumor environments [5]. Furthermore, the inclusion of metallic nanoparticles, such as gold or iron oxide, within inulin-based systems adds capabilities for imaging or hyperthermia, expanding their applications beyond drug delivery [106]. The goal for inulin-based nanoparticles is **clinical translation**, bridging the gap between bench research and bedside applications. Achieving this requires addressing regulatory, manufacturing, and scalability challenges while ensuring reproducibility and safety in clinical trials. Collaborative efforts between researchers, pharmaceutical companies, and regulatory agencies are crucial for establishing standardized protocols for nanoparticle production, characterization, and evaluation. Additionally, advancements in scalable green synthesis methods and cost-effective manufacturing processes are critical to making inulin-based nanoparticles viable for large-scale clinical use. Preclinical and clinical studies must also provide robust data on the efficacy, toxicity, and pharmacokinetics of these nanoparticles to gain regulatory approval. The emerging trends in the development of inulin-based nanoparticles highlight their vast potential to transform cancer therapy. From leveraging 3D printing and AI for personalized and efficient designs to creating hybrid systems with enhanced functionality, these innovations are setting the stage for their clinical success. With sustained research efforts and interdisciplinary collaborations, inulin-based nanoparticles are poised to become a cornerstone in precision oncology, addressing unmet needs in cancer therapeutics and improving patient outcomes.

3.10 Conclusion

Inulin-based nanoparticles have emerged as a versatile and promising platform in cancer therapeutics, offering innovative solutions to the challenges of traditional treatments. Their unique properties, including biocompatibility, biodegradability, and functional versatility, make them ideal for advanced drug delivery systems. By leveraging their ability to target tumor-specific microenvironments, sustain drug release, and co-deliver multiple therapeutic agents, inulin nanoparticles address critical issues such as systemic toxicity, poor drug solubility, and MDR. The mechanisms through which inulin-based nanoparticles exert their therapeutic effects, including ROS generation, apoptosis induction, and mitochondrial dysfunction, highlight their potential to selectively and effectively combat cancer cells. Furthermore, their immunomodulatory capabilities and ability to restore gut microbiota balance add a unique dimension to their application, particularly in cancers of the gastrointestinal tract.

Emerging trends, such as the integration of 3D printing for personalized medicine, AI-guided design, and hybrid systems combining inulin with other biopolymers, are paving the way for more sophisticated and effective cancer therapies. These advancements not only enhance the precision and efficacy of inulin-based systems but also contribute to the broader goal of personalized and precision oncology. However, challenges remain, including stability, scalability in production, and regulatory hurdles, which require concerted efforts from researchers, industry stakeholders, and regulatory agencies. As research continues to refine inulin nanoparticle formulations and address these challenges, their potential for clinical translation becomes increasingly tangible. With their adaptability and compatibility with advanced technologies, inulin-based nanoparticles are poised to play a transformative role in the future of cancer therapy. Their ability to provide targeted, efficient, and less invasive treatment options holds the promise of significantly improving patient outcomes and quality of life. In summary, inulin-based nanoparticles exemplify the convergence of natural materials and nanotechnology to address some of the most pressing challenges in oncology. Their integration into mainstream cancer treatment protocols is not only a possibility but an inevitability as research and innovation continue to push the boundaries of what is achievable in modern medicine.

AI disclosure statement: The author acknowledges the use of AI-based tools for minor language editing or grammatical correction. However, all intellectual contributions, analyses, and conclusions presented in this chapter are entirely the author's own.

References

1. Pucci, C., Martinelli, C., Ciofani, G., Innovative Approaches for Cancer Treatment: Current Perspectives and New Challenges. *Ecancermedicalscience, 13*, 961, 2019, https://doi.org/10.3332/ecancer.2019.961.
2. Markman, J.L., Rekechenetskiy, A., Holler, E., Ljubimova, J.Y., Nanomedicine Therapeutic Approaches to Overcome Cancer Drug Resistance. *Adv. Drug Deliv. Rev., 65*, 13–14, 1866–1879, 2013, https://doi.org/10.1016/j.addr.2013.09.019.
3. Reddy, K.T.K. and Reddy, A.S., Recent Breakthroughs in Drug Delivery Systems for Targeted Cancer Therapy: An Overview. *Cell. Mol. Biomed. Rep., 5*, 1, 13–27, 2025, https://doi.org/10.55705/cmbr.2025.456494.1246.
4. Wang, C., Gao, X., Chen, Z., Chen, Y., Chen, H., Preparation, Characterization and Application of Polysaccharide-Based Metallic Nanoparticles: A Review. *Polymers (Basel), 9*, 12, 689, 2017, https://doi.org/10.3390/polym9120689.
5. Akram, W., Pandey, V., Sharma, R., Joshi, R., Mishra, N., Garud, N., Haider, T., Inulin: Unveiling Its Potential as a Multifaceted Biopolymer in Prebiotics, Drug Delivery, and Therapeutics. *Int. J. Biol. Macromol., 259*, 129131, 2024, https://doi.org/10.1016/j.ijbiomac.2023.129131.
6. El-Nashar, H.A.S., Taleb, M., El-Shazly, M., Zhao, C., Farag, M.A., Polysaccharides (Pectin, Mucilage, and Fructan Inulin) and Their Fermented Products: A Critical Analysis of Their Biochemical, Gut Interactions, and Biological Functions as Antidiabetic Agents. *Phytother. Res., 38*, 2, 662–693, 2024, https://doi.org/10.1002/ptr.8067.
7. Chauhan, D.S., Vashisht, P., Bebartta, R.P., Thakur, D., Chaudhary, V., Jerusalem Artichoke: A Comprehensive Review of Nutritional Composition, Health Benefits and Emerging Trends in Food Applications. *Compr. Rev. Food Sci. Food Saf., 24*, 1, 2025, https://doi.org/10.1111/1541-4337.70114.
8. Giri, S., Dutta, P., Giri, T.K., Inulin-Based Carriers for Colon Drug Targeting. *J. Drug Deliv. Sci. Technol., 64*, 102595, 2021, https://doi.org/10.1016/j.jddst.2021.102595.
9. Aziz, T., Ullah, A., Ali, A., Shabeer, M., Shah, M.N., Haq, F., Iqbal, M., Ullah, R., Khan, F.U., Manufactures of Bio-degradable and Bio-based Polymers for Bio-materials in the Pharmaceutical Field. *J. Appl. Polym. Sci., 139*, 29, 2022, https://doi.org/10.1002/app.52624.
10. Udaipuria, N. and Bhattacharya, S., Novel Carbohydrate Polymer-Based Systems for Precise Drug Delivery in Colon Cancer: Improving Treatment

Effectiveness With Intelligent Biodegradable Materials. *Biopolymers, 116*, 1, 2025, https://doi.org/10.1002/bip.23632.

11. Afinjuomo, F., Abdella, S., Youssef, S.H., Song, Y., Garg, S., Inulin and Its Application in Drug Delivery. *Pharmaceuticals, 14*, 9, 855, 2021, https://doi.org/10.3390/ph14090855.
12. Kumar, S., Dilbaghi, N., Saharan, R., Bhanjana, G., Nanotechnology as Emerging Tool for Enhancing Solubility of Poorly Water-Soluble Drugs. *Bionanoscience, 2*, 4, 227–250, 2012, https://doi.org/10.1007/s12668-012-0060-7.
13. Jangid, A.K., Noh, K.M., Kim, S., Kim, K., Engineered Inulin-Based Hybrid Biomaterials for Augmented Immunomodulatory Responses. *Carbohydr. Polym., 340*, 122311, 2024, https://doi.org/10.1016/j.carbpol.2024.122311.
14. Qiao, Y., Wan, J., Zhou, L., Ma, W., Yang, Y., Luo, W., Yu, Z., Wang, H., Stimuli-responsive Nanotherapeutics for Precision Drug Delivery and Cancer Therapy. *WIREs Nanomed. Nanobiotechnol., 11*, 1, 2019, https://doi.org/10.1002/wnan.1527.
15. Hou, Y., Jin, J., Duan, H., Liu, C., Chen, L., Huang, W., Gao, Z., Jin, M., Targeted Therapeutic Effects of Oral Inulin-Modified Double-Layered Nanoparticles Containing Chemotherapeutics on Orthotopic Colon Cancer. *Biomaterials, 283*, 121440, 2022, https://doi.org/10.1016/j.biomaterials.2022.121440.
16. Jiang, Y., Yan, C., Li, M., Chen, S., Chen, Z., Yang, L., Luo, K., Delivery of Natural Products *via* Polysaccharide-Based Nanocarriers for Cancer Therapy: A Review on Recent Advances and Future Challenges. *Int. J. Biol. Macromol., 278*, 135072, 2024, https://doi.org/10.1016/j.ijbiomac.2024.135072.
17. Wang, X., Zhang, H., Chen, X., Drug Resistance and Combating Drug Resistance in Cancer. *Cancer Drug Resist.*, 2, 2, 141–160, 2019, https://doi.org/10.20517/cdr.2019.10.
18. Zhang, Y., Zhang, X., Lv, L., Gao, S., Li, X., Wang, R., Wang, P., Shi, F., She, J., Wang, Y., Versatile Inulin/Trans-Ferulic Acid/Silk Sericin Nanoparticles-Nourished Probiotic Complex with Prolonged Intestinal Retention for Synergistic Therapy of Inflammatory Bowel Disease. *Carbohydr. Polym., 350*, 123063, 2025, https://doi.org/10.1016/j.carbpol.2024.123063.
19. Ashrafizadeh, M., Zarrabi, A., Hushmandi, K., Hashemi, F., Rahmani Moghadam, E., Raei, M., Kalantari, M., Tavakol, S., Mohammadinejad, R., Najafi, M., Tay, F.R., Makvandi, P., Progress in Natural Compounds/SiRNA Co-Delivery Employing Nanovehicles for Cancer Therapy. *ACS Comb. Sci., 22*, 12, 669–700, 2020, https://doi.org/10.1021/acscombsci.0c00099.
20. Shi, X., Wang, X., Yao, W., Shi, D., Shao, X., Lu, Z., Chai, Y., Song, J., Tang, W., Wang, X., Mechanism Insights and Therapeutic Intervention of Tumor Metastasis: Latest Developments and Perspectives. *Signal Transduct. Target. Ther., 9*, 1, 192, 2024, https://doi.org/10.1038/s41392-024-01885-2.
21. Chadha, S., Kumar, A., Srivastava, S.A., Behl, T., Ranjan, R., Inulin as a Delivery Vehicle for Targeting Colon-Specific Cancer. *Curr. Drug Deliv., 17*, 8, 651–674, 2020, https://doi.org/10.2174/1567201817666200527133719.

22. Ghali, E.N.H.K., Pranav; Chauhan, S. C.; Yallapu, M. M. Inulin-Based Formulations as an Emerging Therapeutic Strategy for Cancer: A Comprehensive Review. *Int. J. Biol. Macromol.*, *259*, 129216, 2024, https://doi.org/10.1016/j.ijbiomac.2024.129216.
23. Cho, Y.S., Han, K., Xu, J., Moon, J.J., Novel Strategies for Modulating the Gut Microbiome for Cancer Therapy. *Adv. Drug Deliv. Rev.*, *210*, 115332, 2024, https://doi.org/10.1016/j.addr.2024.115332.
24. Ren, Y., Nie, L., Luo, C., Zhu, S., Zhang, X., Advancement in Therapeutic Intervention of Prebiotic-Based Nanoparticles for Colonic Diseases. *Int. J. Nanomed.*, *17*, 6639–6654, 2022, https://doi.org/10.2147/IJN.S390102.
25. Cooper, P.D. and Petrovsky, N., Delta Inulin: A Novel, Immunologically Active, Stable Packing Structure Comprising -D-[2 -< 1] Poly(Fructo-Furanosyl) -D-Glucose Polymers. *Glycobiology*, *21*, 5, 595–606, 2011, https://doi.org/10.1093/glycob/cwq201.
26. Usman, M., Zhang, C., Patil, P.J., Mehmood, A., Li, X., Bilal, M., Haider, J., Ahmad, S., Potential Applications of Hydrophobically Modified Inulin as an Active Ingredient in Functional Foods and Drugs - A Review. *Carbohydr. Polym.*, *252*, 117176, 2021, https://doi.org/10.1016/j.carbpol.2020.117176.
27. Seuring, J. and Agarwal, S., Polymers with Upper Critical Solution Temperature in Aqueous Solution. *Macromol. Rapid Commun.*, *33*, 22, 1898–1920, 2012, https://doi.org/10.1002/marc.201200433.
28. Charoenwongpaiboon, T., Wangpaiboon, K., Panpetch, P., Field, R.A., Barclay, J.E., Pichyangkura, R., Kuttiyawong, K., Temperature-Dependent Inulin Nanoparticles Synthesized by Lactobacillus Reuteri 121 Inulosucrase and Complex Formation with Flavonoids. *Carbohydr. Polym.*, *223*, 115044, 2019, https://doi.org/10.1016/j.carbpol.2019.115044.
29. Banerjee, A., Pathak, S., Subramanium, V.D., G., D., Murugesan, R., Verma, R.S., Strategies for Targeted Drug Delivery in Treatment of Colon Cancer: Current Trends and Future Perspectives. *Drug Discov. Today*, *22*, 8, 1224–1232, 2017, https://doi.org/10.1016/j.drudis.2017.05.006.
30. Poshina, D.N., Rakshina, A.D., Skorik, Y.A., Hydrophobic Chitosan Derivatives for Gene and Drug Delivery in Cancer Therapies. *Polysaccharides*, *6*, 1, 11, 2025, https://doi.org/10.3390/polysaccharides6010011.
31. Dou, Y., Li, C., Li, L., Guo, J., Zhang, J., Bioresponsive Drug Delivery Systems for the Treatment of Inflammatory Diseases. *J. Control. Release*, *327*, 641–666, 2020, https://doi.org/10.1016/j.jconrel.2020.09.008.
32. Garanger, E., Boturyn, D., Dumy, P., Tumor Targeting with RGD Peptide Ligands-Design of New Molecular Conjugates for Imaging and Therapy of Cancers. *Anti-Cancer Agents Med. Chem.*, *7*, 5, 552–558, 2007, https://doi.org/10.2174/187152007781668706.
33. Gómez-Guillén, M.C. and Montero, M.P., Enhancement of Oral Bioavailability of Natural Compounds and Probiotics by Mucoadhesive Tailored Biopolymer-Based Nanoparticles: A Review. *Food Hydrocolloids*, *118*, 106772, 2021, https://doi.org/10.1016/j.foodhyd.2021.106772.

34. Gupta, N., Jangid, A.K., Pooja, D., Kulhari, H., Inulin: A Novel and Stretchy Polysaccharide Tool for Biomedical and Nutritional Applications. *Int. J. Biol. Macromol.*, *132*, 852–863, 2019, https://doi.org/10.1016/j.ijbiomac.2019.03.188.
35. Tiwari, R., Sethi, P., Rudrangi, S.R.S., Padarthi, P.K., Kumar, V., Rudrangi, S., Vaghela, K., Inulin: A Multifaceted Ingredient in Pharmaceutical Sciences. *J. Biomater. Sci., Polym. Ed.*, *35*, 16, 2570–2595, 2024, https://doi.org/10.1080/09205063.2024.2384276.
36. Bakshi, H.A., Quinn, G.A., Aljabali, A.A.A., Hakkim, F.L., Farzand, R., Nasef, M.M., Abuglela, N., Ansari, P., Mishra, V., Serrano-Aroca, A., Tambuwala, M.M., Exploiting the Metabolism of the Gut Microbiome as a Vehicle for Targeted Drug Delivery to the Colon. *Pharmaceuticals*, *14*, 12, 1211, 2021, https://doi.org/10.3390/ph14121211.
37. Huang, W., Jiang, T., He, J., Ruan, J., Wu, B., Tao, R., Xu, P., Wang, Y., Chen, R., Wang, H., Yang, Q., Zhang, K., Jin, L., Sun, D., You, J., Modulation of Intestinal Flora: A Novel Immunotherapeutic Approach for Enhancing Thyroid Cancer Treatment. *Probiotics Antimicrob. Proteins*, 17, 3, 1038–1063, 2025, https://doi.org/10.1007/s12602-025-10471-z.
38. Gupta, S.K. and Verma, A., Toxicity and Safety Aspects of Inulin, in: *Inulin for Pharmaceutical Applications*, pp. 169–187, Springer Nature Singapore, Singapore, 2025, https://doi.org/10.1007/978-981-97-9056-2_9.
39. Scimeca, J.C. and Verron, E., Nano-Engineered Biomaterials: Safety Matters and Toxicity Evaluation. *Mater. Today Adv.*, *15*, 100260, 2022, https://doi.org/10.1016/j.mtadv.2022.100260.
40. Moradi Kashkooli, F., Soltani, M., Souri, M., Controlled Anti-Cancer Drug Release through Advanced Nano-Drug Delivery Systems: Static and Dynamic Targeting Strategies. *J. Control. Release*, *327*, 316–349, 2020, https://doi.org/10.1016/j.jconrel.2020.08.012.
41. Behera, S., Mohapatra, S., Behera, B.C., Thatoi, H., Recent Updates on Green Synthesis of Lignin Nanoparticle and Its Potential Applications in Modern Biotechnology. *Crit. Rev. Biotechnol.*, *44*, 5, 774–794, 2024, https://doi.org/10.1080/07388551.2023.2229512.
42. Sahiner, N., Sagbas, S., Yoshida, H., Lyon, L.A., Synthesis and Properties of Inulin Based Microgels. *Colloids Interface Sci. Commun.*, *2*, 15–18, 2014, https://doi.org/10.1016/j.colcom.2014.08.003.
43. Dima, S., Dima, C., Iordăchescu, G., Encapsulation of Functional Lipophilic Food and Drug Biocomponents. *Food Eng. Rev.*, *7*, 4, 417–438, 2015, https://doi.org/10.1007/s12393-015-9115-1.
44. Desai, N., Sainaga Jyothi, V.G.S., Benival, D., Salave, S., Khunt, D., Inulin: A Versatile Polymer in Colon Drug Targeting, in: *Inulin for Pharmaceutical Applications*, pp. 263–288, Springer Nature Singapore, Singapore, 2025, https://doi.org/10.1007/978-981-97-9056-2_12.
45. Lu, X., Chen, J., Guo, Z., Zheng, Y., Rea, M.C., Su, H., Zheng, X., Zheng, B., Miao, S., Using Polysaccharides for the Enhancement of Functionality of

Foods: A Review. *Trends Food Sci. Technol.*, *86*, 311–327, 2019, https://doi.org/10.1016/j.tifs.2019.02.024.
46. Chidambaram, M., Manavalan, R., Kathiresan, K., Nanotherapeutics to Overcome Conventional Cancer Chemotherapy Limitations. *J. Pharm. Pharm. Sci.*, *14*, 1, 67, 2011, https://doi.org/10.18433/J30C7D.
47. Ganie, S.A., Rather, L.J., Li, Q., Recent Innovations in the Strategies for the Functionalization of Chitosan, Pectin, Alginate, Hyaluronic Acid, Dextran and Inulin Biomaterials for Anticancer Applications-A Review. *J. Polym. Environ.*, *31*, 1, 13–35, 2023, https://doi.org/10.1007/s10924-022-02547-6.
48. Logesh, D., Vallikkadan, M.S., Leena, M.M., Moses, J.A., Anandharamakrishnan, C., Advances in Microfluidic Systems for the Delivery of Nutraceutical Ingredients. *Trends Food Sci. Technol.*, *116*, 501–524, 2021, https://doi.org/10.1016/j.tifs.2021.07.011.
49. Jaradat, E., Weaver, E., Meziane, A., Lamprou, D.A., Microfluidics Technology for the Design and Formulation of Nanomedicines. *Nanomaterials*, *11*, 12, 3440, 2021, https://doi.org/10.3390/nano11123440.
50. Jia, F., Liu, X., Li, L., Mallapragada, S., Narasimhan, B., Wang, Q., Multifunctional Nanoparticles for Targeted Delivery of Immune Activating and Cancer Therapeutic Agents. *J. Control. Release*, *172*, 3, 1020–1034, 2013, https://doi.org/10.1016/j.jconrel.2013.10.012.
51. Piñón-Balderrama, C.I., Leyva-Porras, C., Terán-Figueroa, Y., Espinosa-Solís, V., Álvarez-Salas, C., Saavedra-Leos, M.Z., Encapsulation of Active Ingredients in Food Industry by Spray-Drying and Nano Spray-Drying Technologies. *Processes*, *8*, 8, 889, 2020, https://doi.org/10.3390/pr8080889.
52. Liang, X., Lin, D., Zhang, W., Chen, S., Ding, H., Zhong, H.-J., Progress in the Preparation and Application of Inulin-Based Hydrogels. *Polymers (Basel)*, *16*, 11, 1492, 2024, https://doi.org/10.3390/polym16111492.
53. Shi, D., Beasock, D., Fessler, A., Szebeni, J., Ljubimova, J.Y., Afonin, K.A., Dobrovolskaia, M.A., To PEGylate or Not to PEGylate: Immunological Properties of Nanomedicine's Most Popular Component, Polyethylene Glycol and Its Alternatives. *Adv. Drug Deliv. Rev.*, *180*, 114079, 2022, https://doi.org/10.1016/j.addr.2021.114079.
54. Liu, X., Chen, Y., Li, H., Huang, N., Jin, Q., Ren, K., Ji, J., Enhanced Retention and Cellular Uptake of Nanoparticles in Tumors by Controlling Their Aggregation Behavior. *ACS Nano*, *7*, 7, 6244–6257, 2013, https://doi.org/10.1021/nn402201w.
55. Tacias-Pascacio, V.G., García-Parra, E., Vela-Gutiérrez, G., Virgen-Ortiz, J.J., Berenguer-Murcia, A., Alcántara, A.R., Fernandez-Lafuente, R., Genipin as An Emergent Tool in the Design of Biocatalysts: Mechanism of Reaction and Applications. *Catalysts*, *9*, 12, 1035, 2019, https://doi.org/10.3390/catal9121035.
56. Gao, Y., Peng, K., Mitragotri, S., Covalently Crosslinked Hydrogels *via* Step-Growth Reactions: Crosslinking Chemistries, Polymers, and Clinical Impact. *Adv. Mater.*, *33*, 25, 2021, https://doi.org/10.1002/adma.202006362.

57. Kumar, J.A., Krithiga, T., Manigandan, S., Sathish, S., Renita, A.A., Prakash, P., Prasad, B.S.N., Kumar, T.R.P., Rajasimman, M., Hosseini-Bandegharaei, A., Prabu, D., Crispin, S.A., Focus to Green Synthesis of Metal/Metal Based Oxide Nanoparticles: Various Mechanisms and Applications towards Ecological Approach. *J. Clean. Prod.*, *324*, 129198, 2021, https://doi.org/10.1016/j.jclepro.2021.129198.
58. Zhang, W., Sun, J., Li, Q., Liu, C., Niu, F., Yue, R., Zhang, Y., Zhu, H., Ma, C., Deng, S., Free Radical-Mediated Grafting of Natural Polysaccharides Such as Chitosan, Starch, Inulin, and Pectin with Some Polyphenols: Synthesis, Structural Characterization, Bioactivities, and Applications—A Review. *Foods*, *12*, 19, 3688, 2023, https://doi.org/10.3390/foods12193688.
59. Petrovic, S., Bita, B., Barbinta-Patrascu, M.-E., Nanoformulations in Pharmaceutical and Biomedical Applications: Green Perspectives. *Int. J. Mol. Sci.*, *25*, 11, 5842, 2024, https://doi.org/10.3390/ijms25115842.
60. Fan, W., Yung, B., Huang, P., Chen, X., Nanotechnology for Multimodal Synergistic Cancer Therapy. *Chem. Rev.*, *117*, 22, 13566–13638, 2017, https://doi.org/10.1021/acs.chemrev.7b00258.
61. Wu, Q., Hu, Y., Yu, B., Hu, H., Xu, F.-J., Polysaccharide-Based Tumor Microenvironment-Responsive Drug Delivery Systems for Cancer Therapy. *J. Control. Release*, *362*, 19–43, 2023, https://doi.org/10.1016/j.jconrel.2023.08.019.
62. Scialabba, C., Licciardi, M., Mauro, N., Rocco, F., Ceruti, M., Giammona, G., Inulin-Based Polymer Coated SPIONs as Potential Drug Delivery Systems for Targeted Cancer Therapy. *Eur. J. Pharm. Biopharm.*, *88*, 3, 695–705, 2014, https://doi.org/10.1016/j.ejpb.2014.09.008.
63. Zare, I., Zirak Hassan Kiadeh, S., Varol, A., Ören Varol, T., Varol, M., Sezen, S., Zarepour, A., Mostafavi, E., Zahed Nasab, S., Rahi, A., Khosravi, A., Zarrabi, A., Glycosylated Nanoplatforms: From Glycosylation Strategies to Implications and Opportunities for Cancer Theranostics. *J. Control. Release*, *371*, 158–178, 2024, https://doi.org/10.1016/j.jconrel.2024.05.032.
64. Gong, T., Liu, X., Wang, X., Lu, Y., Wang, X., Applications of Polysaccharides in Enzyme-Triggered Oral Colon-Specific Drug Delivery Systems: A Review. *Int. J. Biol. Macromol.*, *275*, 133623, 2024, https://doi.org/10.1016/j.ijbiomac.2024.133623.
65. Hu, T., Li, Z., Gao, C.-Y., Cho, C.H., Mechanisms of Drug Resistance in Colon Cancer and Its Therapeutic Strategies. *World J. Gastroenterol.*, *22*, 30, 6876, 2016, https://doi.org/10.3748/wjg.v22.i30.6876.
66. Kolhatkar, R., Lote, A., Khambhati, H., Active Tumor Targeting of Nanomaterials Using Folic Acid, Transferrin and Integrin Receptors. *Curr. Drug Discov. Technol.*, *8*, 3, 197–206, 2011, https://doi.org/10.2174/157016311796799044.
67. Kemp, J.A., Shim, M.S., Heo, C.Y., Kwon, Y.J., "Combo" Nanomedicine: Co-Delivery of Multi-Modal Therapeutics for Efficient, Targeted, and

Safe Cancer Therapy. *Adv. Drug Deliv. Rev.*, *98*, 3–18, 2016, https://doi.org/10.1016/j.addr.2015.10.019.

68. Khan, I.U., Khan, R.U., Asif, H., Alamgeer, Khalid, S.H., Asghar, S., Saleem, M., Shah, K.U., Shah, S.U., Rizvi, S.A.A., Shahzad, Y., Co-Delivery Strategies to Overcome Multidrug Resistance in Ovarian Cancer. *Int. J. Pharm.*, *533*, 1, 111–124, 2017, https://doi.org/10.1016/j.ijpharm.2017.09.060.
69. Deshmukh, R., Sethi, P., Singh, B., Shiekmydeen, J., Salave, S., Patel, R.J., Ali, N., Rashid, S., Elossaily, G.M., Kumar, A., Recent Review on Biological Barriers and Host–Material Interfaces in Precision Drug Delivery: Advancement in Biomaterial Engineering for Better Treatment Therapies. *Pharmaceutics*, *16*, 8, 1076, 2024, https://doi.org/10.3390/pharmaceutics16081076.
70. Abdel-Wahhab, M.A., El-Nekeety, A.A., Salman, A.S., Abdel-Aziem, S.H., Mehaya, F.M., Hassan, N.S., Protective Capabilities of Silymarin and Inulin Nanoparticles against Hepatic Oxidative Stress, Genotoxicity and Cytotoxicity of Deoxynivalenol in Rats. *Toxicon*, *142*, 1–13, 2018, https://doi.org/10.1016/j.toxicon.2017.12.045.
71. Saraswat, I. and Goel, A., Therapeutic Modulation of the Microbiome in Oncology: Current Trends and Future Directions. *Curr. Pharm. Biotechnol.*, *26*, 2024, https://doi.org/10.2174/0113892010353600241109132441.
72. Zhu, R., Lang, T., Yan, W., Zhu, X., Huang, X., Yin, Q., Li, Y., Gut Microbiota: Influence on Carcinogenesis and Modulation Strategies by Drug Delivery Systems to Improve Cancer Therapy. *Adv. Sci.*, *8*, 10, 2021, https://doi.org/10.1002/advs.202003542.
73. Sanati, M., Afshari, A.R., Kesharwani, P., Sukhorukov, V.N., Sahebkar, A., Recent Trends in the Application of Nanoparticles in Cancer Therapy: The Involvement of Oxidative Stress. *J. Control. Release*, *348*, 287–304, 2022, https://doi.org/10.1016/j.jconrel.2022.05.035.
74. Rahmati, S. and David, A.E.A., Review of Design Criteria for Cancer-Targeted, Nanoparticle-Based MRI Contrast Agents. *Appl. Mater. Today*, *37*, 102087, 2024, https://doi.org/10.1016/j.apmt.2024.102087.
75. Zhang, X., Yi, X., Gao, X., Li, Y., Shen, X., Liver-Targeted Nanoparticles Loaded with Cannabidiol Based on Redox Response for Effective Alleviation of Acute Liver Injury. *Foods*, *13*, 15, 2464, 2024, https://doi.org/10.3390/foods13152464.
76. Pucci, C., Degl'Innocenti, A., Belenli Gümüş, M., Ciofani, G., Superparamagnetic Iron Oxide Nanoparticles for Magnetic Hyperthermia: Recent Advancements, Molecular Effects, and Future Directions in the Omics Era. *Biomater. Sci.*, *10*, 9, 2103–2121, 2022, https://doi.org/10.1039/D1BM01963E.
77. Ashrafizadeh, M., Zarrabi, A., Hashemi, F., Zabolian, A., Saleki, H., Bagherian, M., Azami, N., Bejandi, A.K., Hushmandi, K., Ang, H.L., Makvandi, P., Khan, H., Kumar, A.P., Polychemotherapy with Curcumin and Doxorubicin *via* Biological Nanoplatforms: Enhancing Antitumor Activity. *Pharmaceutics*, *12*, 11, 1084, 2020, https://doi.org/10.3390/pharmaceutics12111084.

78. Zhu, R., Yuan, W., Xia, A., Sun, X., Yan, W., Wu, T., Wang, G., Li, Y., Yin, Q., Li, Y., Inulin-Based Nanoparticle Modulates Gut Microbiota and Immune Microenvironment for Improving Colorectal Cancer Therapy. *Adv. Funct. Mater.*, *34*, 46, 2024, https://doi.org/10.1002/adfm.202407685.
79. Man, S.M., Inflammasomes in the Gastrointestinal Tract: Infection, Cancer and Gut Microbiota Homeostasis. *Nat. Rev. Gastroenterol. Hepatol.*, *15*, 12, 721–737, 2018, https://doi.org/10.1038/s41575-018-0054-1.
80. Zhang, S., Song, Z., Shi, L., Zhou, L., Zhang, J., Cui, J., Li, Y., Jin, D.-Q., Ohizumi, Y., Xu, J., Guo, Y.A., Dandelion Polysaccharide and Its Selenium Nanoparticles: Structure Features and Evaluation of Anti-Tumor Activity in Zebrafish Models. *Carbohydr. Polym.*, *270*, 118365, 2021, https://doi.org/10.1016/j.carbpol.2021.118365.
81. Shi, L., Li, Y., Zhang, S., Gong, X., Xu, J., Guo, Y., Construction of Inulin-Based Selenium Nanoparticles to Improve the Antitumor Activity of an Inulin-Type Fructan from Chicory. *Int. J. Biol. Macromol.*, *210*, 261–270, 2022, https://doi.org/10.1016/j.ijbiomac.2022.04.125.
82. Shao, T., Liu, W., Yuan, P., Li, X., Xu, H., Liu, C., Chen, K., Li, L., Han, J., Wang, G., Enhanced Antitumor Activity of Inulin-Capped Se Nanoparticles Synthesized Using Jerusalem Artichoke Tubers. *Glycoconj. J.*, *38*, 5, 599–607, 2021, https://doi.org/10.1007/s10719-021-10011-1.
83. Hu, N., Gao, Z., Cao, P., Song, H., Hu, J., Qiu, Z., Chang, C., Zheng, G., Shan, X., Meng, Y., Uniform and Disperse Selenium Nanoparticles Stabilized by Inulin Fructans from Codonopsis Pilosula and Their Anti-Hepatoma Activities. *Int. J. Biol. Macromol.*, *203*, 105–115, 2022, https://doi.org/10.1016/j.ijbiomac.2022.01.140.
84. Mauro, N., Utzeri, M.A., Cillari, R., Scialabba, C., Giammona, G., Cavallaro, G., Cholesterol-Inulin Conjugates for Efficient SN38 Nuclear Delivery: Nanomedicines for Precision Cancer Therapy. *Cancers (Basel)*, *14*, 19, 4857, 2022, https://doi.org/10.3390/cancers14194857.
85. Vatansever, O., Bahadori, F., Bulut, S., Eroglu, M.S., Coating with Cationic Inulin Enhances the Drug Release Profile and *in Vitro* Anticancer Activity of Lecithin-Based Nano Drug Delivery Systems. *Int. J. Biol. Macromol.*, *237*, 123955, 2023, https://doi.org/10.1016/j.ijbiomac.2023.123955.
86. Jangid, A.K., Solanki, R., Patel, S., Pooja, D., Kulhari, H., Genistein Encapsulated Inulin-Stearic Acid Bioconjugate Nanoparticles: Formulation Development, Characterization and Anticancer Activity. *Int. J. Biol. Macromol.*, *206*, 213–221, 2022, https://doi.org/10.1016/j.ijbiomac.2022.02.031.
87. Kim, S.E., Yoon, J.C., Jang, S.R., Yoo, Y.-J., Tae, H.-J., Park, C.H., Kim, C.S., Muthurasu, A., Kim, H.Y., *In Vivo* and *In Vitro* Biodistribution of Inulin-Tethered Boron-Doped Amine-Functionalized Carbon Dots. *ACS Biomater. Sci. Eng.*, *9*, 2, 1002–1010, 2023, https://doi.org/10.1021/acsbiomaterials.2c01256.
88. Kourani, K., Jain, P., Kumar, A., Jangid, A.K., Swaminathan, G., Durgempudi, V.R., Jose, J., Reddy, R., Pooja, D., Kulhari, H., Kumar, L.D., Inulin Coated

Mn3O4 Nanocuboids Coupled with RNA Interference Reverse Intestinal Tumorigenesis in Apc Knockout Murine Colon Cancer Models. *Nanomed. Nanotechnol. Biol. Med.*, *40*, 102504, 2022, https://doi.org/10.1016/j.nano.2021.102504.
89. Han, L., Sun, J., Williams, P.A., Yang, J., Zhang, S., Octenyl-Succinylated Inulins for the Delivery of Hydrophobic Drug. *Int. J. Biol. Macromol.*, *221*, 1112–1120, 2022, https://doi.org/10.1016/j.ijbiomac.2022.09.068.
90. Ayala-Fuentes, J.C., Gallegos-Granados, M.Z., Villarreal-Gómez, L.J., Antunes-Ricardo, M., Grande, D., Chavez-Santoscoy, R.A., Optimization of the Synthesis of Natural Polymeric Nanoparticles of Inulin Loaded with Quercetin: Characterization and Cytotoxicity Effect. *Pharmaceutics*, *14*, 5, 888, 2022, https://doi.org/10.3390/pharmaceutics14050888.
91. Joseph, S., Jadav, M., Solanki, R., Patel, S., Pooja, D., Kulhari, H., Synthesis, Characterization, and Application of Honey Stabilized Inulin Nanoparticles as Colon Targeting Drug Delivery Carrier. *Int. J. Biol. Macromol.*, *263*, 130274, 2024, https://doi.org/10.1016/j.ijbiomac.2024.130274.
92. Jangid, A.K., Patel, K., Jain, P., Patel, S., Gupta, N., Pooja, D., Kulhari, H., Inulin-Pluronic-Stearic Acid Based Double Folded Nanomicelles for PH-Responsive Delivery of Resveratrol. *Carbohydr. Polym.*, *247*, 116730, 2020, https://doi.org/10.1016/j.carbpol.2020.116730.
93. Lunawat, A.K., Vishwakarma, N., Raikwar, S., Future Prospects in Inulin Research, in: *Inulin for Pharmaceutical Applications*, pp. 325–341, Springer Nature Singapore, Singapore, 2025, https://doi.org/10.1007/978-981-97-9056-2_15.
94. Desu, B.S.R., Biradar, R.M., Vijaykanth, M.S., Sethi, P., Krishnan, K., Prema, S., Kallur, H.J., Senthamaraikannan, A., Inulin as Stabilizer, in: *Inulin for Pharmaceutical Applications*, pp. 73–90, Springer Nature Singapore, Singapore, 2025, https://doi.org/10.1007/978-981-97-9056-2_4.
95. Jadhav, K., Kole, E., Singh, R., Rout, S.K., Verma, R.K., Chatterjee, A., Mujumdar, A., Naik, J., A Critical Review on Developments in Drying Technologies for Enhanced Stability and Bioavailability of Pharmaceuticals. *Dry. Technol.*, *42*, 9, 1415–1441, 2024, https://doi.org/10.1080/07373937.2024.2357181.
96. Pandey, S., Nayak, P., Malaiya, A., Paliwal, R., Alam, M.I., Kashid, S., Yadav, A.K., Paliwal, S.R., Colloidal Drug Delivery System: An Overview, in: *Novel Carrier Systems for Targeted and Controlled Drug Delivery*, pp. 339–390, Springer Nature Singapore, Singapore, 2024, https://doi.org/10.1007/978-981-97-4970-6_15.
97. Huang, J., Zhu, Y., Xiao, H., Liu, J., Li, S., Zheng, Q., Tang, J., Meng, X., Formation of a Traditional Chinese Medicine Self-Assembly Nanostrategy and Its Application in Cancer: A Promising Treatment. *Chin. Med.*, *18*, 1, 66, 2023, https://doi.org/10.1186/s13020-023-00764-2.

98. Tian, Y., Lei, Y., Wang, Y., Lai, J., Wang, J., Xia, F., Mechanism of Multidrug Resistance to Chemotherapy Mediated by Pglycoprotein (Review). *Int. J. Oncol.*, *63*, 5, 119, 2023, https://doi.org/10.3892/ijo.2023.5567.
99. Zhu, J., Lee, H., Huang, R., Zhou, J., Zhang, J., Yang, X., Zhou, W., Jiang, W., Chen, S., Harnessing Nanotechnology for Cancer Treatment. *Front. Bioeng. Biotechnol.*, *12*, 2025, https://doi.org/10.3389/fbioe.2024.1514890.
100. Bhuskute, H., Shende, P., Prabhakar, B., 3D Printed Personalized Medicine for Cancer: Applications for Betterment of Diagnosis, Prognosis and Treatment. *AAPS PharmSciTech*, *23*, 1, 8, 2021, https://doi.org/10.1208/s12249-021-02153-0.
101. Alzoubi, L., Aljabali, A.A.A., Tambuwala, M.M., Empowering Precision Medicine: The Impact of 3D Printing on Personalized Therapeutic. *AAPS PharmSciTech*, *24*, 8, 228, 2023, https://doi.org/10.1208/s12249-023-02682-w.
102. Guptha, P.M., Deepan, T., Alekkhya, V., Gunda, R.K., Babu, M.R., Pamu, S., Potential of Inulin to Revolutionize Pharmaceutical Industries, in: *Inulin for Pharmaceutical Applications*, pp. 343–369, Springer Nature Singapore, Singapore, 2025, https://doi.org/10.1007/978-981-97-9056-2_16.
103. Heydari, S., Masoumi, N., Esmaeeli, E., Ayyoubzadeh, S.M., Ghorbani-Bidkorpeh, F., Ahmadi, M., Artificial Intelligence in Nanotechnology for Treatment of Diseases. *J. Drug Target.*, *32*, 10, 1247–1266, 2024, https://doi.org/10.1080/1061186X.2024.2393417.
104. Zheng, J.-J., Li, Q.-Z., Wang, Z., Wang, X., Zhao, Y., Gao, X., Computer-Aided Nanodrug Discovery: Recent Progress and Future Prospects. *Chem. Soc. Rev.*, *53*, 18, 9059–9132, 2024, https://doi.org/10.1039/D3CS00575E.
105. Adir, O., Poley, M., Chen, G., Froim, S., Krinsky, N., Shklover, J., Shainsky-Roitman, J., Lammers, T., Schroeder, A., Integrating Artificial Intelligence and Nanotechnology for Precision Cancer Medicine. *Adv. Mater.*, *32*, 13, 2020, https://doi.org/10.1002/adma.201901989.
106. Mauro, N., Li Volsi, A., Scialabba, C., Licciardi, M., Cavallaro, G., Giammona, G., Photothermal Ablation of Cancer Cells Using Folate-Coated Gold/Graphene Oxide Composite. *Curr. Drug Deliv.*, *14*, 3, 433–443, 2017, https://doi.org/10.2174/1567201813666160520113804.

4

Chitosan: Biomedical Applications and Cancer Therapeutic Potential

Md Aamir Aftab, Iftkhar Ahmad*, Asma Fatima and Saiqa Ikram†

Department of Chemistry, Jamia Millia Islamia, New Delhi, India

Abstract

Chitosan (CS), the natural biopolymer derived from crustacean exoskeletons and fungi, has garnered significant interest in healthcare research owing to its remarkable biodegradability, biological suitability, and versatility. These attributes have enabled its application across diverse domains, including drug delivery, tissue engineering, gene therapy, and cancer therapeutics. CS has plenty of advantages with its suitability across various fields of medicine as a natural biopolymer. CS is synonymous with the innovation in nanotechnology facilitating the creation of nanoparticles that enhances ways to administer drugs, specifically for diseases like cancer. The application of stimuli-responsive CS nanoparticles (CS-NPs) featuring pH, redox, or thermo-sensitive CS-NPs allows for resistance to drugs in chemotherapy to be reduced. In addition to improving the biological accessibility of medications, the ability to target certain regions boosts their efficacy and transforms the cancer treatment industry. Further expansion into transforming the delivery system for doxorubicin into doxorubicin CS polymer conjugates can show immense potential in long-term, tumor-targeted treatment because it enhances cellular absorption while lowering the chance of developing resistance. The function of CS, functionalized CS, and their composite in the delivery of drugs, tissue engineering, gene therapy, and cancer therapy has been thoroughly addressed in the present chapter.

***Keywords*:** Chitosan, gene therapy, siRNA delivery, wound healing, tissue regeneration, metastasis, angiogenesis, immunomodulator

**Corresponding author*: iftkharwani32@gmail.com

†*Corresponding author*: sikram@jmi.ac.in

Luqman Jameel Rather, Showkat Ali Ganie and Mohammed A. Assiri (eds.) Polysaccharide Biomaterials in Cancer Research and Therapy: From Lab to Life, (87–120) © 2026 Scrivener Publishing LLC

4.1 Introduction

Biopolymers utilized in means of medicine administration enclose diverse array of materials that serve as pivotal carriers for active pharmaceutical ingredients and are distinguished by their harmless, sustainable, and environment-friendly nature. The latter two attributes are instrumental in ensuring the safe elimination of the carrier following drug administration. Biopolymers offer an important role in the fabrication of a wide range of administrative methods, such as hydrocolloids, liposomes, dietary supplements, and granular structures, including nanoparticles (NPs), pellets, and microparticles [1]. Though the next most often occurring polymer after cellulose is chitin, its practical exploitation remains markedly constrained owing to its inherently semi-crystalline architecture and the prevalence of robust intermolecular hydrogen bonds, which confer substantial insolubility in conventional solvents. Nevertheless, technological advancements have facilitated the partial N-deacetylation of chitin, thereby converting it into its soluble counterpart, chitosan (CS), which exhibits enhanced applicability. This process, typically performed in strong alkaline conditions, makes CS soluble in acidic environments [2]. As a result, CS, a synthetically deacetylated form of chitin, has found diverse applications across various industries. It finds extensive utilization across a plethora of industries, including the fabrication of edible and biodegradable packaging films within the food sector, the prolongation of food shelf life, the pharmaceutical domain, the remediation of water and wastewater, the formulation of cosmetics, the establishment of advanced bandage for external injuries, and an array of other multifaceted applications [3, 4]. CS, which is mostly derived from insects, crabs, clams, algal species, and fungus, is classified into three categories according to its molar mass (Mm): light, moderate, and heavy Mm CS. High Mm CS features longer chains and a higher number of hydroxyl groups [5]. Structurally, CS is a polycationic straight carbohydrate made up of N-acetyl-glucosamine and D-glucosamine monomer linked together by β-1-4 glycosidic bonds (Figure 4.1).

Esteemed as one of the most ubiquitously employed biopolymers within the pharmaceutical sector, CS, a derivative of chitin, demonstrates a broad spectrum of bioactivities, encompassing antiproliferative, antimicrobial, immunostimulatory, and hypocholesterolemic properties, phytoalexin production, antihypertensive, neuroprotective, wound-healing, and antiulcer properties [6]. Endowed with exceptional biocompatibility, CS serves as an optimal vector for the administration of nucleic acids, anticancer compounds, and chemotherapeutics, while its chemically modified

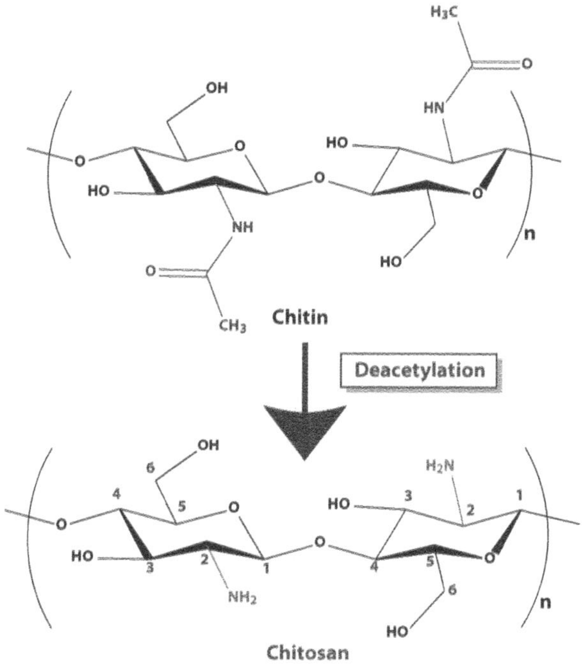

Figure 4.1 Generation of CS from chitin; removal of an acetyl group.

derivatives exhibit potent antiproliferative activity, either as standalone therapeutics or in synergistic conjunction with other anticancer modalities. For instance, CS-based glycoconjugates can target altered glycosylation in cancer cells, enhancing the penetration of anticancer agents [7]. As previously emphasized, the primary origin of chitin and CS includes insects, crabs, clams, algal species, and fungus (Figure 4.2), with industrial-scale extraction primarily focusing on crab and shrimp shells, transforming these waste materials into high-value byproducts for medical and pharmaceutical applications [8]. The journey to obtain chitin begins with its extraction from shellfish waste, which contains chitin, lipids, inorganic salts, and proteins. To liberate chitin from these components, two main methods are employed: chemical and biological.

The chemical route uses strong alkaline solutions (greater than 1M sodium hydroxide) and acids (greater than 3M hydrochloride) under warmth to break down the structural elements, converting chitin into CS or fragmenting it partially. Acids such as sulfuric, nitric, formic, acetic, and particularly dilute hydrochloric acid are commonly utilized for demineralization. Meanwhile, proteins and pigments like carotenoids are

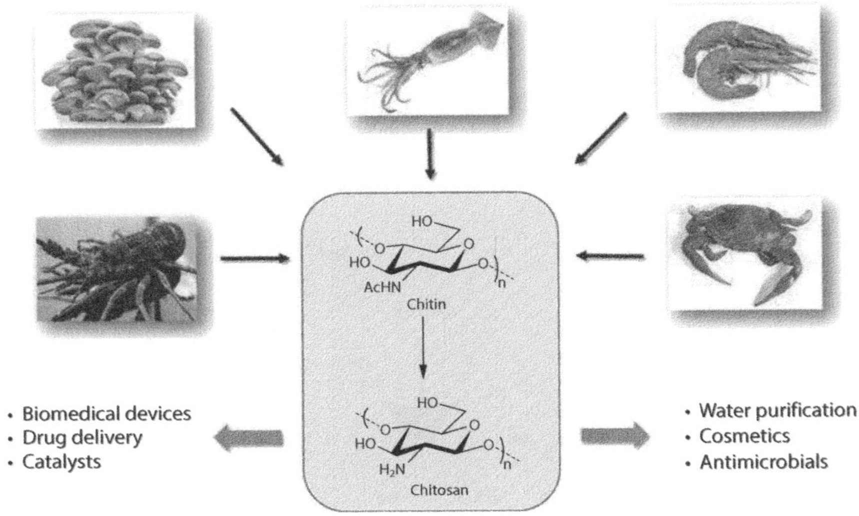

Figure 4.2 Source and application of chitin and CS [11].

removed with the help of dilute sodium hydroxide and organic solvents like acetone [9]. On the other hand, biological processes, celebrated for their eco-friendliness, lower energy consumption, and cost efficiency, offer a gentler alternative. These methods leverage enzymatic reactions and microbial fermentation, resulting in chitin with superior molecular weight and crystalline structure [9, 10]. Unlike their chemical counterparts, these processes rely on the natural metabolites of microorganisms to generate the necessary acidic and alkaline environments for chitin extraction [9].

4.2 CS as Stabilizer for NPs

Natural polymers are often favored as adjusting component to alter the chemical and physical properties in the synthesis of metal NPs owing to their inherent biocompatibility and widespread availability. Among these, CS stands out due to its high positive charge density and exceptional biocompatibility, making it an ideal candidate for NP stabilization. As depicted in Figure 4.3a, uncoated metal NPs are prone to aggregation in solution, driven by van der Waals forces acting upon their exposed metallic surfaces. Conversely, CS functions as an efficient steric and electrostatic adjusting component, encapsulating the NPs with a positively charged layer that mitigates aggregation. This robust electrostatic interaction facilitates the

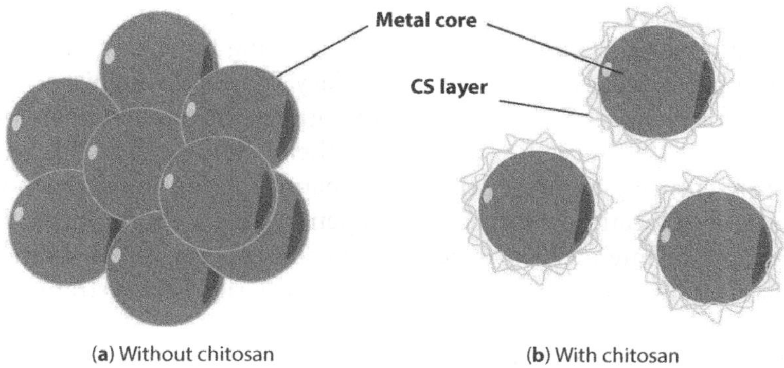

Figure 4.3 (a) Metal NPs aggregate in absence of CS capping agent. (b) Metal NPs disperse well with a CS capping agent [15].

establishment of homogeneously dispersed metal NPs, as illustrated in Figure 4.3b. Numerous investigations have underscored the stabilizing prowess of CS in the synthesis of metal NPs. As an instance, CS has been used as a regulating agent in the sustainable production of AgNPs *via* an electrolytic oxidation–complexation process alongside UV-induced suppression [12].

Similarly, AuNPs developed in an environment of CS as well as citric acid show exceptional stability in aqueous solutions with no agglomeration [13]. In addition, CS oligosaccharide (COS), a water-soluble derivative of CS, is increasingly being utilized as a coating substance for metal NPs in varied fields of medicine such as medication and gene transfer, phototherapy, and reconstruction of tissues [12]. In one prominent case, COS functioned as both a green-reducing agent and regulator in the single-pot production of AuNPs for transmission of genes, where its electro-positive amine groups dramatically increased its bonding strength to extrachromosomal DNA [14].

4.3 Biomedical Applications of CS

4.3.1 Drug Delivery System

Drug delivery systems (DDSs) are innovative formulations that optimize the administration of medicinal substances. DDS improves medication stability, controlled release, and specific administration by combining active medicinal agents with tailored carriers, such as environment-friendly polymers.

These advanced platforms dramatically increase bioavailability, reduce side effects, and maximize therapeutic results, resulting in a paradigm shift in current pharmacology [1, 16]. An exemplary DDS is distinguished by its capacity for controlled release, maintaining the plasma concentration of the therapeutic agent within the optimal therapeutic range, while simultaneously ensuring targeted delivery by channeling the active compound to the desired location of impact [1]. Depending on the route of administration and the intended site of action, different delivery vehicles—such as tablets, capsules, or hydrogels—are used [16]. Drug administration may occur *via* invasive methods, such as parenteral routes, or non-invasive pathways, including mucosal delivery through oral, buccal, nasal, pulmonary, or rectal routes, with mucosal strategies being extensively employed in DDS to augment mucoadhesion and facilitate superior drug release [1]. Comprehensive studies have underscored the efficacy of chitin and CS as efficacious drug delivery agents, with CS being particularly prominent in hydrogel development. Its remarkable attributes, including bioadhesive properties, a multi-cationic surface enabling formation of hydrogen and electrostatic interactions, and exceptional environmental friendliness—ensuring non-toxicity and immunological quiescence upon contact with biological tissues or fluids—render it an invaluable component in sophisticated DDSs [16, 17].

Nanotechnology has emerged as a prominent approach in drug administration, particularly through the usage of nanomaterials, which are characterized by their nanoscale size (1–100 nm) and unique quantum mechanical properties [17, 18]. This technology enhances precision in imaging and drug delivery applications. CS-designed NPs are notably effective in the mucosal delivery route, facilitating drug transport to the brain and eyes and treating various diseases, including cancer, gastrointestinal disorders, and pulmonary conditions [19, 20]. The extent of medicine discharge out of these NPs is governed by their solubility, diffusion, and size, typically ranging from 100 to 400 nm. Photon correlation spectroscopy is employed to measure their size by analyzing Brownian motion [21]. Topical medicines are used to treat a variety of ocular illnesses; however, due to ocular defensive mechanisms, fewer than 5% of these treatments penetrate the cornea and reach the intraocular tissues. CS-based NPs provide a viable alternative for improving medication bioavailability and extending retention in ocular tissues [22, 23]. Silva *et al.* conducted research using nanotechnology in which eye drops containing polymer-based NPs loaded with the antibiotic ceftazidime were employed to address ocular illnesses caused by *P. aeruginosa*. Their analysis of mucoadhesion, the interaction between NPs and ocular mucosal tissue, revealed that these polymeric NPs improved drug transport through the ocular mucosal barrier, enhancing bioavailability and protecting the drug from degradation. Substantial ionic interactions among CS's amino group and the o-hydroxybenzoic acid component of mucin enable extended drug retention in the eye, as the study showed that CS's structural properties lengthen the time that antibiotics reach ocular mucosal tissue. Moreover, CS's hydrophilicity, biodegradability, and inherent antimicrobial activity underscore its significant prospective for application in drug-administration systems [24].

Cánepa *et al.* conducted a groundbreaking study on administering IFN-alpha using CS-based NPs for oral delivery. This approach addresses the challenges of decreased absorption due to brush border enzyme deterioration and liver metabolism, which often hinder oral drug bioavailability [25]. IFNα, employed in the treatment of cancer and viral infections, necessitates frequent dosing owing to its abbreviated half-life, thereby contributing to side effects and patient compliance difficulties [26]. Cánepa *et al.* demonstrated that IFNα encapsulated within CS-based NPs exhibited antiviral efficacy on par with that of commercially available IFNα, while significantly enhancing its bioavailability in the gastrointestinal tract, a result attributable to the ionic interactions between chemical groups of CS and mucin's salicylic acid component. This interaction resulted in an increase in the NP size upon mucin adsorption and a drop of NP surface charge, which improved drug retention and absorption [25].

4.3.2 Tissue Engineering and Regenerative Medicine

Biomaterials function as scaffolds that emulate the natural cellular matrix outside the cell and surroundings, thereby augmenting laboratory methodologies and facilitating effective tissue regeneration, while simultaneously addressing the limitations of cell therapy by providing an optimal milieu for 3D cellular growth and integration; for *in vitro* applications, these polymeric materials must demonstrate exceptional biocompatibility and possess intricate porous architectures to foster cell proliferation and differentiation. In regenerative medicine, biomaterials must provide robust mechanical support for neurite extension while promoting tissue regeneration through differentiating somatic cells and seamless incorporation into host tissue [27]. Mitigating inflammatory responses post-implantation is paramount, rendering attributes such as environmental friendliness, sustainability, tensile integrity, architectural design, and cell attachment capability indispensable for the efficacy of biomaterials.

The prospect of CS-based scaffolds for neurological system rejuvenation has been meticulously examined, highlighting the adaptable physicochemical properties of CS and its derived materials, which promote the scaffolds engineering with precisely calibrated structural configurations. Biomaterial scaffolds intended for central nervous system (CNS) regeneration are principally classified into hydrogels and biodegradable constructs [28]. CS hydrogels, formed through physical or chemical crosslinking, vary in stability and uniformity. Physical interactions, such as ionic and hydrogen bonds, create fewer stable structures, while covalent bonds yield more uniform properties. Faster biodegradation can be achieved using labile bonds that degrade under physiological conditions [29]. *In situ* gelling through physical interactions facilitates cell delivery without pre-shaped hydrogel structures, offering a less invasive implantation process [30]. Hydrogels derived from CS and its derived material, including carboxymethyl-CS (CMC) and CS lactate, as well as hybrid formulations with other biopolymers like gelatin, have been extensively explored for CNS applications, while biodegradable scaffolds, predominantly fabricated through advanced methodologies such as freeze-drying, supercritical carbon dioxide processing, electrospinning, 3D bioprinting and solvent evaporation, provide crucial architectural support for tissue regeneration. These porous scaffolds, made from CS blends with materials like gelatin, collagen, and Poly(3,4-ethylenedioxythiophene) (PEDOT), offer customizable porous structures with varying size ranges and mechanical properties, promoting effective cell integration and tissue repair [31, 32].

In non-CNS tissue engineering applications, the Mm and extent of deacetylation (EoD) of CS are paramount in governing its biodegradability and rheological properties, with elevated Molecular weight (Mw) conferring retarded biodegradation and augmented viscosity, while EoD values ranging from 65% to 82% expedite biodegradation [33]. Notably, the reviewed studies exhibit considerable heterogeneity in the chemical characteristics of the initial CS, with Mm ranging from 1 to 550 kDa and EoD values spanning from 75% to 95% [34]. Interestingly, CNS-focused tissue engineering and regenerative medicine studies seldom evaluate variations in Mw or EoD of their CS sources. Many do not even report these critical characteristics. The primary distinctions among these studies lie in the utilization of various polymeric composites and their respective ratios as precursor materials. Implantation of CS-based biomaterials within the CNS presents promising approach to mitigate its inherently limited regenerative capacity by facilitating tissue reconstruction and neuronal process reconnection. Furthermore, the integration of somatic cells and bioactive molecules into these frameworks has recognized as a highly promising technique to augment rejuvenation treatment [35]. Biomaterials function as sophisticated delivery vehicles that not only sustain cell viability and engraftment but also create a controlled microenvironment conducive to cell differentiation and proliferation, thus deviating from the natural injury response mechanisms [31].

4.3.3 Gene Therapy and siRNA Delivery

Gene therapy is progressively emerging as a paradigm of therapeutic delivery, leveraging the modulation of cellular machinery to elicit remedial effects. Analogous to conventional DDSs, the deployment of genetic treatments within the CNS encounters formidable impediments, including limited penetration of the barrier between blood and brain, the inherent heterogeneity of neural tissue, invasive or suboptimal administration methodologies, and complexities associated with precise dosing. Various vectors, predominantly viral, have been used to address these barriers [36]. Nevertheless, the potential hazards of human illness and immunogenic reactions linked with viral vectors catalyzed the pursuit of safer, non-viral alternatives. CS's intrinsic polycationic nature facilitates robust electrostatic interactions with anionic biomolecules such as DNA and RNA, rendering it a highly promising candidate for gene delivery systems. A multitude of CS-based platforms have been engineered for nucleic acid delivery, with Mao *et al.* investigating the formulation parameters influencing siRNA and DNA administration efficacy and transmission effectiveness. Their findings revealed that CS with intermediate Mm and EoD yields complexes exhibiting optimal physicochemical stability and superior transfection performance [37].

CS and its derived materials have been extensively exploited in gene administration applications, with PEGylation demonstrating remarkable efficacy in augmenting the environmental friendliness and structural firmness of siRNA-stacked compounds [38]. Moreover, polyethylene glycol (PEG) functions as a molecular connection among CS and targeting molecules, facilitating the formation of nucleic acid complexes and enhancing the cellular internalization of CS gene administration mechanism. Despite the multifaceted utility of CS, NPs have emerged as superior platforms for addressing an array of neurological pathologies, including diseases such as Alzheimer (AD), Parkinson, glioblastoma, encephalomyelitis disseminata, medulloblastoma, and even neurotropic viral infections such as HIV within the brain [39]. The pursuit of minimally invasive therapeutic strategies has recently driven the creation of advanced compositions for administration of gene from the nasal cavity to the brain. Rassu *et al.* pioneered CS-coated solid-lipid NPs encapsulating BACE1 siRNA for intranasal administration, aimed at combating AD. In a comparable manner,

Van Woensel *et al.* engineered siRNA-loaded CS-NPs hitting Gal-1, which, upon intranasal delivery in murine models, elicited profound modifications within the tumor microenvironment (TME) of glioblastoma multiforme [40]. Expanding on these innovations, Sánchez-Ramos and colleagues devised a CS-Manganese_fodipir_chelate-based intranasal nanocarrier platform for the administration of siRNA as well as dsDNA, exemplifying a cutting-edge approach to gene therapy. They demonstrated the effectiveness of anti-eGFP siRNA-loaded NPs in reducing GFP mRNA expression across different brain regions in Tg GFP+ mice [41]. These advancements signal a promising step toward overcoming the challenges that currently hinder CNS-directed gene therapy.

4.3.4 Wound Healing and Antibacterial Properties

The skin, as the body's protective layer, shields against physical, mechanical, and chemical damage and pathogens. Wound healing involves granulation and scar tissue formation, driven by activated stem cells releasing cytokines and growth factors at the wound site [42]. Factors like injuries, blister, and illness like hypoglycemia can compromise skin barrier, leading to water and protein loss and heightened bacterial infection risk. Bacterial infections in the dermis slow the healing process due to delayed dermal cell migration and collagen synthesis [43]. While minor skin damage heals naturally, severe cases often require enhanced interventions to restore structural integrity. Biomaterials play a vital role in engineered skin tissue, with functional wound dressings designed to be porous for oxygen permeability and protective against external elements. These dressings also accelerate healing by minimizing bleeding and maintaining moisture [44]. Research into wound healing has primarily concentrated on water-friendly polymeric hydrocolloids, emulating the outside cell by maintaining a high water-retention capacity. CS has exhibited remarkable efficacy in expediting wound healing through its ability to enhance hemostasis by stimulating collagen synthesis in fibroblasts. This hemostatic activity is further reinforced by its capacity to form coagulum with erythrocytes and its modulatory effects on blood clotting pathways [44].

Additionally, chitin-derived polymers, when synergistically integrated with other polymers, yield advanced injury treatment that enhances the growth of cells as well as provides robust protection against microbial infections. These polymers exhibit anti-infective properties, enhance growth factor activity, and facilitate cell regeneration and migration, making them highly effective for wound care [45]. CS further stimulates macrophage activation, inducing an upregulated secretion of growth factors, phagocytic swelling protein-2 (MIP-2), and cytokines. This activation boosts collagen production, exerts antibacterial effects, and stimulates epithelial tissue proliferation *via* MIP-2 [27]. Antimicrobial properties of CS allow its combination with antimicrobial agents for treating acute skin injuries. However, lipid-based carriers, such as liposomes, are favored for topical skin disorders because of their improved skin contact and capacity to transport poorly soluble medicines. CS-coated liposomes improve antibacterial activity while treating epidermal and delicate tissue illnesses. Hemmingsen *et al.* found that integrating antimicrobial medications like chlorhexidine (CHX) into CS-based hydrocolloids increased spherosomes preservation and long-term release of medicines. Chitosomes with CHX showed greater and prolonged CHX release compared to formulations without chitosomes. This research underscores CS's role in enhancing long-term drug retention for skin injury treatments [46].

4.3.5 CS in Tissue Regeneration

4.3.5.1 Applications in Bone and Cartilage Regeneration

This evolving interdisciplinary domain integrates knowledge from life sciences, engineering, and chemistry to design 3D scaffolds featuring complex, interwoven porous architectures. These scaffolds are meticulously engineered to emulate the characteristics of mechanical integrity and natural tissues, including biocompatibility and osteoinductivity, with the primary objective of regenerating or substituting defective or lost bone cells [47]. CS and its derivatives have emerged as pivotal materials in scaffold fabrication given their outstanding characteristics. To optimize the physical characteristics and biocompatibility of these scaffolds, CS is frequently combined with artificial polymers such as polylactide, caprolactam homopolymer, PEG, and polymethyl methacrylate. These composites are meticulously engineered for osseous tissue generation, fulfilling the complex requirements of the final framework material [48]. Tanatsaparn *et al.*, for example, designed scaffolds made of composite materials by incorporating $(\text{methyl-methacrylate})_n$-CS-graft with mineral ions coupled hydroxyapatite. This pioneering approach yielded a microporous architecture with exceptional compressive strength, making it highly conducive to bone cell proliferation and drug delivery in the context of bone repair [49]. In addition to synthetic polymers, natural biopolymers including alginate, fibroin, gelatin, and hyaluronic acid are frequently synergized alongside CS to engineer sophisticated frameworks for rejuvenation of osseous tissue. Moreira *et al.* innovatively introduced an on-site formation of hybrid hydrocolloid comprising CS and gelatin, augmented with glass-based bioactive nanomaterials [50]. This injectable hydrocolloid demonstrates cytocompatibility, ensuring the survival of human osteosarcoma cells, and undergoes *in situ* gelation at physiological temperature, thereby enabling seamless syringe-based administration. Moreover, carbonaceous nanomaterials are being effectively integrated with CS to fabricate advanced scaffolds for enhancing bone tissue engineering outcomes. These carbon nanomaterials offer remarkable mechanical stability, strengthening organic–inorganic hybrid scaffolds and enhancing their potential in bone repair applications [51].

Chondrocytes, the cornerstone of cartilage tissue, play a vital role in synthesizing outside cell proteins. Hyaline cartilage, identified to exhibit impressive biomechanical attributes such as resilience to shock, stress allocation, and abrasion resistance, facilitates seamless joint articulation. CS, a versatile biopolymer, offers unique orthopedic tissue development for its adaptability in forming sponges, hydrogels, and fibers [52]. Its structural kinship with glycosaminoglycans, integral to the extracellular matrix, underscores its potential in cartilage regeneration. The fusion of CS with other biopolymers has captivated attention, given their biocompatibility and non-toxic profiles [53]. Shen *et al.* showcased a CS-gelatin hydrogel's highly porous architecture promoted cell growth and nutrient exchange, fostering remarkable rapid growth and attachment of human laryngeal prominence cells. Impressively, 65.9% hydrogel has been degraded over 70 days, aligning with cartilage regeneration timelines and highlighting its promise in tissue engineering [54]. Explorations into protein-based hydrogels like collagen combined with CS have further advanced cartilage repair strategies. Kaviani *et al.* developed a hydrocolloid blend of collagen, CS, and tribasic calcium phosphate *via* cryodesiccation, leveraging collagen's essential role in the cartilage beyond the cell for bone development and maintenance of cartilage-producing cells. CS's inclusion mitigated collagen's inherent weaknesses—its rapid degradation and limited mechanical strength—resulting in improved structural integrity, cell proliferation, and attachment. Byu Choi *et al.* delved into incorporating type II collagen and chondroitin sulfate into methacrylated glycol CS hydrocolloid using visible blue light and riboflavin [55]. Histological assessments revealed denser cell clusters on the hydrogel's outer regions, with fewer cells internally due to restricted nutrient and oxygen diffusion. The Col II and CS additives enhanced cellular condensation, chondrogenesis, and chondroid cluster formation, likely through integrin $\alpha 10\beta 1$–Col II interactions. These findings spotlight CS-based hydrogels, enriched with Col II, as a formidable contender for injectable scaffolds in cartilage repair.

4.3.5.2 Cardiac and Neural Tissue Engineering

CS hydrogels have emerged as a potent resource in neurovascular manufacturing, excelling in facilitating cellular attachments, association, viability, and neurite extension. Furthermore, 3D CS scaffolds, enriched with nerve growth factor (NGF), exhibit a cooperative effect that enhances the generation of neurons, demonstrating considerable promise for the repair of CNS as well as PNS [56]. In many instances, CS significantly enhanced the environment-friendly nature of PVA in nanofiber frameworks, thereby boosting PC12 cell viability and proliferation *in vitro*. In PVA/single-walled carbon nanotube (SWCNT) composites, CS fostered enhanced proliferation and incorporation of U373 belonging to human brain cells. In compliance polycaprolactone (PCL)/CS fibers facilitated robust PC12 cell adhesion and promoted neuronal processes following the fiber path, while PLGA/CS frameworks directed generation of neurons, proving effective in peripheral nerve rejuvenation in laboratory as well as living models [57]. Chemical versatility of CS facilitates its interaction with cell-attachment molecules, which bind to Schwann cell surface proteins. This interaction promotes enhanced cell adhesion and proliferation, a critical process for driving peripheral nerve regeneration. CS-based microparticles and NPs have been precisely developed to transport anticancer drugs, developmental characteristics, and other medications to the CNS. For instance, Skop *et al.* developed CS microspheres capable of transporting neurons as well as developmental characteristics to sites of CNS injury [58]. Similarly, Elnaggar *et al.* developed CS-NPs crafted piperine, a neuron guarding compound for Alzheimer's disease, enabling specific delivery to the brain. Furthermore, CS-NPs have been optimized for intranasal delivery, efficiently crossing the boundary associated to blood and brain to administer therapeutic chemicals directly to the CNS [59].

4.4 CS in Cancer Therapeutics

The anticancer efficacy of CS across various cell lines is principally attributed to its capacity to induce apoptosis, a process initiated by the activation of procaspase, setting off a cascade that amplifies cell death signaling. The cytotoxic potency of CS is modulated by its molecular mass and EoD [60]. LMMC exhibits pronounced cytotoxicity against oral squamous cell carcinoma (SCC) Ca9-22 cells in laboratory, initiating apoptosis *via* caspase-3 activation and cell division inhibition *via* external cell programmed cell death triggered by caspase-8. The augmented cytotoxicity of LMMC, compared to its high Mm counterpart, is largely due to increased cations, providing enhanced affinity for the anionic membranes of cancer cells [61]. This heightened interaction enables LMMC to target tumors *via* ionic interaction to the cancerous cell membrane or *via* endocytic mechanisms [60].

Antiproliferative effects of CS on urinary bladder tumor cell T24, demonstrated by cell sorting *via* fluorescence activation as well as DNA fragmentation assays, are linked to apoptosis. Flow cytometry analysis of CS's impact on T24 cell cycle distribution revealed a DNA content increment till the G2 phase and a decrement as the S phase ends, leading to cell membrane disruption and necrosis [62]. CS-NPs have revealed the prevention of human hepatoma cell BEL7402 rapid growth through mechanisms involving surface charge neutralization, membrane permeation, mitochondrial membrane potential reduction, and lipid peroxidation induction. CS-NPs also impede cellular viability in colon carcinoma cell HT-29. Their specific aggregation within cancer cells is facilitated by the enhanced penetrating and holding effect, coupled with the attenuation of P-glycoprotein facilitated multiple medication resistance, thereby bolstering their anticancer efficacy [63].

LMMC precipitates an S phase blockade in carcinoma cells *via* cytokine-mediated signaling, subsequently impeding DNA synthesis and frequently triggering cellular senescence, a pivotal mechanism in oncological therapies. This cell cycle disruption is intricately linked to the formation of ROS and activation of complex signaling involving TGF-β, Smad proteins, and cyclin-dependent kinase inhibitors. Research suggests that LMMC's ability to halt the cell cycle in the G1 phase may involve protein production changes independent of p53, with implications for DNA damage response mechanisms. Further investigation into this pathway is necessary to elucidate the complete anticancer mechanism of LMMC [64].

COS has been shown to inhibit cell proliferation, reduce S phase cell numbers, and decrease DNA synthesis in Lewis lung carcinoma (LLC) cells by modulating p21, cyclin A, and CDK-2 levels [65]. COS also exhibits its antiangiogenic properties, likely due to heparanase inhibition, and reduces tumor size in colorectal adenocarcinoma HT-29 cells by decreasing MMP-2 secretion. The antitumor effects of COS are also attributed to its ability to inhibit MMPs, ODC activity, COX-2 expression, and NO production, thereby reducing tumor growth, vascular invasion, and metastatic potential [66]. The anticancer potential of CS and its derivatives, particularly regarding Mm and EoD, has been demonstrated across various cancer cell lines, including PC3, A549, and HepG2. The results suggest that lower Mm CS derivatives like COS are more effective than higher Mm CS, though the exact antitumor mechanisms of high molecular weight chitosan (HMWC) remain unclear [60]. Additional study is required to totally comprehend and optimize the therapeutic uses of CS in cancer therapy.

4.4.1 Inhibition of Metastasis and Angiogenesis

CS-NPs carrying siRNA are being demonstrated to affect tumor cell migration, similar to their effect on cancer cell proliferation. Identifying key factors involved in cancer cell migration is essential for developing targeted therapies. For instance, BRAF undergoes mutations in cancer cells, driving malignancy and metastasis [67, 68]. Targeting the BRAF oncogene has demonstrated promise in curtailing cancer metastasis, and CS-NPs, engineered with a 350-nm diameter, have been innovatively designed to facilitate the targeted delivery of BRAF-siRNA in gastric carcinoma cells. Upon treatment with these siRNA-loaded NPs, a notable suppression of metastasis was evident, attributable to the downregulation of BRAF expression [69]. Insulin-like growth factor receptor-1 (IGF-1R) plays a critical role in modulating oncogenic progression. As a receptor tyrosine kinase, IGF-1R engages with multiple signaling cascades, including the epidermal growth factor receptor, to exacerbate cancerous malignancy. IGF-1R activates signal transducers and trigger for transcription 3 (STAT3) in metastatic breast carcinoma cells, resulting in the elevated levels of metal metalloproteinases within the matrix and vascular endothelial growth factor; either of these two facilitates the metastatic dissemination of tumor cells [70]. Therefore, down-regulating IGF-1R is critical for inhibiting cancer metastasis. To address this, CS-NPs incorporating IGF-1R-siRNA and docetaxel (DTX) were created. Additionally, surface modification of CS nanocarriers with aptamers, such as anti-MUC1 aptamers, has been employed to selectively target breast cancer cells. Aptamers offer advantages including low cost, high specificity, small size, and low immunogenicity [71]. The use of anti-MUC1 aptamers enhances the selective targeting of breast cancer cells, reducing IGF-1R expression and down-regulating downstream targets like STAT3, VEGF, and MMP-9, ultimately inhibiting metastasis [45].

In addition to this, the trimethylation of CS has been shown to improve its solubility, and the conjugation with hyaluronate (HA) allows for specific focus on cancer cells overexpressing CD44. N,N,N-trimethyl@ Hyaluronate-CS-NPs have been fabricated for siRNA administration, particularly to suppress IL-6 and STAT 3 expressions. These HA-conjugated NPs facilitate cellular uptake and exhibit minimal harmful effects, excellent transfection potency, and sustained release, offering a promising solution for suppressing cancer cell migration [72]. Despite the promising potential of CS-NPs, challenges such as their limited membrane penetration and inadequate buffering capacity persist; to overcome these obstacles, poly(histidine-arginine)6 (H6R6) peptides have been integrated into the NPs, enhancing both cellular uptake and endosomal escape. These improved CS-NPs hold promise for efficient siRNA delivery and metastasis inhibition. CS-NPs also demonstrate high loading efficiency for β-catenin-siRNA (β-CT-siRNA) with reported values as high as 97%. β-CT, a component of the regulatory system, contributes significantly to carcinoma spread. Activating β-CT and promoting its nuclear migration increase metastasis-related genes. PEGylated CS-NPs can efficiently distribute β-catenin-siRNA and prevent carcinoma spread [73].

Epithelial-to-mesenchymal transition (EMT), a critical mechanism that drives the spread of cancerous cells, is a prime target for CS-NPs. During EMT, epithelial markers like E-cadherin are reduced, while mesenchymal markers like N-cadherin and vimentin are increased. Recent advancements have led to the development of snail-siRNA-CS-NPs for the therapeutic management of prostate cancer. When PC-3 cells were exposed to these NPs, a significant suppression of metastasis was observed, mediated through the downregulation of snail expression, alongside an elevation in the appearance of E-cadherin and Claudin-1 [74]. These studies collectively demonstrate that CS-NPs offer a powerful platform for metastasis inhibition through targeted delivery of siRNA, providing significant potential for cancer therapy. CS exerts its antitumor activity through an antiangiogenic mechanism, disrupting the delicate balance between pro- and anti-angiogenic mechanism beneath clinical circumstances. In 2009, Y. Xu and colleagues demonstrated that CS-NPs effectively inhibited the progression of hepatoma by impeding tumor angiogenesis, a process closely linked to the suppression of vascular permeability factor 2 (VPF2) expression [75].

4.4.2 CS-Based Therapeutic Administration Technologies for Malignancy Therapies

Despite significant advancements, drug forbearance remains a prime hurdle, leading to the failure of current therapeutic approaches [76]. In response, Boroujeni *et al.* created curcumin-folate-CS-NPs for breast tumor treatment. Their extensive evaluations demonstrated that these NPs serve as effective carriers, delivering curcumin directly to cancer cells [77]. Similarly, Vignesh *et al.* formulated ascorbate-CS-NPs aimed at inhibiting cervical cancer. Through a series of in-laboratory and on-site studies, they observed a considerable reduction in cervical cancer cell viability, with minimal impact on normal human cells, highlighting the prospective application of these NPs for cervical cancer therapy. Glycol CS-based NPs also show remarkable tumor-targeting efficiency, leveraging the heightened passive tumor targeting outcome to advance therapeutic outcomes [78]. Ana Vanessa and colleagues explored EGFR-targeted CS-NPs for therapeutic administration, further highlighting versatility and efficacy of CS-based methods in malignancy therapy. CS biological degradation allows for the prolonged and regulated release of encapsulated agents, reducing dosing frequency and enhancing patient compliance, particularly in infectious disease therapies. Consequently, CS-based constituents are being extensively applied in the therapy of diabetes, cancer, and other conditions. CS-NPs are gaining popularity as attractive medicinal product delivery carriers due to their capacity to increase the dissolution of water-resistant medicines, regulate release of medications, reduce harmful effects, and improve the efficacy of treatment. These NPs also protect inconstant therapeutics from proteolytic degradation within the digestive tract, as evidenced by numerous publications on CS-based DDSs [79].

Derivatives such as trimethyl CS, renowned for its solubility at neutral pH, are synthesized through the reaction of CS with CH_3-I in the presence of NaOH. Trimethyl CS NPs have outstanding penetration capabilities, either by passing through cells or easily moving across the regions outside of cell [80]. Chen *et al.* synthesized trimethyl CS-CSK peptide conjugates using electrically charged gel formation, resulting in substance with an average size of 173.6 ± 6.8 nm. These conjugates considerably increased bioavailability of Gemzar when consumed and its permeability across porcine intestinal epithelial membranes, demonstrating promising therapeutic potential in breast cancer care [81]. Gao *et al.* explored NPs of CS derivatives for oral antigen delivery in fish vaccination, synthesizing carboxymethyl-CS-NPs encapsulating products outside the cell of *Vibrio anguillarum via* ionic gelation; these NPs safeguarded the antigen in the stomach and facilitated its regulated discharge in the intestinal tract, thereby augmenting innate as well as adaptive defensive responses more effectively than antigen solutions, establishing them as a potent antigen delivery system [82]. Additionally, CS NPs have been used to deliver doxorubicin, with enhanced absorption in the ileum and jejunum compared to conventional doxorubicin-loaded NPs.

Thiolated CS derivatives have shown significant potential in oral medication governance, owing to mucoadhesive characteristics, which are facilitated by the disulfide linking between thiolated polysaccharides and mucosal glycoproteins. George *et al.* synthesized an ecological nanocomposite hydrocolloid incorporating light-induced synthesized ZnO NPs and *Cucumis melo* seed concentrates, interconnected with aldehydic cellulose, for the governance of curcumin, exhibiting enhanced anticancer efficacy and biocompatibility *in vitro* [83]. Meanwhile, M.M. Martinez *et al.* engineered an ionic hydrocolloid interconnected with D-gluconate 6-phosphate trisodium salt, which demonstrated non-toxicity, no dermal irritation, and sufficient adhesion, making it suitable for wound healing applications [84].

4.4.3 Immunomodulatory Potential of CS in Cancer Therapy

The immune system is indispensable in identifying and eradicating neoplastic cells, with immune cells constituting crucial elements within the TME. In individuals without malignancies, cells harboring mutations that evade endogenous repair mechanisms are promptly recognized and eliminated by the immune system, thereby forestalling tumorigenesis. Antigen-presenting cells, such as phagocytes and dendrites, orchestrate immune surveillance by detecting tumor-associated antigens and then activating specialized immune cell subsets, including helper T cells, killer T cells, and NK cells, to mount a precise antitumor response. Nevertheless, tumor cells may evade immunological detection by establishing a tolerogenic or immunosuppressive milieu, ushering in a period known as "tumor escape," in which immune efficiency is reduced, promoting tumor development [85].

Recognizing that immune cells can occasionally adopt immunosuppressive and tumor-promoting roles, therapeutic approaches designed to reinvigorate these cells toward an immunostimulatory phenotype have garnered significant attention. Furthermore, augmenting the vulnerability of cancer cells to immune recognition serves to enhance immune system efficacy. This paradigm underpins the burgeoning field of immunotherapy that has come to prominence as a critical technique in the treatment for advanced tumors in the past few years. Immunotherapy encompasses a broad spectrum of modalities, like as cytokine therapies, immunoglobulin-based interventions, and agents aimed at mitigating immunosuppressive mechanisms [86]. Current immunotherapeutic techniques include monoclonal antibodies (mAbs) therapies addressing inhibitors of immune checkpoints, receptive cell treatment with modified T cells, and vaccines to prevent cancer. Nonetheless, such treatments have constraints and negative consequences, which may include the emergence of autoimmune disorders, immunological-mediated injury to natural tissues, and inflammation-related syndromes caused by complex immune hyper-activation [87]. Moreover, resistance mechanisms in certain patients can precipitate relapse, while others may exhibit a lack of therapeutic response. Factors such as mutational burden, neoantigen presence, and the extent of tumor immune infiltration play pivotal roles in determining patient outcomes.

Biomaterial-based strategies have emerged as promising methods to enhance the efficacy of immunotherapy and mitigate its side effects, serving as both immune adjuvants and drug delivery vehicles. These systems not only improve drug loading and release control, protecting sensitive molecules such as antigens from premature degradation, but also enable conjugation with intended components to enhance particularity of tissues and minimize comprehensive toxicity or immunological responses, while facilitating the co-delivery of drugs with complementary mechanisms of action for a more efficient therapeutic approach [88]. CS owing to its immunomodulatory properties can steer immune cell polarization toward an anti-/pro-inflammatory response, positioning itself as a potent contender for oncological therapeutics. Its versatility has been harnessed in a variety of expressions for the administration of cytokines (e.g., IL-12, IL-21, and γ-interferon), tumor cell lysates, nucleic acids (such as mRNA and siRNA), and chemoimmunotherapeutic agents, in addition to its native form [89]. CS-based systems, including NPs, gels, microneedles, and films, have been engineered to facilitate the development and stimulation of immune cells within the TME.

In a clinical trial with lung cancer patients, oral administration of water-soluble-CS alongside local radiotherapy was evaluated for 60 patients each in experimental and control, which led to a notable increase in blood CD3 and CD4 cell populations within the investigational cohort, resulting in a heightened ratio of CD4:CD8 compared to radiation therapy alone. Additionally, the expansion of NK cells and enhanced secretion of IL-6 and TNFα were observed. However, the impact of these immunological changes on patient survival and progression of disease was not investigated [90]. In a separate therapeutic investigation, glycated-CS (Gly-CS) was utilized as an addition to laser therapy and indocyanine green (ICYG), a photosensitive means, to induce discerning thermal effects in a cohort of 10 breast cancer patients (with 2 patients withdrawing prior to study completion). Gly-CS was delivered locally in combination alongside laser immunotherapy (LIT), resulting in positive responses in all local lesions in 8 patients. Surprisingly, one patient had total reduction of lung metastatic tumors, while others showed significant decreases in lung, lymph node, and liver metastases. Of the 8 patients, 1 achieved a thorough response, 4 demonstrated limited responses, 1 exhibited constant illness, and 2 showed illness progression [91].

4.5 Modifications of CS and their Therapeutic Application

CS is gaining increasing attention in the medicinal and pharmacological fields owing to its abundant existence and advantageous ecological qualities, including low immunity, biological compatibility, eco-friendliness, and mucosal adhesivity [92]. Structurally, CS contains three distinctive active sites: amine group at the 2nd carbon and hydroxyl group at the 3rd and 6th carbon (Figure 4.1). While modifications at the amine group at the 2nd carbon or hydroxyl group at the 6th carbon are relatively simple, altering the hydroxyl group at the 3rd carbon is challenging to modify because of strong steric hindrance. The amino groups, owing to their high reactivity, are most frequently modified, enabling efficient grafting reactions. Although the amino groups exhibit higher reactivity in nucleophilic reactions than the alcoholic groups, each of them can readily interact with positively charged compounds such as halogen-based alkanes, ethanoyl chlorides, and acidic substances, leading to nonselective functionalization [93].

The diverse array of active functional groups in CS facilitates its binding with proteins, imparting a positive charged nature, which enhances cellular interaction and promotes diversification. Despite these advantages, CS's poor solubility, especially at physiological pH 7.4, poses a significant limitation in its biomedical applications, rendering it an inefficient absorption enhancer [94]. Additionally, natural CS exhibits relatively low transfection efficiency and lacks certain functionalities crucial for specific applications. Consequently, the modification and functionalization of CS have garnered substantial interest. These alterations not only increase CS's solubility, expanding its biomedical applications, but also introduce novel biochemical reactions and improve its physical qualities [51]. Surprisingly, structural alterations of CS have no effect on its fundamental properties but rather provide fresh qualities.

The distinct structural morphology of CS enables its involvement in a broad spectrum of chemical reactions, including reduction, oxidation, complexation, acylation, cross-linking, phosphorylation, and halogenation, culminating in the synthesis of novel derivatives [93]. Over the last decade, CS and its derivatives have received a lot of interest because they

Table 4.1 Derivatives of CS and their distinctive characteristics.

S. no.	Derivatives of CS	Distinctive characteristics	Reference
1	Carboxymethyl CS-graft-cetylacetic acid	Serves as an excellent vehicle for administering clarithromycin to the bacteria that cause diarrhea	[96]
2	Modified CS coated-$ZnFe_2O_4$	Acts as a sustainable DDS	[97]
3	Galactosylated-CS	Enhances hepatocyte attachment and DNA synthesis	[98]
4	Lectin-CS–sugar blend	Demonstrates increased antibacterial actions	[40]
5	CS-graft-polyimine	Functions as a potential uninfected-viral genetic transporter	[99]
6	Trimethyloctyl ammonium-CS	Excellent drug integration ability improves delivery and release properties	[100]
7	MethoxyPEG-Capryl sulfate-CS	Enhances the dissolution of paclitaxel, a water-resistant oncology medication, in amphiphilic medium	[101]
8	CS-graft-PCL	Appropriate in multiple biological purposes	[102]
9	CS having warfarin	Exhibits reduction in oxidative stress, metallic ion retention, inhibition of the degradation of lipids, as well as collecting free radicals	[97]
10	CS-L_Arg and CS-PEG	Effective in live administration of medicinal siRNAs, lowers RBC hemorrhaging, and improves the survival of cells	[103]
11	ALP embedded CS	Increases ALP activity, encouraging accumulation of calcium and bone marrow cells growth	[104]

have better biochemical capabilities than unmodified CS, particularly while having aspects such as developing gels, dissolution, and the capacity to assemble themselves into nanomaterials. Furthermore, their introduction of water-resistant derivatives with divalent properties, together with the chemical conjugation to a variety of medicinal and bioactive agents, has significantly enhanced DNA binding capacities and biocompatibility [95]. The numerous chemically modified derivatives of CS and their distinctive functions and properties are summarized in Table 4.1.

Currently, quaternized CS-NPs) are extensively utilized in vaccine development. These CS-NPs serve as vaccine adjuvants by enhancing macrophage distribution in tissues that secrete chemokines. Upon initial administration, quaternized CS-NPs induce the aggregation of monocytes, thereby augmenting the immunogenic response of antigens. When employed as an adjuvant in H5N1 vaccines, quaternized CS-NPs significantly elevate specific antibody titers in a serum from a mouse while also activating CD8+ and CD4+ T lymphocyte populations. Furthermore, CS-NPs facilitate the enhanced absorption of antigens by myelogenous dendrites, thereby stimulating cells representing antigens. For example, BVA protein encapsulated in HTCC and sodium TPP NPs exhibits a first fast ejection, afterward developing a persistent and regulated drug delivery profile [105].

4.6 Strategies for Enhancing Bioavailability

The assembly of polymer and peptide function as highly effective therapeutics transporters, markedly enhancing oral bioavailability by shielding the drug from degradation and metabolic processes. Owing to their nanoscale dimensions, these NPs can traverse the mucosal boundary and adhering to fundamental epithelial cells, consequently extending the drug's occupancy duration within the gastrointestinal tract and facilitating improved absorption. The efficacy of these conjugates is profoundly influenced by the specific polymer chosen for their formulation. CS composed of irregularly dispersed β-1-4-linked deacetylated D-glucosamine as well as acetylated N-acetyl-D-glucosamine part entities is extremely sustainable and environment-friendly, making it an attractive choice for improved therapeutic administration platform [106]. CS-based carriers have demonstrated high drug encapsulation efficiency and desirable mucoadhesive properties [95]. Furthermore, CS can enhance permeability by opening intercellular tight junctions through interactions between its cationic molecular groups and anionic tight junction proteins. However, CS's solubility in only acidic environments due to deprotonation limits its absorption potential as the drug may become trapped within the carrier [107].

N-trimethyl CS (TMC), a moderately quaternized CS derivative, offers improved solubility in neutral and basic medium, maintaining its functionality as a permeation enhancer under physiological conditions [80, 106]. TMC-NPs exhibit superior absorption efficiency over CS-NPs, primarily due to enhanced interactions with intestinal epithelial cells and increased mucoadhesion. This characteristic facilitates both transcellular and paracellular pathways, thereby improving the efficacy of drug delivery [108]. Furthermore, TMC can be combined with such ligands exhibiting discreet correspondence for specific cell types of intestines. One such ligand, CSK, a peptide that is of natural origin, targets goblet cells (Gc), which are the subsequent most numerous kinds of epithelial cells in the intestine and perform a significant function in mucus formation inside the gastrointestinal tract. CSK pairing improves NP absorption *via* caveolae and endocytosis through clathrin [108]. Studies by Tian *et al.* demonstrated that modified CSK-lipid-NPs (modified) displayed a pronounced interaction with intestinal Gc, suggesting their potential as effective carriers for drug transport across intestinal barriers. Additionally, Jin *et al.* revealed that CSK significantly augmented NP uptake in Gc-like, mucus-secreting HT29-MTX cells. On-site research involving insulin@CSK-NPs (modified) reported an increase of 1.7-fold in ileal permeation and enhancement of about 1.5-fold in oral bioavailability contrasted to unchanged NPs [106].

4.7 Challenges and Future Prospects

CS has distinguished itself as a multifaceted pharmaceutical excipient, serving as a permeation enhancer and a hemostatic agent, with diverse applications spanning wound healing, advanced dressings, weight management, and cholesterol modulation. However, the landscape of cancer treatment presents formidable challenges, as various malignant cells exhibit resistance to standard chemotherapeutic agents including docetaxel, 5-FU, cisplatin, methotrexate, and procarbazine. These drugs are often associated with severe acute and chronic toxicities affecting the gastrointestinal tract, reticuloendothelial system, bone marrow, and gonads [3]. CS and derivatives, particularly CS-nanocomposites, have emerged as promising candidates in antitumor therapy. The specific antitumor activity, combined with their inherent non-toxicity, biocompatibility, and biodegradability, positions them as natural alternatives to mitigate the adverse effects of conventional chemotherapy. Despite the significant global burden of cancer and decades of intensive research into more effective anticancer strategies, the clinical application of CS in oncology remains relatively underexplored [32]. The fabrication of CS-based therapeutics, which exhibit minimal toxicity to non-cancerous cells, is critical in this context.

The FDA has labelled CS as a Generally Recognized as Safe chemical. It has been authorized for treatments for wounds and judged safe for normal oral ingestion at dosages of no more than 4.5 g per day during a period of 12 weeks, with only mild adverse effects such as nausea and constipation observed. However, chemical modifications of CS-NPs and derivatives can alter their pharmacokinetics and toxicity profiles, necessitating comprehensive toxicity evaluations for each derivative. Improving CS's solubility and biological activity through increased deacetylation and strategic chemical modifications can lead to the development of more efficacious derivatives [95]. The therapeutic efficacy of CS-based anticancer formulations is often impeded by suboptimal drug accumulation within target cells and the hostile TME, characterized by inadequate perfusion, arteriovenous shunting, hypoxic and necrotic zones, and heightened interstitial fluid pressure. Nonetheless, encapsulating anticancer drugs within CS-NPs significantly improves targeted delivery by using the increased EPR effect. For instance, dextran-conjugated doxorubicin enclosed in 100-nm CS-NPs demonstrates higher accumulation and therapeutic effectiveness within cancer cells [24].

Although only a limited number of CS-based formulations are presently in clinical trials, they exhibit substantial potential to transform cancer diagnosis, treatment, and pain management, offering the prospect of a paradigm shift in the therapeutic landscape of this formidable disease. CS and its derivatives demonstrate superior permeation capabilities through the negatively charged tumor cell membranes, significantly enhancing their bioavailability within tumor cells [109]. Exploring the relationship between their structural characteristics and their efficacy in inhibiting tumor growth and metastasis across diverse cellular pathways could unveil novel insights into their anticancer mechanisms. Advanced chemical modifications, complex formation, and graft polymerization of CS offer promising avenues for the design and development of tailored hybrid materials for innovative anticancer therapeutic applications.

4.8 Conclusion

CS, a biopolymer obtained from natural sources, has rapidly gained importance in the biomedical and pharmaceutical industries because of its flexibility and biocompatibility. In addition, some structural characteristics of CS accompanied by modifiable functional groups permit the production and modification of sufficient derivatives with diverse properties, such as increased solubility, improved bioactivity, and enhanced targeting ability. This has increased its usage in therapeutic administration, tissue engineering, cancer treatment, wound healing, and genetic administration. CS-based NPs offer significant prospects in cancer treatment. These could tackle many challenges that are typically associated with the TME, such as poor vascularization and hypoxia. As a result of such properties, combined with mucoadhesion, biodegradability, and the ability to encapsulate hydrophobic drugs, CS formulations can improve the targeted delivery of chemotherapeutic agents and enhance their bioavailability. In addition, CS-based materials have immune modulatory properties and are thus significant in immunotherapy as they provide novel ways to reactivate immune cells and improve antigen presentation. While CS formulations have shown encouraging results in both preclinical and clinical studies, there are still challenges to overcome, such as scaling up production, variability in pharmacokinetics, and the necessity for personalized toxicity assessments of chemically modified derivatives. Tackling these issues through advanced synthesis methods and comprehensive clinical evaluations could facilitate wider clinical use. The unique properties of CS, along with its adaptability for specific biomedical applications, make it a groundbreaking material in contemporary therapeutics. Continued research and clinical progress in CS-based formulations are anticipated to not only improve the effectiveness of current therapies but also create new opportunities for innovative treatment approaches, especially in combating cancer and other chronic illnesses.

AI disclosure statement: The author acknowledges the use of AI-based tools for minor language editing or grammatical correction. However, all intellectual contributions, analyses, and conclusions presented in this chapter are entirely the author's own.

References

1. Parhi, R., Drug delivery applications of chitin and chitosan: a review. *Environ. Chem. Lett.*, 18, 3, 577–94, 2020 May.
2. Rasti, H., Parivar, K., Baharara, J., Iranshahi, M., Namvar, F., Chitin from the Mollusc Chiton: Extraction, Characterization and Chitosan Preparation. *Iran. J. Pharm. Res.*, 16, 1, 366–79, 2017.

3. Joseph, S.M., Krishnamoorthy, S., Paranthaman, R., Moses, J.A., Anandharamakrishnan, C., A review on source-specific chemistry, functionality, and applications of chitin and chitosan. *Carbohydr. Polym. Technol. Appl.*, 2, 100036, 2021 Dec.
4. Tissera, W.M.J.C., Rathnayake, S.I., Abeyrathne, E.D.N.S., Nam, K.C., An improved extraction and purification method for obtaining high-quality chitin and chitosan from blue swimmer (Portunus pelagicus) crab shell waste. *Food Sci. Biotechnol.*, 30, 13, 1645–55, 2021 Dec.
5. Ang, L.F., Por, L.Y., Yam, M.F., Study on Different Molecular Weights of Chitosan as an Immobilization Matrix for a Glucose Biosensor. *PLoS One*, 8, 8, e70597, 2013 Aug 5, Pandit A, editor.
6. Shakil, MdS., Hasan, MdA., Uddin, MdF., Islam, A., Nahar, A., Das, H., *et al.*, *In Vivo* Toxicity Studies of Chitosan-Coated Cobalt Ferrite Nanocomplex for Its Application as MRI Contrast Dye. *ACS Appl. Bio Mater.*, 3, 11, 7952–64, 2020 Nov 16.
7. Adhikari, H.S. and Yadav, P.N., Anticancer Activity of Chitosan, Chitosan Derivatives, and Their Mechanism of Action. *Int. J. Biomater.*, 2018, 1–29, 2018 Dec 30.
8. Islam, S., Bhuiyan, M.A.R., Islam, M.N., Chitin and Chitosan: Structure, Properties and Applications in Biomedical Engineering. *J. Polym. Environ.*, 25, 3, 854–66, 2017 Sep.
9. Özel, N. and Elibol, M., A review on the potential uses of deep eutectic solvents in chitin and chitosan related processes. *Carbohydr. Polym.*, 262, 117942, 2021 Jun.
10. Pachapur, V.L., Guemiza, K., Rouissi, T., Sarma, S.J., Brar, S.K., Novel biological and chemical methods of chitin extraction from crustacean waste using saline water: Novel biological and chemical methods of chitin extraction. *J. Chem. Technol. Biotechnol.*, 91, 8, 2331–9, 2016 Aug.
11. Jardine, A. and Sayed, S., Valorisation of chitinous biomass for antimicrobial applications. *Pure Appl. Chem.*, 90, 2, 293–304, 2018 Feb 23.
12. Bharathiraja, S., Bui, N.Q., Manivasagan, P., Moorthy, M.S., Mondal, S., Seo, H., *et al.*, Multimodal tumor-homing chitosan oligosaccharide-coated biocompatible palladium nanoparticles for photo-based imaging and therapy. *Sci. Rep.*, 8, 1, 500, 2018 Jan 11.
13. Esther, J. and Sridevi, V., Synthesis and characterization of chitosan-stabilized gold nanoparticles through a facile and green approach. *Gold Bull.*, 50, 1, 1–5, 2017 Mar.
14. Abrica-González, P., Zamora-Justo, J.A., Sotelo-López, A., Vázquez-Martínez, G.R., Balderas-López, J.A., Muñoz-Diosdado, A., *et al.*, Gold nanoparticles with chitosan, N-acylated chitosan, and chitosan oligosaccharide as DNA carriers. *Nanoscale Res. Lett.*, 14, 1, 258, 2019 Dec.
15. Phan, T.T.V., Phan, D.T., Cao, X.T., Huynh, T.C., Oh, J., Roles of Chitosan in Green Synthesis of Metal Nanoparticles for Biomedical Applications. *Nanomaterials*, 11, 2, 273, 2021 Jan 21.

16. Chitin and Chitosan in Drug Delivery, in: *Sustainable Agriculture Reviews* [Internet], pp. 175–239, Springer International Publishing, Cham, 2019 [cited 2025 Jan 14], Available from: http://link.springer.com/10.1007/978-3-030-16581-9_6.
17. Ahmad, A., Mubarak, N.M., Naseem, K., Tabassum, H., Rizwan, M., Najda, A., *et al.*, Recent advancement and development of chitin and chitosan-based nanocomposite for drug delivery: Critical approach to clinical research. *Arabian J. Chem.*, 13, 12, 8935–64, 2020 Dec.
18. Sim, S. and Wong, N., Nanotechnology and its use in imaging and drug delivery (Review). *Biomed. Rep.*, 14, 5, 2021 Mar 5 [cited 2025 Jan 14]. Available from: http://www.spandidos-publications.com/10.3892/br.2021.1418.
19. Mohammed, M., Syeda, J., Wasan, K., Wasan, E., An Overview of Chitosan Nanoparticles and Its Application in Non-Parenteral Drug Delivery. *Pharmaceutics*, 9, 4, 53, 2017 Nov 20.
20. Garg, U., Chauhan, S., Nagaich, U., Jain, N., Current Advances in Chitosan Nanoparticles Based Drug Delivery and Targeting. *Adv. Pharm. Bull.*, 9, 2, 195–204, 2019 Jun 1.
21. Naskar, S., Sharma, S., Kuotsu, K., Chitosan-based nanoparticles: An overview of biomedical applications and its preparation. *J. Drug Deliv. Sci. Technol.*, 49, 66–81, 2019 Feb.
22. Shinde, U.A., Joshi, P.N., Jain, D.D., Singh, K., Preparation and Evaluation of N-Trimethyl Chitosan Nanoparticles of Flurbiprofen for Ocular Delivery. *Curr. Eye Res.*, 44, 5, 575–82, 2019 May 4.
23. Zhao, R., Li, J., Wang, J., Yin, Z., Zhu, Y., Liu, W., Development of Timolol-Loaded Galactosylated Chitosan Nanoparticles and Evaluation of Their Potential for Ocular Drug Delivery. *AAPS PharmSciTech*, 18, 4, 997–1008, 2017 May.
24. Silva, M., Calado, R., Marto, J., Bettencourt, A., Almeida, A., Gonçalves, L., Chitosan Nanoparticles as a Mucoadhesive Drug Delivery System for Ocular Administration. *Mar. Drugs*, 15, 12, 370, 2017 Dec 1.
25. Cánepa, C., Imperiale, J.C., Berini, C.A., Lewicki, M., Sosnik, A., Biglione, M.M., Development of a Drug Delivery System Based on Chitosan Nanoparticles for Oral Administration of Interferon-α. *Biomacromolecules*, 18, 10, 3302–9, 2017 Oct 9.
26. Lombardi, A., Tsomos, E., Hammerstad, S.S., Tomer, Y., Interferon alpha: The key trigger of type 1 diabetes. *J. Autoimmun.*, 94, 7–15, 2018 Nov.
27. Boni, R., Ali, A., Shavandi, A., Clarkson, A.N., Current and novel polymeric biomaterials for neural tissue engineering. *J. Biomed. Sci.*, 25, 1, 90, 2018 Dec.
28. Gnavi, S., Barwig, C., Freier, T., Haastert-Talini, K., Grothe, C., Geuna, S., The Use of Chitosan-Based Scaffolds to Enhance Regeneration in the Nervous System, in: *International Review of Neurobiology* [Internet], pp. 1–62, Elsevier, 2013 [cited 2025 Jan 15], Available from: https://linkinghub.elsevier.com/retrieve/pii/B9780124200456000018.

29. Pellá, M.C.G., Lima-Tenório, M.K., Tenório-Neto, E.T., Guilherme, M.R., Muniz, E.C., Rubira, A.F., Chitosan-based hydrogels: From preparation to biomedical applications. *Carbohydr. Polym.*, 196, 233–45, 2018 Sep.
30. Shariatinia, Z. and Jalali, A.M., Chitosan-based hydrogels: Preparation, properties and applications. *Int. J. Biol. Macromol.*, 115, 194–220, 2018 Aug.
31. Wang, Y., Tan, H., Hui, X., Biomaterial Scaffolds in Regenerative Therapy of the Central Nervous System. *Biomed Res. Int.*, 2018, 1–19, 2018 Apr 1.
32. Xu, C., Guan, S., Wang, S., Gong, W., Liu, T., Ma, X., *et al.*, Biodegradable and electroconductive poly(3,4-ethylenedioxythiophene)/carboxymethyl chitosan hydrogels for neural tissue engineering. *Mater. Sci. Eng.: C*, 84, 32–43, 2018 Mar.
33. Rodríguez-Vázquez, M., Vega-Ruiz, B., Ramos-Zúñiga, R., Saldaña-Koppel, D.A., Quiñones-Olvera, L.F., Chitosan and Its Potential Use as a Scaffold for Tissue Engineering in Regenerative Medicine. *Biomed Res. Int.*, 2015, 1–15, 2015.
34. Chedly, J., Soares, S., Montembault, A., Von Boxberg, Y., Veron-Ravaille, M., Mouffle, C., *et al.*, Physical chitosan microhydrogels as scaffolds for spinal cord injury restoration and axon regeneration. *Biomaterials*, 138, 91–107, 2017 Sep.
35. Ricks, C., Shin, S., Becker, C., Grandhi, R., Extracellular matrices, artificial neural scaffolds and the promise of neural regeneration. *Neural Regener. Res.*, 9, 17, 1573, 2014.
36. Choudhury, S.R., Hudry, E., Maguire, C.A., Sena-Esteves, M., Breakefield, X.O., Grandi, P., Viral vectors for therapy of neurologic diseases. *Neuropharmacology*, 120, 63–80, 2017 Jul.
37. Mao, S., Sun, W., Kissel, T., Chitosan-based formulations for delivery of DNA and siRNA. *Adv. Drug Deliv. Rev.*, 62, 1, 12–27, 2010 Jan.
38. Gao, S., Zhao, P., Lin, C., Sun, Y., Wang, Y., Zhou, Z., *et al.*, Differentiation of Human Adipose-Derived Stem Cells into Neuron-Like Cells Which Are Compatible with Photocurable Three-Dimensional Scaffolds. *Tissue Eng. Part A*, 20, 7–8, 1271–84, 2014 Apr.
39. Gu, J., Al-Bayati, K., Ho, E.A., Development of antibody-modified chitosan nanoparticles for the targeted delivery of siRNA across the blood-brain barrier as a strategy for inhibiting HIV replication in astrocytes. *Drug Deliv. Transl. Res.*, 7, 4, 497–506, 2017 Aug.
40. Van Woensel, M., Wauthoz, N., Rosière, R., Mathieu, V., Kiss, R., Lefranc, F., *et al.*, Development of siRNA-loaded chitosan nanoparticles targeting Galectin-1 for the treatment of glioblastoma multiforme *via* intranasal administration. *J. Control. Release*, 227, 71–81, 2016 Apr.
41. Sanchez-Ramos, J., Song, S., Kong, X., Foroutan, P., Martinez, G., Dominguez-Viqueria, W., *et al.*, Chitosan-Mangafodipir nanoparticles designed for intranasal delivery of siRNA and DNA to brain. *J. Drug Deliv. Sci. Technol.*, 43, 453–60, 2018 Feb.

42. Liu, Y., Liu, Y., Wu, M., Zou, R., Mao, S., Cong, P., *et al.*, Adipose-derived mesenchymal stem cell-loaded β-chitin nanofiber hydrogel promote wound healing in rats. *J. Mater. Sci.: Mater. Med.*, 33, 2, 12, 2022 Feb.
43. Ma, M., Zhong, Y., Jiang, X., Thermosensitive and pH-responsive tannin-containing hydroxypropyl chitin hydrogel with long-lasting antibacterial activity for wound healing. *Carbohydr. Polym.*, 236, 116096, 2020 May.
44. Jones, M., Kujundzic, M., John, S., Bismarck, A., Crab vs. Mushroom: A Review of Crustacean and Fungal Chitin in Wound Treatment. *Mar. Drugs*, 18, 1, 64, 2020 Jan 18.
45. Jafari, H., Bernaerts, K.V., Dodi, G., Shavandi, A., Chitooligosaccharides for wound healing biomaterials engineering. *Mater. Sci. Eng.: C*, 117, 111266, 2020 Dec.
46. Hemmingsen, L.M., Julin, K., Ahsan, L., Basnet, P., Johannessen, M., Škalko-Basnet, N., Chitosomes-In-Chitosan Hydrogel for Acute Skin Injuries: Prevention and Infection Control. *Mar. Drugs*, 19, 5, 269, 2021 May 12.
47. Prabaharan, M. and Sivashankari, P.R., Prospects of Bioactive Chitosan-Based Scaffolds in Tissue Engineering and Regenerative Medicine, in: *Chitin and Chitosan for Regenerative Medicine* [Internet], P.K. Dutta (Ed.), pp. 41–59, Springer India, New Delhi, 2016 [cited 2025 Jan 18], (Springer Series on Polymer and Composite Materials). Available from: https://link.springer.com/10.1007/978-81-322-2511-9_2.
48. Rogina, A., Pribolšan, L., Hanžek, A., Gómez-Estrada, L., Gallego Ferrer, G., Marijanović, I., *et al.*, Macroporous poly(lactic acid) construct supporting the osteoinductive porous chitosan-based hydrogel for bone tissue engineering. *Polymer*, 98, 172–81, 2016 Aug.
49. Tithito, T., Suntornsaratoon, P., Charoenphandhu, N., Thongbunchoo, J., Krishnamra, N., Tang, I.M., *et al.*, Fabrication of biocomposite scaffolds made with modified hydroxyapatite inclusion of chitosan-grafted-poly(methyl methacrylate) for bone tissue engineering. *Biomed. Mater.*, 14, 2, 025013, 2019 Feb 25.
50. Moreira, C.D.F., Carvalho, S.M., Sousa, R.G., Mansur, H.S., Pereira, M.M., Nanostructured chitosan/gelatin/bioactive glass *in situ* forming hydrogel composites as a potential injectable matrix for bone tissue engineering. *Mater. Chem. Phys.*, 218, 304–16, 2018 Oct.
51. Sivashankari, P.R. and Prabaharan, M., Chitosan/carbon-based nanomaterials as scaffolds for tissue engineering, in: *Biopolymer-Based Composites* [Internet], pp. 381–97, Elsevier, 2017 [cited 2025 Jan 19], Available from: https://linkinghub.elsevier.com/retrieve/pii/B9780081019146000120.
52. Azeez, M.A., Lateef, A., TB, A., *et al.*, Biomedical Applications of Cocoa Bean Extract-Mediated Silver Nanoparticles as Antimicrobial, Larvicidal and Anticoagulant Agents. *J. Cluster Sci.*, 28, 1, 149–64, 2017 Jan 1.
53. Kuo, C.Y., Chen, C.H., Hsiao, C.Y., Chen, J.P., Incorporation of chitosan in biomimetic gelatin/chondroitin-6-sulfate/hyaluronan cryogel for cartilage tissue engineering. *Carbohydr. Polym.*, 117, 722–30, 2015 Mar.

54. Shen, Z.S., Cui, X., Hou, R.X., Li, Q., Deng, H.X., Fu, J., Tough biodegradable chitosan–gelatin hydrogels *via in situ* precipitation for potential cartilage tissue engineering. *RSC Adv.*, 5, 69, 55640–55647, 2015. https://doi.org/10.1039/C5RA06835E.
55. Choi, B., Kim, S., Lin, B., Wu, B.M., Lee, M., Cartilaginous Extracellular Matrix-Modified Chitosan Hydrogels for Cartilage Tissue Engineering. *ACS Appl. Mater. Interfaces*, 6, 22, 20110–21, 2014 Nov 26.
56. Li, G., Xiao, Q., Zhang, L., Zhao, Y., Yang, Y., Nerve growth factor loaded heparin/chitosan scaffolds for accelerating peripheral nerve regeneration. *Carbohydr. Polym.*, 171, 39–49, 2017 Sep.
57. Xue, C., Hu, N., Gu, Y., Yang, Y., Liu, Y., Liu, J., *et al.*, Joint Use of a Chitosan/PLGA Scaffold and MSCs to Bridge an Extra Large Gap in Dog Sciatic Nerve. *Neurorehabil. Neural Repair*, 26, 1, 96–106, 2012 Jan.
58. Skop, N.B., Calderon, F., Levison, S.W., Gandhi, C.D., Cho, C.H., Heparin crosslinked chitosan microspheres for the delivery of neural stem cells and growth factors for central nervous system repair. *Acta Biomater.*, 9, 6, 6834–43, 2013 Jun.
59. Elnaggar, Y.S., Etman, S.M., Abdelmonsif, D.A., Abdallah, O.Y., Intranasal piperine-loaded chitosan nanoparticles as brain-targeted therapy in Alzheimer's disease: optimization, biological efficacy, and potential toxicity. *J. Pharmaceut. Sci.*, 104, 10, 3544–3556, 2015. DOI: 10.1002/jps.24557.
60. Park, J.K., Chung, M.J., Choi, H.N., Park, Y.I., Effects of the Molecular Weight and the Degree of Deacetylation of Chitosan Oligosaccharides on Antitumor Activity. *IJMS*, 12, 1, 266–77, 2011 Jan 6.
61. Zhang, J., Xia, W., Liu, P., Cheng, Q., Tahi, T., Gu, W., *et al.*, Chitosan Modification and Pharmaceutical/Biomedical Applications. *Mar. Drugs*, 8, 7, 1962–87, 2010 Jun 25.
62. Hasegawa, M., Yagi, K., Iwakawa, S., Hirai, M., Chitosan Induces Apoptosis *via* Caspase-3 Activation in Bladder Tumor Cells. *Jpn. J. Cancer Res.*, 92, 4, 459–66, 2001 Apr.
63. Ramasamy, T., Ruttala, H.B., Chitrapriya, N., Poudal, B.K., Choi, J.Y., Kim, S.T., *et al.*, Engineering of cell microenvironment-responsive polypeptide nanovehicle co-encapsulating a synergistic combination of small molecules for effective chemotherapy in solid tumors. *Acta Biomater.*, 48, 131–43, 2017 Jan.
64. Wimardhani Y, S., Suniarti D, F., Freisleben H, J., Wanandi SI, C., Siregar, N., Ikeda, M.A., Chitosan exerts anticancer activity through induction of apoptosis and cell cycle arrest in oral cancer cells. *J. Oral Sci.*, 56, 2, 119–26, 2014.
65. Shen, K.T., Chen, M.H., Chan, H.Y., Jeng, J.H., Wang, Y.J., Inhibitory effects of chitooligosaccharides on tumor growth and metastasis. *Food Chem. Toxicol.*, 47, 8, 1864–71, 2009 Aug.
66. Nam, K.S., Kim, M.K., Shon, Y.H., Inhibition of proinflammatory cytokine-induced invasiveness of HT-29 cells by chitosan oligosaccharide. *J. Microbiol. Biotechnol.*, 17, 12, 2042–5, 2007 Dec.

67. Caputo, F., Santini, C., Bardasi, C., Cerma, K., Casadei-Gardini, A., Spallanzani, A., *et al.*, BRAF-Mutated Colorectal Cancer: Clinical and Molecular Insights. *IJMS*, 20, 21, 5369, 2019 Oct 28.
68. Croce, L., Coperchini, F., Magri, F., Chiovato, L., Rotondi, M., The multifaceted anti-cancer effects of BRAF-inhibitors. *Oncotarget*, 10, 61, 6623–40, 2019 Nov 12.
69. Huo, J., Effects of chitosan nanoparticle-mediated BRAF siRNA interference on invasion and metastasis of gastric cancer cells. *Artif. Cells Nanomed. Biotechnol.*, 44, 5, 1232–5, 2016 Jul 3.
70. Banerjee, K. and Resat, H., Constitutive activation of STAT 3 in breast cancer cells: A review. *Int. J. Cancer*, 138, 11, 2570–8, 2016 Jun.
71. Taghdisi, S.M., Danesh, N.M., Nameghi, M.A., Bahreyni, A., Ramezani, M., Alibolandi, M., *et al.*, Co-delivery of doxorubicin and α-PCNA aptamer using AS1411-modified pH-responsive nanoparticles for cancer synergistic therapy. *J. Drug Deliv. Sci. Technol.*, 58, 101816, 2020 Aug.
72. Masjedi, A., Ahmadi, A., Atyabi, F., Farhadi, S., Irandoust, M., Khazaei-Poul, Y., *et al.*, Silencing of IL-6 and STAT3 by siRNA loaded hyaluronate-N,N,N-trimethyl chitosan nanoparticles potently reduces cancer cell progression. *Int. J. Biol. Macromol.*, 149, 487–500, 2020 Apr.
73. Rudzinski, W.E., Palacios, A., Ahmed, A., Lane, M.A., Aminabhavi, T.M., Targeted delivery of small interfering RNA to colon cancer cells using chitosan and PEGylated chitosan nanoparticles. *Carbohydr. Polym.*, 147, 323–32, 2016 Aug.
74. Afkham, A., Aghebati-Maleki, L., Siahmansouri, H., Sadreddini, S., Ahmadi, M., Dolati, S., *et al.*, Chitosan (CMD)-mediated co-delivery of SN38 and Snail-specific siRNA as a useful anticancer approach against prostate cancer. *Pharmacol. Rep.*, 70, 3, 418–25, 2018 Jun.
75. Xu, Y., Wen, Z., Xu, Z., Chitosan nanoparticles inhibit the growth of human hepatocellular carcinoma xenografts through an antiangiogenic mechanism. *Anticancer Res.*, 29, 12, 5103–9, 2009 Dec.
76. Ferrara, N. and Adamis, A.P., Ten years of anti-vascular endothelial growth factor therapy. *Nat. Rev. Drug Discov.*, 15, 6, 385–403, 2016 Jun.
77. Esfandiarpour-Boroujeni, S., Bagheri-Khoulenjani, S., Mirzadeh, H., Amanpour, S., Fabrication and study of curcumin loaded nanoparticles based on folate-chitosan for breast cancer therapy application. *Carbohydr. Polym.*, 168, 14–21, 2017 Jul.
78. Sekar, V., Rajendran, K., Vallinayagam, S., Deepak, V., Mahadevan, S., Synthesis and characterization of chitosan ascorbate nanoparticles for therapeutic inhibition for cervical cancer and their *in silico* modeling. *J. Ind. Eng. Chem.*, 62, 239–249, 2018, https://doi.org/10.1016/j.jiec.2018.01.001.
79. Liu, C., Tan, Y., Liu, C., Chen, X., Yu, L., Preparations, characterizations and applications of chitosan-based nanoparticles. *J. Ocean Univ. China*, 6, 3, 237–43, 2007 Jul.

80. Sandri, G., Bonferoni, M.C., Rossi, S., Ferrari, F., Boselli, C., Caramella, C., Insulin-Loaded Nanoparticles Based on N-Trimethyl Chitosan: *In Vitro* (Caco-2 Model) and *Ex Vivo* (Excised Rat Jejunum, Duodenum, and Ileum) Evaluation of Penetration Enhancement Properties. *AAPS PharmSciTech*, 11, 1, 362–71, 2010 Mar.
81. Chen, G., Svirskis, D., Lu, W., Ying, M., Huang, Y., Wen, J., N -trimethyl chitosan nanoparticles and CSKSSDYQC peptide: N -trimethyl chitosan conjugates enhance the oral bioavailability of gemcitabine to treat breast cancer. *J. Control. Release*, 277, 142–53, 2018 May.
82. Gao, P., Xia, G., Bao, Z., Feng, C., Cheng, X., Kong, M., ... & Chen, X., Chitosan based nanoparticles as protein carriers for efficient oral antigen delivery. *Int. J. Biol. Macromolecules,* 91, 716–723, 2016, https://doi.org/10.1016/j.ijbiomac.2016.06.015.
83. George, D., Maheswari, P.U., Sheriffa Begum, K.M.M., Arthanareeswaran, G., Biomass-Derived Dialdehyde Cellulose Cross-linked Chitosan-Based Nanocomposite Hydrogel with Phytosynthesized Zinc Oxide Nanoparticles for Enhanced Curcumin Delivery and Bioactivity. *J. Agric. Food. Chem.*, 67, 39, 10880–90, 2019 Oct 2.
84. Martínez-Martínez, M., Rodríguez-Berna, G., Gonzalez-Alvarez, I., Hernández, M.J., Corma, A., Bermejo, M., *et al.*, Ionic Hydrogel Based on Chitosan Cross-Linked with 6-Phosphogluconic Trisodium Salt as a Drug Delivery System. *Biomacromolecules*, 19, 4, 1294–304, 2018 Apr 9.
85. Bhutia, S.K., Mallick, S.K., Maiti, T.K., Tumour escape mechanisms and their therapeutic implications in combination tumour therapy. *Cell Biol. Int.*, 34, 5, 553–63, 2010 May.
86. Dobosz, P. and Dzieciątkowski, T., The Intriguing History of Cancer Immunotherapy. *Front. Immunol.*, 10, 2965, 2019 Dec 17.
87. Wolf, B., Zimmermann, S., Arber, C., Irving, M., Trueb, L., Coukos, G., Safety and Tolerability of Adoptive Cell Therapy in Cancer. *Drug Saf.*, 42, 2, 315–34, 2019 Feb 8.
88. Yang, F., Shi, K., Peng, J.Y., Hao, Y., Rong, P.J., Yong, Q.Z., Advanced biomaterials for cancer immunotherapy. *Acta Pharmacol. Sin.*, 41, 7, 911–27, 2020 Jul.
89. Li, X., Dong, W., Nalin, A.P., Wang, Y., Pan, P., Xu, B., *et al.*, The natural product chitosan enhances the anti-tumor activity of natural killer cells by activating dendritic cells. *OncoImmunology*, 7, 6, e1431085, 2018 Jun 3.
90. Ma, J.X., Qian, L., Zhou, Y., Stimulation effect of chitosan on the immunity of radiotherapy patients suffered from lung cancer. *Int. J. Biol. Macromol.*, 72, 195–8, 2015 Jan.
91. Li, X., Ferrel, G.L., Guerra, M.C., Hode, T., Lunn, J.A., Adalsteinsson, O., *et al.*, Preliminary safety and efficacy results of laser immunotherapy for the treatment of metastatic breast cancer patients. *Photochem. Photobiol. Sci.*, 10, 5, 817–21, 2011 May.

92. Dimassi, S., Tabary, N., Chai, F., Blanchemain, N., Martel, B., Sulfonated and sulfated chitosan derivatives for biomedical applications: A review. *Carbohydr. Polym.*, 202, 382–96, 2018 Dec.
93. Qin, Y., Li, P., Guo, Z., Cationic chitosan derivatives as potential antifungals: A review of structural optimization and applications. *Carbohydr. Polym.*, 236, 116002, 2020 May.
94. Snyman, D., Hamman, J.H., Kotze, J.S., Rollings, J.E., Kotzé, A.F., The relationship between the absolute molecular weight and the degree of quaternisation of N-trimethyl chitosan chloride. *Carbohydr. Polym.*, 50, 2, 145–50, 2002 Nov.
95. Sarmento, B., Goycoolea, F.M., Sosnik, A., Das Neves, J., Chitosan and Chitosan Derivatives for Biological Applications: Chemistry and Functionalization. *Int. J. Carbohydr. Chem.*, 2011, 1–1, 2011 Dec 15.
96. Cong, Y., Geng, J., Wang, H., Su, J., Arif, M., Dong, Q., *et al.*, Ureido-modified carboxymethyl chitosan-graft-stearic acid polymeric nano-micelles as a targeted delivering carrier of clarithromycin for Helicobacter pylori: Preparation and *in vitro* evaluation. *Int. J. Biol. Macromol.*, 129, 686–92, 2019 May.
97. Liu, H., Liu, J., Xie, X., Li, X., Development of photo-magnetic drug delivery system by facile-designed dual stimuli-responsive modified biopolymeric chitosan capped nano-vesicle to improve efficiency in the anesthetic effect and its biological investigations. *J. Photochem. Photobiol. B: Biol.*, 202, 111716, 2020 Jan.
98. Park, I.K., Yang, J., Jeong, H.J., Bom, H.S., Harada, I., Akaike, T., *et al.*, Galactosylated chitosan as a synthetic extracellular matrix for hepatocytes attachment. *Biomaterials*, 24, 13, 2331–7, 2003 Jun.
99. Li, Z.T., Guo, J., Zhang, J.S., Zhao, Y.P., Lv, L., Ding, C., *et al.*, Chitosan-graft-polyethylenimine with improved properties as a potential gene vector. *Carbohydr. Polym.*, 80, 1, 254–9, 2010 Mar.
100. Zhang, H., Chen, S., Jia, X., Huang, Y., Ji, R., Zhao, L., Comparation of the phytotoxicity between chemically and green synthesized silver nanoparticles. *Sci. Total Environ.*, 752, 142264, 2021 Jan.
101. Yao, Z., Zhang, C., Ping, Q., Yu, L., A series of novel chitosan derivatives: Synthesis, characterization and micellar solubilization of paclitaxel. *Carbohydr. Polym.*, 68, 4, 781–92, 2007 Apr.
102. Wiens, M., Elkhooly, T.A., Schröder, H.C., Mohamed, T.H.A., Müller, W.E.G., Characterization and osteogenic activity of a silicatein/biosilica-coated chitosan-graft-polycaprolactone. *Acta Biomater.*, 10, 10, 4456–64, 2014 Oct.
103. Noh, S.M., Park, M.O., Shim, G., Han, S.E., Lee, H.Y., Huh, J.H., *et al.*, Pegylated poly-l-arginine derivatives of chitosan for effective delivery of siRNA. *J. Control. Release*, 145, 2, 159–64, 2010 Jul.
104. Zheng, D., Neoh, K.G., Kang, E.T., Bifunctional coating based on carboxymethyl chitosan with stable conjugated alkaline phosphatase for inhibiting bacterial adhesion and promoting osteogenic differentiation on titanium. *Appl. Surf. Sci.*, 360, 86–97, 2016 Jan.

105. Xu, Y., Du, Y., Huang, R., Gao, L., Preparation and modification of N-(2-hydroxyl) propyl-3-trimethyl ammonium chitosan chloride nanoparticle as a protein carrier. *Biomaterials*, 24, 27, 5015–22, 2003 Dec.
106. Jin, Y., Song, Y., Zhu, X., Zhou, D., Chen, C., Zhang, Z., *et al.*, Goblet cell-targeting nanoparticles for oral insulin delivery and the influence of mucus on insulin transport. *Biomaterials*, 33, 5, 1573–82, 2012 Feb.
107. Cafaggi, S., Russo, E., Stefani, R., Leardi, R., Caviglioli, G., Parodi, B., *et al.*, Preparation and evaluation of nanoparticles made of chitosan or N-trimethyl chitosan and a cisplatin–alginate complex. *J. Control. Release*, 121, 1–2, 110–23, 2007 Aug.
108. Zhang, J., Zhu, X., Jin, Y., Shan, W., Huang, Y., Mechanism Study of Cellular Uptake and Tight Junction Opening Mediated by Goblet Cell-Specific Trimethyl Chitosan Nanoparticles. *Mol. Pharmaceutics*, 11, 5, 1520–32, 2014 May 5.
109. Zhang, H., Wu, F., Li, Y., Yang, X., Huang, J., Lv, T., *et al.*, Chitosan-based nanoparticles for improved anticancer efficacy and bioavailability of mifepristone. *Beilstein J. Nanotechnol.*, 7, 1861–70, 2016 Nov 28.

5

Gum Acacia Synthetic Routes for Anticancer Treatment Development

Tahira Bashir[1], Muhammad Ahsan Ullah Danish[2], Farhat Bano[3], Tayyaba Ijaz[4], Ji-Xin Tang[5*] and Muhammad Asmat Ullah Saleem[6†]

[1]*Department of Cell Biology, Harbin Medical University, Harbin, China*
[2]*Department of Allied Health Sciences, The University of Agriculture, Dera Ismail Khan, Khyber Pakhtun khwa, Pakistan*
[3]*College of Veterinary Medicine, Northeast Agricultural University, Harbin, China*
[4]*University Institute of Medical Lab Technology, University of Lahore, Punjab, Pakistan*
[5]*Guangdong Provincial Key Laboratory of Autophagy and Major Chronic Noncommunicable Diseases, Key Laboratory of Prevention and Management of Chronic Kidney Diseases of Zhanjiang City, Institute of Nephrology, Affiliated Hospital of Guangdong Medical University, Zhanjiang, Guangdong, China*
[6]*Institute of Nephrology, Affiliated Hospital of Guangdong Medical University, Zhanjiang, Guangdong, China*

Abstract

Cancer remains a major concern worldwide in health aspects, and daily, several types of cancer are increasing across the globe. It has a profound effect on healthcare, families, individuals, and economic status on a huge scale. Advancements in cancer treatment and research have led to innovative strategies and improved outcomes for cancer-affected patients. Several treatments are currently working against cancer, but the gum acacia synthetic route is considered one of the most crucial anticancer treatments. It increased the mucoadhesion, anticancer potential, and mechanical strength, which blocked 60% (cervical type) of cancer in the *in vitro* study. This synthetic route facilitates the silver nanoparticle stabilization in anticancer activities such as nanocarriers. Similarly, gum acacia stabilized the gold nanoparticle position in breast cancer treatment and significantly inhibited tumor growth.

**Corresponding author*: Tangjixin@gdmu.edu.cn
†*Corresponding author*: Dr.asmat_neau@yahoo.com

Luqman Jameel Rather, Showkat Ali Ganie and Mohammed A. Assiri (eds.) Polysaccharide Biomaterials in Cancer Research and Therapy: From Lab to Life, (121–148) © 2026 Scrivener Publishing LLC

Whereas gum acacia called gum arabic has been prepared through several routes by using distinctive applications. Gum acacia as nanoparticles of iron oxide, a natural polymer, also plays a role as a functional group of sulfone for the synthesis of pharmaceutical products. Gum acacia has been modified and its efficient properties have been enhanced. Additionally, microgels made by gum acacia are used for biomedical applications; for example, nanoparticles of silver and cobalt showcase antioxidant and antimicrobial properties. Acacia gum is derived from the acacia plants that contain modern as well as traditional medicinal usage; its demulcent, antiseptic, and astringent properties play a role in sore throat, diarrhea, cough, and diabetes treatment. Moreover, its good prebiotic (Bifidobacteria) source inhibits gut dysbiosis. Researchers have increased their focus on pharmaceutical products by gum acacia, which is used as a medical treatment against several diseases such as nephropathy, bladder abnormality, osteoporosis, and cancer. Acacia plants reveal strong activity against several types of cell lines that represent the broad-spectrum effectiveness of acacia in blocking cancer growth in several organs. Gum acacia-based nanoparticles facilitate drug delivery in several types of tumors; for example, in breast cancer, gold nanoparticles act as carriers for efficient drug delivery with minimalistic toxicity or other side effects. Study outcomes embrace the importance of natural agents like gum acacia due to their effectiveness against tumors, creating new paths for developing novel anticancer therapies with the lowest after-effects but enhanced efficacy. This chapter highlights the versatility of acacia gum through several synthetic routes to provide the latest information related to cancer treatment globally in the current aura. This paper concerns gum acacia collection, purification, and amplification for oncology studies through novel technologies.

Keywords: Medicinal plant, bioactive agents, gum acacia, cancer, anticancer compound, immune cells, nanoparticles

5.1 Introduction

Cancer is a metabolic disorder and is a leading cause of severe death even in the presence of prevention and treatment checkpoints [1–3]. Worldwide, cancer is the hallmark of morbidity and mortality, and average cases might increase around 21 million by 2030 [4, 5]. Studies have found that the USA faced around 600,920 cancer-related deaths in 2017 [6]. The term "cancer" represents the uncontrolled or mismanagement growth of healthy cells that can cause genetic alteration and instabilities gathered within the cells or tissues that can turn healthy cells into a malignant one. Genetic alterations include oncogenes, cell growth metabolic genes, and DNA mutation or damaged genes. Both internal factors (hormonal, immune, and genetic disorders) and external factors (infectious agents, food, tobacco, air, smoking, and radiation) can lead to tumor progression [7]. However, there are several types of tumors in humans, but breast cancer and lung cancer are most common in females and males, respectively [8, 9]. Furthermore, cancer is a huge burden on human health in a society in both underdeveloped and developed countries [10]. Additionally, around 80% of the population is depending on traditional or herbal medicines, and around 60% have been clinically approved against cancer treatment and also medically recommended [11, 12]. Natural gums are used for cancer drug delivery systems due to their availability, acceptance for cell lines and animal models, low immunogenicity, biocompatibility, biodegradability, bioactivity, low cost, and renewability. Yet, to some extent, these natural compounds need certain modifications [13]. Effective medical strategies for the control of cancer mortality are needed. The conventional ways including radiotherapy, chemotherapy, and surgery have been successfully improving the life survival of cancer patients, but their efficacy is limited [14]. However, immunotherapy can tackle the tumor cells at their advanced metastatic level. Though these therapies are non-targeted tumor cells, they can even target normal or healthy cells, which can lead to fatal consequences. Drug delivery for cancer can particularly target the cancerous tissues and enter into the cancer cell [15, 16]. In the last several decades, great research has been achieved in oncology nanomedicine. Several types of nanoparticles (NPs) such as lipid-based, inorganic, and polymeric NPs have been used for cancer therapeutic development. Recent advances in nanotechnology have enhanced nano–bio interactions, improving nanocarrier development and the efficacy of drug delivery systems with reduced toxicity, improving the efficacy of loaded drugs with reduced toxicity [17, 18].

Plants are favorable to producing effective bioactive compounds that can tackle several types of diseases in the current era. Among them, Acacia tree is a huge one and has diverse types of natural compounds and revealed remarkable therapeutic activities against several diseases. This natural source can save human health and protect harmful environments with zero or negligible side effects [19]. Gum acacia, also called gum arabic (GA), is collected from acacia seyal and Senegal trees. Most gum acacia is taken from the arid lands of Senegal, Ethiopia, Nigeria, Chad, and Sudan. However, among others, Sudan and Nigeria are 80% sources of GA. Also, names were taken from Arabian traders who exported this gum to European countries and became popular in this trading system. Gum acacia is considered one of the best gums compared to other available natural gums, and the history of gum acacia is 5000 years back [20]. Around 900 acacia trees produce gum in the current era, and these species are located in tropical areas majorly in Africa; that is why Africa is supposed to have a large production of gum acacia, and traditionally, GA was exuded from

Senegal species [21]. The average production of gum acacia is around 250 g per tree per year, and the annual yield is about 60,000 tons. The production of acacia gum is due to any stress, injury, fungal, bacteria, or insect attacks on trees. It is generally released from damaged sites into the fractures of bark and appears as tears [22–24]. Different types of gums are extracted from different (seeds, leaves, and bark) parts of plants [25]. All gums are polysaccharides in nature, and through hydrolysis, they are converted into (pentosane and hexose) monosaccharides. Furthermore, they contain polyuronides and arabinose or galactose as sugar moiety. Several techniques are used for structural identification [26]. Acacia tree is used as a medicinal plant in several countries, as listed in Table 5.1.

Gum acacia has a broad range of applications in a variety of sectors, is a rich source of dietary fibers that are essential for health benefits, has a key role in gut microbiota yields, is a positive factor for immunomodulation, and blocks the pathogenicity in the host [36]. However, overproduction of immune cells can lead to inflammation, tissue damage, autoimmune diseases, and even cancer growth. Therefore, it is urgent to develop or find natural compounds capable of downregulating inflammation-related

Table 5.1 Medicinal use of acacia tree in some countries.

Part of tree	Countries	Use	Ref.
Roots	Ethiopia	Chest pain	[27]
Roots and leaves	Ethiopia	Intestinal parasites	[28]
Bark, trunk, and stem	Kenya	Pneumonia	[29]
Roots	Kenya	Malaria	[30]
Bark and leaves	Sudan	Leprosy and bleeding	[31]
Wood	Sudan	Rheumatisms, arthritis, and rheumatoid fever	[32]
Bark, leaves, and roots	Uganda	Necrosis nodules and diarrhea	[33]
Seed and gum	Morocco, Egypt, and Algeria	Fever, eyes, respiratory and gastric infection, and rheumatisms	[34, 35]

diseases in the future. Moreover, gum acacia is an edible biomolecule and shows strong immunomodulatory, anti-inflammatory, and antitumor properties. A recent study has found that gums act as drug carriers in the form of hydrogels that facilitate anticancer treatment. Another research revealed that gum acacia plays a fundamental role in silver nanoparticles drug delivery system for fungal and bacterial activities [37, 38]. This chapter aims to provide potential antitumor usage of gum acacia. Biopolymer compounds development for drug delivery is an emerging area in biomedical research. Because tumors are a highly challenging and threatening disease for humans, the cancer ratio is upregulated daily. There are a variety of tumors that lead to different types of body organ cancer including breast cancer, brain cancer, bone cancer, and blood cancer. Triple-negative breast cancer is one of the most aggressive types of tumor growth [39, 40]. Until now, no effective therapy is available for cancer treatment following radiation and chemotherapy.

5.2 Basic of Gum Acacia (Types, Structure, Chemical, and Physical Nature)

Plant-derived gums have various species including gum karaya, gum tragacanth, gum ghatti, and Arabic or acacia gum [41, 42]. Acacia-derived different types of gums have different characteristics, and even from the same species, still gums show differences in their physiochemical nature. Additionally, researchers have found that the same group of trees grown in different areas produced diverse characteristics containing gums [43]. However, acacia-derived gums have hydrocolloid characteristics that make them water-soluble, and they are crucial for food companies to modify and control the rheological characteristics of liquid food things. Gum acacia plays a role as an emulsifier, thickener, film former, suspending agent, flocculant, and stabilizer. Next, they are less colorful in solution form, and due to these characteristics, gum acacia stabilized at high price in international marketing as compared to other gums [44, 45]. From acacia, Senegal-derived GA is widely used due to their low viscosity, high solubility, good emulsification, and zero toxicity properties. In addition to gum Arabic, GA may be used as an alternative, depending on its functional and physicochemical properties [46]. Besides this, for the identification or selection of unique gum from a list of several types of gums, extensive analytical tests are needed. This strategy reveals the chemical nature of each of the gums, and five basic parameters are essential during the identification of a particular gum that includes specific optical rotation, nitrogen contents, ash contents, moisture content, and also absence of tannins. Generally, several gums dissolve in water at different concentrations, but acacia gum can dissolve in hot and cold water up to 50% (W/W) [47, 48] as shown in Table 5.2. Additionally, as listed in Table 5.3, it has a heteropolysaccharide with 2% polypeptide nature, and carbohydrate contains 40% residues of D-galactose, 24% L-arabinose, 13% L-rhamnose, and uronic acid that act as polyanionic activity of acacia gum.

The chemical structure of gum is quite complex (Figure 5.1) and still needs to be studied. However, the major structural backbone is β-galactopyranose

Table 5.2 Quality parameters of gum acacia [49].

Contents	**Range (%)**
Moisture	13–15
Ash	2–4
Internal energy	30–39
Volatile matter	51–65
Optical Degrees	-26 to -34
Nitrogen Content	0.26–0.39

Table 5.3 Physical characteristics of gum acacia [49].

Components	**Acacia seyal (%)**	**Acacia senegal (%)**
Galactose	38	44
Arabinose	46	27
Glucuronic acid	6.5	14.50
Rhamnose	4	13
Nitrogen	0.15	0.36
4-O-meth1 glucuronic acid	5.5	1.5
Molecular weight	850,000	380,000
Specific rotation	51	-30

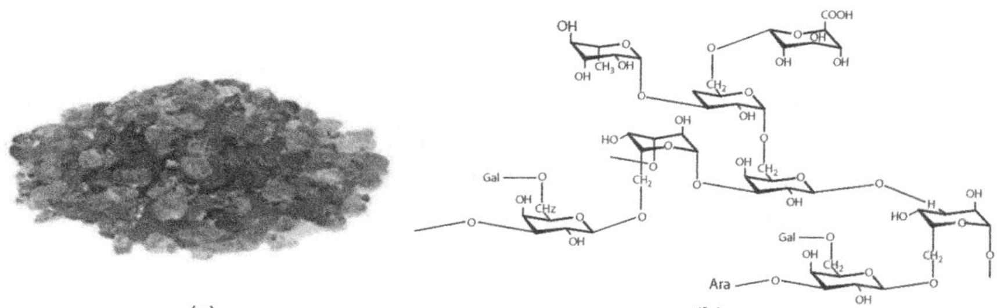

(a) (b)

Figure 5.1 (a) physical and (b) chemical structure of gum acacia [49].

with 1,3 (bonds) and 1,6 (side chain) linkage of galactopyranose, whereas β-D-glucuronopyranose is a terminating point. Moreover, gum acacia is composed of almost 64 subunits of β-homogalactan and has three major molecular groups called arabinogalactan-protein, glycoprotein, and arabinogalactan. The physicochemical nature of gum acacia has significant surface properties; the presence of hydrophobic amino acids and sugar residues at a hydrophilic site in arabinogalactan-protein plays a role in the amphiphilicity of acacia gum that facilitates its adsorption activity [50]. It has been reported that the chemical composition of gum can change due to the half-life of trees, geographical sources, soil conditions, and weather [51]. However, pods, flowers, and leaves have plentiful phytochemical constituents including carbohydrates, anthocyanins, flavonoids, phenolics, saponins, and proteins [52]. The study examined that stem bark of the acacia tree contains tannins, coumarin, phenols, alkaloids, steroids, terpenoids, saponins, and flavonoids [53, 54]. Moreover, the leaves part contains ferulic acid, caffeic acid, p-coumaric acid, salicylic acid, and gallic acid [55–57]. Similarly, oleamide, clionasterol, stigmasterol, campesterol, lupeol, epicatechin, and catechin are detected in stem bark [58]. Besides these, phytoconstituents of gum acacia include magnesium, gallic, chlorogenic, potassium salts, ellagic, and polysaccharides [59].

Gum acacia is a dry exudate spherical- and tear-shaped that is obtained from the stems part of acacia trees; it is friable and amber-yellow [60]. Gum acacia is an arabin called arabinogalactan–protein complex that includes potassium salts, magnesium, and calcium [47]. Karamalla's study reported that gum contains 14.41% moisture content and 3.5% average ash content [61]. Meanwhile, protein constitute is important for emulsification of gum acacia, and about 3% of the protein amount is crucial for a good quality of gum acacia [61]. However, the percentage of protein depends on the collection time, plant species, soil, and geographical source. pH of gum acacia is acidic in nature (4.66) [62]. Although gum acacia is soluble in water and forms an aqueous solution with 50% concentration, gum acacia is insoluble in oil and nonpolar solvent [63]. The concentration and types of the mineral in acacia gum are very crucial, as they play a key role in the polarity of arabin, which, in turn, has great impact on hydration compactness, solubility, and stability of gum colloidal solution [64].

5.3 Immunomodulatory Role of Gum Acacia

Destruction of immune responses can cause severe consequences of cancer development [65]. Particularly, lack of MHC class 1, potential tumor antigen, stimulatory, and costimulatory molecules can lead to failure of antigen presentation, cancer cell elimination, and T-cell recognition [66, 67]. Moreover, chemotherapy-related side effects can cause an extra burden for patients as it reduces the immune tendency of patients [68]. To activate and target the repressed form of immune responses against tumor cells, there is a need for potential delivery of effective strategies. Several therapies are working including dendritic cell vaccination [69], tumor infiltrating lymphocytes [70], and cytokines therapy but have a low therapeutic index with severe side effects [71]. However, in the renal carcinoma study, immunotherapy showed effective results and decreased tumor progression [72]. Antibody therapies that use monoclonal antibodies for the treatment of cancer and output lead to prolonged survival [73]. Ipilimumab monoclonal antibody is FDA-approved for cancer (melanoma) therapy [74].

Similarly, nivolumab improves the survival rate of melanoma patients [75]. Some therapeutic strategies are used to improve immunomodulatory activities and manage multiple myeloma status. Thalidomide drug is one of them that can stimulate T-cell responses in multiple myeloma patients [76, 77]. When checking processes for the immune system are impaired, then cancer immunosurveillance occurs that facilitates lack of exact target, identification, and destruction of cancer cells, which can cause metastasis phase [78]. Immunotherapy is considered a sound target strategy for cancer treatment; plant-derived natural polysaccharide-containing compounds exert great immunomodulatory effects for anticancer activities that increase the survival of cancer patients [79]. Gum acacia is currently used as an anticancer bioactive compound that has negligible side effects on patients with wide availability and low cost. Scientists have revealed that natural agents cure cancer effectively as compared to semi-synthetic or synthetic compounds (chemotherapy and radiotherapy); GA has been examined for its toxicity against hepatocellular carcinoma, lung carcinoma, colorectal, and breast carcinoma cell lines. Cancer patients showed decreased development of tumor growth due to regular consumption of gum acacia. Research has found that inhibition of cancer progression is due to the immunomodulatory role of gum acacia [80]. Studies have found that acacia gum, with other herbal bioactive compounds called polysaccharopeptides, significantly increased T-cell responses. Since GA also contains glycoproteins and polysaccharides, these have been examined as immunomodulation roles.

Moreover, IgM antibody titer was upregulated in the gum acacia–treated group, which indicated that GA enhanced T-cell-dependent B-cell responses [81]. This is because T cells are a crucial part of adaptive immunity, and they can effectively eliminate cancerous cells [82]. The main role of T cells is to activate cytokine secretion rather than direct elimination of tumor cells [83]. Hence, immunotherapy is an emerging strategy for cancer treatment; its effectiveness property is enhancing the transportation of drug-loaded nanoparticles by utilizing T-cell responses [84]. Another study revealed that gum acacia has the ability to activate dendritic cells [85] and showed that it has adaptive and innate immunity activation property and also has anti-parasitic activity. The immunopotentiator property is due to the presence of arabinogalactan protein [86]. In some studies, it has been reported that gum acacia plays a role as vehicle control during the immunological effect of herbal medicine [87, 88]. A combinational study of gum acacia with polysaccharopeptide compound shows significant immunopotentiator activity; glycoprotein-based gum acacia has T-cell stimulatory properties [81].

5.4 Antitumor Properties of Gum Acacia

Carcinogenesis is one of the leading causes of death worldwide, and researchers revealed that due to the continuous rising ratio of cases, it could reach up to 70% within the next 20 years [89]. The conventional approaches for cancer treatment including radiation, surgery, and chemotherapy show cancer recurrence association, the outcome of severe side effects, and lead to the emergence of tumor resistance [90]. However, plant-derived or natural medicinal strategies have been used as an essential route for various diseases and of course for cancer study as well. Historically, this was the most popular therapeutic method among ancient Egyptians, and about 700 medicinal plants are used [91]. Additionally, due to low efficacy with severe side effects of conventional cancer treatments, scientists focused on plant-derived therapeutic antitumor development agents with cost effects and low side effects [92]. Research has found that more than 60% of antitumor compounds were obtained from aquatic organisms, microorganisms, and plants. Therapeutic effects of these compounds are initiated through various pathways including activation of immune systems, inhibition of angiogenesis, and apoptosis induction [93]. Sustainable and controlled drug delivery procedures are a fundamental part of an effective anticancer compound formation that will overcome the consequences related to conventional anticancer approaches [94]. For suitable and slow anticancer agent delivery, polymeric hydrogels are considered the best strategy [95], a site-specific drug carrier for long periods of compound delivery during tumor treatment [96, 97]. Studies have reported that several polymeric gels are used for oral cavity tumor growth inhibition [98]. Moreover, hydrogels derived from gum have been reported for colon cancer treatment and used as a drug delivery route. The swelling effects of hydrophilic gums were reduced by interlinking gum with other polymers to improve the mechanical properties of gum drug delivery. Polymers have a strong potential for intermolecular interaction formation between the chain of various polymers that facilitate the antitumor compound protection during its delivery [99]. However, natural or plant-derived gums are widely involved in pharmaceutical industries as a dosage form [100]. Gum acacia treatment is upgraded at the transcription level of several cell proliferation genes in colonic tissues including interleukin 18, sulfatase 1, vav 3 oncogene, ubiquitin D, and CD38 antigen [101–105]. This natural gum therapy

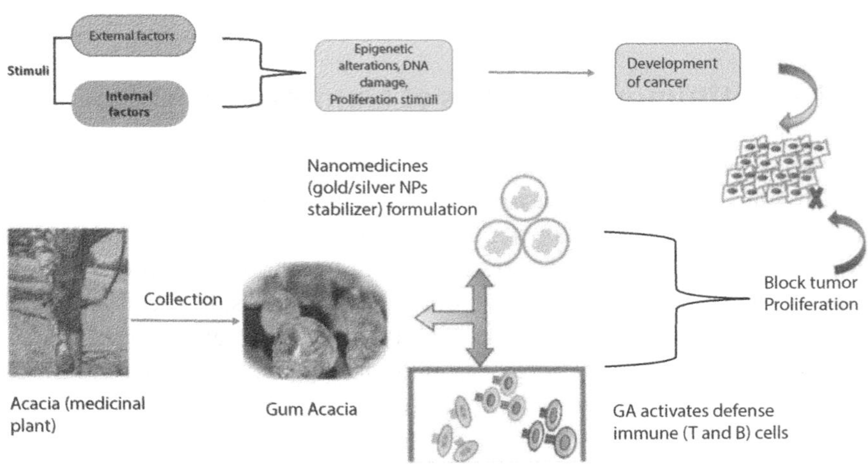

Figure 5.2 Graphical mechanism of gum acacia inhibits tumor growth by utilizing nanomedicines and immunomodulatory effects.

downregulates the overexpression of ß-catenin protein that has a strong role in pro-oncogenic and GA treatment; the tumor cell growth was potentially inhibited [106, 107], as presented in Figure 5.2.

5.5 Advancement in Gum Acacia Applications

5.5.1 Improvement in Cancer Therapies

Gum acacia nanoparticles have been widely studied for the treatment of cancer patients, and they are considered to biologically safe because GA provides strong stability to gold nanoparticles (Figure 5.2) during breast carcinoma treatment. GA-base nanoparticles have no interaction with blood components, which indicates that it is a promising drug delivery route for oncology study [108]. Furthermore, gum polymer-based synthesis of microspheres can particularly target the aggressive form of tumor cells; it might be considered a novel type of therapy for cancer cell diagnosis and treatment [109]. Gum acacia-based polymers are isolated from acacia plant then loaded with microspheres with folic acid and curcumin, facilitating tumor-microspheres attachment. Then this process blocks the tumor progression through the activation or initiation of apoptosis. Under the tumor microenvironment phase, microspheres release curcumin, which inhibits the anti-apoptotic protein through the activation of certain types of enzymes. Microspheres have the ability to reduce the size of cancer cell and enhance the life span of healthy cells, as studied in the mice model [110]. Gum acacia effectively delivers the potential natural anticancer drug curcumin to the triple negative breast cancer cell lines. These targeted bio polymeric microspheres can be deployed as an effective vehicle for the delivery of different anticancer drugs particularly, which are hydrophobic in nature, to the various folate receptor overexpressing cancer cells circumventing any systemic toxicity to the normal cells [109].

5.5.2 Novel Delivery Routes or Formulations

- **Liquid exfoliation method:** This method is applicable for the transition metal dichalcogenide (TMD) nanosheets formation where gum acacia acts as a stabilizing and exfoliating agent. Furthermore, it induced an apoptosis pathway and enhanced inhibition of cell proliferation [111]. TMDs received considerable research attention for anticancer therapeutic potential. TMD-mediated nanosheets embrace cost-effective and simple route for more assembly, and various types of nanosheets, including WSe_2, WS_2, MoS_2, and $MoSe_2$, were developed through gum acacia. These nanosheets show remarkable absorption capacity of photo-thermal rays, and antitumor activity was examined by flow cytometry after the drug was loaded. Collectively, a study indicated that this is a potentially valuable strategy for cancer therapeutic roles [111]. TMD routes have been discovered for oncology research due to potential absorbance of radiation and the production of heat for ablation [112, 113]. However, a variety of plant-derived polymeric compounds are used for TMD exfoliation of nanosheets, but according to current research, gum acacia is one of the finest liquid exfoliating and stabilizer agents. It is an anionic type of polysaccharide with 90% arabinogalactan [114]. Moreover, gum acacia has been comprehensively studied for drug delivery, food applications, biosensors, and tissue engineering because gum has low viscosity, biocompatibility, and other functional properties [115–118].

- **As a hydrogel agent:** a modified form of gum acacia functions effectively in nanoparticle formation and supports magnetic biomaterial activity. Efficient hydrogel formation requires characterization using resonance spectroscopy and related techniques. This unique hydrogel formation from GA can be effectively used in tissue engineering in the form of biomaterial [119].
- **Tumor imaging and sensor:** Gum acacia has water-soluble radical, fabricated, electrically active, and redox properties. Additionally, having a strong or high-end battery with shelf-life, technical characterization, and electrical conductivity was supervised. Later, this might be applicable as a sensor device in the fabrication of semiconductors [120]. Gum acacia coating facilitates the coupling of bioactive compounds by increasing the colloidal stability of reactive functional groups. Similarly, MRI outcomes revealed that gum acacia with magnetic nanoparticles accumulated at the glioma tumor site [121].
- **As nanoparticle stabilizer in tumor study:** Multiple types of research have been conducted for the effective use of gum acacia in the field of molecular imaging and nano-constructs because gum acacia plays a role in the form of oxidizing or

reducing agent that is crucial to detecting the molecular functionality of nanomaterials. This phenomenon has been examined to eliminate toxicity and for stability improvement, pathogen detection, and dispersion improvement of nanoparticles. The characterization of nanoparticles was done through transmission electron microscopy and DLS called dynamic light scattering for the analysis of morphology and size distribution of nanoparticles, respectively. However, DLS results showed that gum acacia-treated nanoparticles have smaller agglomerates within 30 h as compared to the untreated groups. Moreover, thermogravimetric results found that an average decrease in weight was around 23%, indicating that gum acacia possesses a potential affinity for iron oxide-containing surfaces. Therefore, GA strongly or effectively dispersed nanoparticles in aqueous solution. However, gum acacia-treated gold nanoparticles have strong stabilization properties against oxidation [122]. Gum acacia acts as an antioxidant agent for the preparation of biocompatible nanoparticles, which is further used for therapeutic and diagnostic applications in the field of nanomedicine. The study has investigated that in gamma-Al_2O_3 (nanoparticles) preparation and modification, gum acacia is used to avoid the clustering of nanoparticles in aqueous solutions. After gum modification, nanoparticles dispersed properly, and their bio-desulfurization and adsorptive desulfurization capacity was increased [123, 124].

Similarly, the adsorption property of GA has been investigated in magnetic and hydroxyapatite nanoparticles [125]. The better bimolecular attachment of nanoparticles in oncology studies have been examined after NPs modification through gum acacia treatment [126]. Furthermore, breast cancer is considered to be the leading cause of women's death worldwide. Recent research has been conducted on letrozole (LTZ), an anticancer drug. The drug delivery system uses nanoscale carriers (polysaccharides and metal nanoparticles) that are widely used to target cancerous cells. However, to reduce the toxicity of the drug, green synthesis of nanoparticles is preferred in research field as compared to a chemically fabricated method. The study has prepared LTZ-GA gold nanoparticles, which are considered a rapid and safe method for the characterization and synthesis of gum acacia gold nanoparticles. Morphological and structural properties are stable and have significant therapeutic efficacy. Hence, the gum

Table 5.4 FDA-approved nanomedicines for cancer therapy [130–133].

Product	Component	Compound	Company	Treatment	Years
Onivyde	Liposome	Irinotecan	Janssen Limited	Prostate cancer	2015
Genexol PM	PEG-PLA	Paclitaxel	Tolmar Limited	Breast cancer	2007
Abraxane	Albumin	Paclitaxel	Celgene Limited	Breast cancer	2005
Eligard	PLGA	Leuprolide	Samyang Limited	Pancreatic cancer	2002
Doxil	Liposome-PEG	Doxorubicin	Merrimack Limited	Ovarian cancer	1995

acacia-based NPs drug delivery process is considered a reliable and better strategy for cancer treatment [108]. Scientists are working on a vehicle that would effectively facilitate the delivery of drugs to the target site. A mechanism that induces cellular entrance or permeates to the outer membrane of mitochondria is being invented that activates apoptosis. The drug delivery process targeted by nanoparticles has gained substantial consideration. Nanoparticles in nanomedicine are being developed at a large scale with their unique characteristics (functioning, composition, and size alteration) [127–129]. Several nanomedicines work against the tumor cells effectively and efficiently; some approved drugs are listed in Table 5.4.

5.5.3 Focus on Bioavailability and Antitumor Therapeutic Potential

The active part of gum acacia has been used as a stabilizing compound that is important for blocking the aggregation step during nanoparticle formation or preparation. This is the reason why gum acacia is the most popular in nanoparticle preparation [134]. Hence, gum acacia is also used as an anti-inflammatory, antimicrobial, and antioxidant agent [118]. Nanoprism substances were coated with gum acacia, and the later photothermal effect was examined in an *in vitro* study. Due to the addition of gum acacia, the photothermal and biocompatibility impact of nanoprisms has been significantly increased on tumor cells [135]. Gum acacia forms a complex with several other polymeric agents and is molded into nanoparticles that actively play a role in drug delivery process. Furthermore, nanoparticles containing gum acacia, carboxymethylcellulose, and *Stauntonia brachyanthera* compounds were used for the lutein delivery system [136]. GA was used as a stabilizer during selenium nano-rods preparation [137]. Their stability was enhanced after the addition of gum acacia polysaccharides [138]. Studies have revealed that gold nanoparticles with the combination of gum acacia were used for cancer treatment [139]. *In vivo*, the study has examined that GA enhanced the bioavailability of a compound called curcumin that potentially blocks tumor cell proliferation [136]. Similarly, gum acacia with starch nanocrystals were developed for hydroxyurea drug delivery [137]. Hence, plant-derived polysaccharides in natural agents such as gum acacia for micro- and nanoparticles development have a strong existence as carriers during drug delivery pathway because gum has uniqueness in its abundance, biocompatibility, and biodegradability [140, 141]. One of the advanced properties is microspheres, which make gum acacia superior in the drug delivery process, with more loading capability, small size, constant and controlled release of a drug, and penetration capacity toward capillary vessels [142].

5.6 Current Challenges and Future Prospective

Collectively, cancer cases are growing day by day due to lifestyle changes, life expectancy, and developing urbanization. Additionally, cancer stages are developing at an advanced level just because of insufficient public awareness, care physicians, and lack of diagnostic facilities (imaging, geographic distances, and pathology) in cancer hospitals that offer special services for cancer patients. The implementation of conventional screening protocols is challenging due to poor expertise and resources. There is a need to conduct advanced research to enhance awareness in the public, combat stigma, and educate health practitioners; these checkpoints might reduce cancer diagnostic errors or delays. Further study is needed to understand health behavior properly that can lead to participants in early screening of tumor growth. The regular approval for commercially available gum acacia is the main hurdle; it changes the functional activities and molecular parameters of gum. Additionally, fluctuating prices at high levels and irregularity in supply can lead to down-marketing of gum acacia popularity. However, gum acacia is an ideal bioactive compound for nano-conjugation properties. The above discussion regarding GA has a role in cancer treatment, and it clearly exhibits that gum acacia is a fundamental component of an abundance of polysaccharides for stable dispersion of nanoparticle formulation. Gum acacia has a crucial role during the preparation of several types of nanoparticles for nano-medicinal functional tumor handling. From a future view, gum acacia seems pivotal and bright for the medical industries, especially in oncology. This will shed light on health-related country economics for cancer assessment of interventions, financing methods, value-related care system, and other tumor assessment technologies. Furthermore, scale up quality research that could be implementable and lead to better improvement in tumor control. Developing scientifically proven technologies can enable innovation, and research could address particularly cancer-related challenges. There is a need to introduce solution-oriented research that could improve affordability, access, and outcomes related to tumors.

5.7 Conclusion

Plant-derived bioactive compounds have effective therapeutic properties against tumor diseases. The major advantages of natural compounds such as anticancer include cost-effectiveness, diversity in their mechanism of action, and negligible toxicity. However, low solubility, low bioavailability, low stability, and high toxicity can decrease the medicinal use of these compounds. Advanced technology is used for pharmaceutical modifications or convenient effectiveness of bioactive compounds, and outcomes revealed the improvement in anticancer activities. Gum acacia is considered as the most effective plant-derived natural agent with high solubility, anticorrosive potential, antioxidant, chelating ability, and commercially available and non-bioaccumulative properties. Natural gum acacia has shown strong activity in both cell and animal models; unfortunately, there is still a lack of research on its role as an anticancer agent. Anticancer therapeutic investigation for GA should be further studied, which will provide a high level of anticancer treatment options.

AI disclosure statement: The author acknowledges the use of AI-based tools for minor language editing or grammatical correction. However, all intellectual contributions, analyses, and conclusions presented in this chapter are entirely the author's own.

References

1. He, L., Gu, J., Lim, L.Y., Yuan, Z.X., Mo, J., Nanomedicine-Mediated Therapies to Target Breast Cancer Stem Cells. *Front. Pharmacol.*, 7, 313, 2016.

2. Qin, W., Huang, G., Chen, Z., Zhang, Y., Nanomaterials in Targeting Cancer Stem Cells for Cancer Therapy. *Front. Pharmacol.*, 18, 8, 2017.
3. Zhang, L.Q., Lv, R., Qu, X.D., Chen, X., Lu, H.S., Wang, Y., Aloesin Suppresses Cell Growth and Metastasis in Ovarian Cancer SKOV3 Cells through the Inhibition of the MAPK Signaling Pathway. *Anal. Cell Pathol. (Amst.)*, 2017, 8158254, 2017.
4. Byers, T.E., Wender, R.C., Jemal, A., Baskies, A.M., Ward, E.E., Brawley, O.W., The American Cancer Society challenge goal to reduce US cancer mortality by 50\% between 1990 and 2015: Results and reflections. *CA Cancer J. Clin.*, 66, 359–369, 2016.
5. Smith, R.A., Andrews, K.S., Brooks, D.D., DeSantis, C.E., Fedewa, S.A., Lortet-Tieulent, J., *et al.*, Cancer screening in the United States, 2016: A review of current American Cancer Society guidelines and current issues in cancer screening. *CA Cancer J. Clin.*, 66, 95–114, 2016.
6. Siegel, R.L., Miller, K.D., Fedewa, S.A., Ahnen, D.J., Meester, R.G.S., Barzi, A., *et al.*, Colorectal cancer statistics, 2017. *CA Cancer J. Clin.*, 67, 3, 177–193, 2017.
7. de Visser, K.E. and Joyce, J.A., The evolving tumor microenvironment: From cancer initiation to metastatic outgrowth. *Cancer Cell*, 41, 3, 374–403, 2023.
8. Loudon, J.R., Thorburn, J.R., Graham, J., Vallance, R., Mcgarrity, G., Neoplasms of the lung. *Br. Med. J.*, 1, 1551, 1978.
9. Zhou, Z.L., Tang, M., Liu, Y., Zhang, Z., Lu, R., Lu, J., Apigenin inhibits cell proliferation, migration, and invasion by targeting Akt in the A549 human lung cancer cell line. *Anticancer Drugs*, 28, 446–456, 2017.
10. Shaikh, A.M., Shrivastava, B., Apte, K.G., Navale, S., Medicinal Plants as Potential Source of Anticancer Agents: A Review. *J. Pharma. Phyto.*, 5, 291–295, 2016.
11. Cragg, G.M., Newman, D.J., Yang, S.S., Natural product extracts of plant and marine origin having antileukemia potential. The NCI experience. *J. Nat. Prod.*, 69, 3, 488–98, 2006.
12. Khan, H., Medicinal Plants in Light of History: Recognized Therapeutic Modality. *J. Evid.-Based Integr. Med.*, 19, 216–9, 2014.
13. Soleimani, K., Derakhshankhah, H., Jaymand, M., Samadian, H., Stimuli-responsive natural gums-based drug delivery systems for cancer treatment. *Carbohydr. Polym.*, 254, 117422, 2021.
14. Gotwals, P.J., Cameron, S., Cipolletta, D., Cremasco, V., Crystal, A.S., Hewes, B., *et al.*, Prospects for combining targeted and conventional cancer therapy with immunotherapy. *Nat. Rev. Cancer*, 17, 286–301, 2017.

15. Nam, J., Son, S., Park, K.S., Zou, W., Shea, L.D., Moon, J.J., Cancer nanomedicine for combination cancer immunotherapy. *Nat. Rev. Mater.* , 4, 398–414, 2019.
16. Riley, R.S., June, C.H., Langer, R.S., Mitchell, M.J., Delivery technologies for cancer immunotherapy. *Nat. Rev. Drug Discov.*, 18, 175–96, 2019.
17. Manzari, M.T., Shamay, Y., Kiguchi, H., Rosen, N., Scaltriti, M., Heller, D.A., Targeted drug delivery strategies for precision medicines. *Nat. Rev. Mater.*, 6, 351–70, 2021.
18. Mitchell, M.J., Billingsley, M.M., Haley, R.M., Wechsler, M., Peppas, N.A., Langer, R.S., Engineering precision nanoparticles for drug delivery. *Nat. Rev. Drug Discov.*, 20, 101–24, 2020.
19. Batiha, G.E.S., Akhtar, N., Alsayegh, A.A., Abusudah, W.F., Almohmadi, N.H., Shaheen, H.M., *et al.*, Bioactive Compounds, Pharmacological Actions, and Pharmacokinetics of Genus Acacia. *Mol.*, 27, 21, 2022.
20. Nasir, O., Umbach, A.T., Rexhepaj, R., Ackermann, T.F., Bhandaru, M., Ebrahim, A., *et al.*, Effects of gum arabic (Acacia senegal) on renal function in diabetic mice. *Kidney Blood Press. Res.*, 35, 5, 365–72, 2012.
21. Wekesaa, C., Luvandaa, A. M., Mugaa, M. O., Chikamaia,B. N., Makenzib,P. M., Market chain analysis of gum arabic trade in kenya. *Oct. Jour. Env. Res.* 12, 93–106, 2013.
22. Seigler, D.S., Economic potential from Western Australian Acacia species: secondary plant products. 4, 3, 109–116, 2002.
23. Bemiller, J.N., Whistler, R., Barkalow, D.G., Chen, C.C., Chapter 9 - Aloe, chia, flaxseed, okra, psyllium seed, quince seed, and tamarind gums, in: *Industrial Gums*, Third Edition, R. Whistler and J.N. Bemiller (Eds.), pp. 227–56, Academic Press, London, 1993.
24. Evert, R.F., *Esau's Plant Anatomy,: Meristems, Cells and Tissues of The Plant Body- Their Structure, Function and Development*, 99, 4, 785–786, 2005.
25. Avachat, A.M., Dash, R.R., Shrotriya, S.N., Recent Investigations of Plant Based Natural Gums, Mucilages and Resins in Novel Drug Delivery Systems. *J. Pharm. Res.*, 45, 1, 2011.
26. Prajapati, V.D., Jani, G.K., Moradiya, N.G., Randeria, N.P., Pharmaceutical applications of various natural gums, mucilages and their modified forms. *Carbohydr. Polym.*, 92, 2, 685–99, 2013.
27. Lulekal, E., Kelbessa, E., Bekele, T., Yineger, H., An Ethnobotanical Study of Medicinal Plants in Mana Angetu District, Southeastern Ethiopia. *J. Ethnobiol. Ethnomed.*, 4, 10, 2008.
28. Teklehaymanot, T., An ethnobotanical survey of medicinal and edible plants of Yalo Woreda in Afar regional state, Ethiopia. *J. Ethnobiol. Ethnomed.*, 13, 1–40, 2017.

29. Mutai, M., Njeru, E.M., Ntabo, R.M., Ethnobotanical Survey of Medicinal Plants Used By the Marakwet Community in Cherangani Forest, Kenya. *J. Med. Chem. Sci.*, 136, 2, 347–54, 2021.
30. Nguta, J.M., Mbaria, J.M., Gakuya, D.W., Gathumbi, P.K., Kiama, S.G., Traditional antimalarial phytotherapy remedies used by the South Coast community, Kenya. *J. Ethnopharmacol.*, 131, 2, 256–67, 2010.
31. Yagi, S.M., Ethnobotanical Survey of Medicinal Plants in West Kordofan (Western Sudan). *Ethnobot. Leafl.*, 2009, 8, 2009.
32. El Ghazali, G., Tohami, M., Elegami, A., Abdalla, W., Mohammed, M., *Medicinal Plants of the Sudan, part IV, "Medicinal Plants of Northern Kordofan,"* 1997.
33. Gradé, J.T., Tabuti, J.R.S., Van Damme, P., Ethnoveterinary knowledge in pastoral Karamoja, Uganda. *J. Ethnopharmacol.*, 122, 2, 273–93, 2009.
34. Hammiche, V. and Maiza, K., Traditional medicine in Central Sahara: pharmacopoeia of Tassili N'ajjer. *J. Ethnopharmacol.*, 105, 3, 358–67, 2006.
35. Batanouny, K.H., The wild medicinal plants in North Africa: History and present status, 26, 500, 1999.
36. Barkeer, S., Pothuraju, R., Malakar, P., Pimentel, T.C., Siddiqui, J.A., Nair, S.A., Gum acacia dietary fiber: Significance in immunomodulation, inflamatory diseases, and cancer. *Phytother. Res.*, 38, 3, 1509–21, 2024.
37. Singh, B., Sharma, K., Rajneesh, Dutt, S., Dietary fiber tragacanth gum based hydrogels for use in drug delivery applications. *Bioact. Carbohydr. Dietary Fibre.*, 21, 100208, 2020.
38. Sharma, S., Virk, K., Sharma, K., Bose, S.K., Kumar, V., Sharma, V., *et al.*, Preparation of gum acacia-poly(acrylamide-IPN-acrylic acid) based nanocomposite hydrogels *via* polymerization methods for antimicrobial applications. *J. Mol. Struct.*, 1215, 128298, 2020.
39. Torre, L.A., Bray, F., Siegel, R.L., Ferlay, J., Lortet-Tieulent, J., JJemal, A., Global cancer statistics, 2012. *CA Cancer J. Clin.*, 65, 2, 87–108, 2015.
40. Costa, R.L.B. and Gradishar, W.J., Triple-Negative Breast Cancer: Current Practice and Future Directions. *J. Oncol. Pract.*, 13, 5, 301–3, 2017.
41. Jani, G.K., Shah, D.P., Prajapati, V.D., Jain, V.C., Gums and mucilages: versatile excipients for pharmaceutical formulations. *Asian J. of Pharma. Sci.*, 5, 309–323, 2009.
42. Choudhary, P.D. and Pawar, H.A., Recently Investigated Natural Gums and Mucilages as Pharmaceutical Excipients: An Overview. *J. Pharm.*, 2014, 204849, 2014.

43. Yebeyen, D., Lemenih, M., Feleke, S., Characteristics and quality of gum arabic from naturally grown Acacia senegal (Linne) Willd. trees in the Central Rift Valley of Ethiopia. *Food Hydrocolloids.*, 23, 1, 175–80, 2009.
44. Elmanan, M., Al-Assaf, S., Phillips, G.O., Williams, P.A., Studies on Acacia exudate gums: Part VI. Interfacial rheology of Acacia senegal and Acacia seyal. *Food Hydrocolloids.*, 22, 4, 682–9, 2008.
45. Vanloot, P., Dupuy, N., Guiliano, M., Artaud, J., Characterisation and authentication of A. senegal and A. seyal exudates by infrared spectroscopy and chemometrics. *Food Chem.*, 135, 4, 2554–60, 2012.
46. Taha, K., Elmahi, H., Hassan, E., Shayoub, M., Analytical Study On Three Types Of Gum From Sudan. *J. For. Prod. Ind.*, 1, 11–6, 2012.
47. Prasad, N., Thombare, N., Sharma, S.C., Kumar, S., Gum arabic – A versatile natural gum: A review on production, processing, properties and applications. *Ind. Crops Prod.*, 187, 115304, 2022.
48. Randall, R.C., Phillips, G.O., Williams, P.A., Fractionation and characterization of gum from Acacia senegal. *Food Hydrocolloids*, 3, 1, 65–75, 1989.
49. Dauqan, E. and Abdullah, A., Utilization of gum Arabic for industries and human health. *Am. J. Appl. Sci.*, 10, 10, 1270–9, 2013.
50. Sanchez, C., Renard, D., Robert, P., Schmitt, C., Lefebvre, J., Structure and rheological properties of acacia gum dispersions. *Food Hydrocolloids*, 16, 3, 257–67, 2002.
51. Azzaoui, K., Hammouti, B., Lamhamdi, A., Mejdoubi, E.M., Berrabah, M., The Gum Arabic in the southern region of Morocco. *Morrocan J. Chem.*, 3, 99–107, 2014.
52. Abdel-Farid, I.B., Sheded, M.G., Mohamed, E.A., Metabolomic profiling and antioxidant activity of some Acacia species. *Saudi J. Biol. Sci.*, 21, 5, 400–8, 2014.
53. Abdllha, H.B., Mohamed, A.I., Almoniem, K.A., Adam, N.I., Alhaadi, W., Elshikh, A., *et al.*, Evolution of Antimicrobial, Antioxidant Potentials and Phytochemical Studies of Three Solvent Extracts of Five Species from Acacia Used in Sudanese Ethnomedicine. *AI Mag.*, 06, 691–8, 2016.
54. Sadiq, G.U., Dibal, F.S., Abdullahi, Y., Anticonvulsant Screening of Ethanol and N-Hexane Extracts of Acacia seyal Del. (Stem Bark) in Rats. 3, 1, 17–21, 2018.
55. Mekbib, S.B., Regnier, T., Sivakumar, D., Korsten, L., Evaluation of Ethiopian plant extracts, Acacia seyal and Withania somnifera, to control green mould and ensure quality maintenance of citrus (Citrus sinensis L.). *Fruits.*, 64, 285–94, 2009.
56. Mekbib, S.B., *In vitro* antimicrobial assay of selected medicinal plants against medically important plant and food-borne pathogens. *J. Med. Plants Stud.*, 4, 163–9, 2016.

57. Magnini, R.D., Hilou, A., Millogo-Koné, H., Compaoré, S., P, J.-M., Davin-Régli, A., A Review on ethnobotanical uses, biological activities and phytochemical aspects of Acacia senegal (L.) Willd. and Acacia seyal Delile. (Fabaceae)., 2, 32–55, 2020.
58. Elmi, A., Spina, R., Risler, A., Philippot, S., Mérito, A., Duval, R.E., *et al.*, Evaluation of Antioxidant and Antibacterial Activities, Cytotoxicity of Acacia seyal Del Bark Extracts and Isolated Compounds. *Mol.*, 25, 2392, 2020.
59. Nie, S., Wang, C.S., Cui, S.W., Wang, Q., Xie, M., Phillips, G.O., A further amendment to the classical core structure of gum arabic (Acacia senegal). *Food Hydrocolloids.*, 31, 42–8, 2013.
60. Awad, S.S., Rabah, A.A., Ali, H.I., Mahmoud, T.E., 1 - Acacia Seyal Gums in Sudan: Ecology and Economic Contribution, in: *Gum Arabic,* A.A. Mariod (Ed.), Academic Press, 3–11, 2018.
61. Li, J., Deng, Q., Yu, X., Wang, W., Structural studies of a new fraction obtained by gradient ethanol precipitation from Acacia seyal gum. *Food Hydrocolloids.*, 107, 105932, 2020.
62. Idris, O.M.I. and Haddad, G.M., Gum Arabic's (Gum Acacia's) Journey from Tree to End User, 3, 17, 372, 2011.
63. Idris, O., What is gum Arabic? An overview. *Int. J. Sudan Res.*, 7, 1–14, 2017.
64. Mariod, A.A., 24 - Functional Properties of Gum Arabic, in: Gum Arabic, A.A. Mariod (Ed.)., Academic Press, 283–295, 2018.
65. Hanahan, D. and Weinberg, R.A., Hallmarks of Cancer: The Next Generation. *Cell.*, 144, 5, 646–74, 2011.
66. Dunn, G.P., Old, L.J., Schreiber, R.D., The Immunobiology of Cancer Immunosurveillance and Immunoediting. *Immun.,* 21, 2, 137–48, 2004.
67. Mittal, D., Gubin, M.M., Schreiber, R.D., Smyth, M.J., New insights into cancer immunoediting and its three component phases—elimination, equilibrium and escape. *Curr. Opin. Immunol.*, 27, 16–25, 2014.
68. Ashfaq, M., Haider, G., Ather, T., Ahsan, M., Khan, M.E., Seher, S., The current spectrum of infections in cancer patients with chemotherapy related neutropenia. *Infect. Dis. J. Pak.*, 32, 4, 147–53, 2023.
69. Anguille, S., Smits, E.L.J., Lion, E., Van Tendeloo, V.F.I., Berneman, Z.N., Clinical use of dendritic cells for cancer therapy. *Lancet Oncol.*, 15, 7, e257–67, 2014.
70. Rosenberg, S.A., Yang, J.C.H., Sherry, R.M., Kammula, U.S., Hughes, M., Phan, G.Q., *et al.*, Durable Complete Responses in Heavily Pretreated Patients with Metastatic Melanoma Using T-Cell Transfer Immunotherapy. *Clin. Cancer Res.*, 17, 4550–7, 2011.

71. Lasek, W., Zagożdżon, R., Jakóbisiak, M., Interleukin 12: still a promising candidate for tumor immunotherapy? *Cancer Immunol. Immunother.*, 63, 419–35, 2014.
72. Hanzly, M.I., Aboumohamed, A., Yarlagadda, N.K., Creighton, T., Digiorgio, L., Fredrick, A., *et al.*, High-dose interleukin-2 therapy for metastatic renal cell carcinoma: a contemporary experience. *Urol.*, 83, 5, 1129–34, 2014.
73. Ribatti, D., From the discovery of monoclonal antibodies to their therapeutic application: an historical reappraisal. *Immunol. Lett.*, 161, 1, 96–9, 2014.
74. Acharya, U.H. and Jeter, J.M., Use of ipilimumab in the treatment of melanoma. *Clin. Pharmacol.*, 5, 21–7, 2013.
75. Mamalis, A., Garcha, M.K., Jagdeo, J., Targeting the PD-1 pathway: a promising future for the treatment of melanoma. *Arch. Dermatol. Res.*, 306, 511–9, 2014.
76. Sze, D., Brown, R., Yang, S., Ho, P., Gibson, J., Joshua, D., The Use of Thalidomide in Myeloma Therapy as an Effective Anticancer Drug. *Curr. Cancer Drug Targets*, 6, 325–31, 2006.
77. Brown, R.D., Spencer, A., P.J.H., N.K., K.K., S.Y., D.M.S., E.A., J.G., Joshua, D.E., Prognostically significant cytotoxic T cell clones are stimu-lated after thalidomide therapy in patients with multiple myeloma. *Leuk. Lymphoma.*, 50, 11, 1860–4, 2009.
78. Dunn, G.P., Old, L.J., Schreiber, R.D., The Three Es of Cancer Immunoediting. *Annu. Rev. Immunol.*, 22, 329–60, 2004.
79. Eliza, W.L.Y., Fai, C.K., Chung, L.P., Efficacy of Yun Zhi (Coriolus versicolor) on survival in cancer patients: systematic review and meta-analysis. *Recent Pat. Inflamm. Allergy Drug Discov.*, 6, 1, 78–87, 2012.
80. Ahmad, R., Ahmad, N., Naqvi, A., Shehzad, A., Al-Ghamdi, M., Role of traditional Islamic and Arabic plants in cancer therapy. *J. Tradit. Complement. Med.*, 7, 2, 195–204, 2016.
81. Sekhon, B.K., Roubin, R.H., Li, Y., Devi, P., Nammi, S., Fan, K., *et al.*, Evaluation of Selected Immunomodulatory Glycoproteins as an Adjunct to Cancer Immunotherapy. *PLoS One.*, 22, 11, e0146881, 2016.
82. Restifo, N.P., Dudley, M.E., Rosenberg, S.A., Adoptive immunotherapy for cancer: harnessing the T cell response. *Nat. Rev. Immunol.*, 12, 269–81, 2012.
83. Waldman, A.D., Fritz, J.M., Lenardo, M.J., A guide to cancer immunotherapy: from T cell basic science to clinical practice. *Nat. Rev. Immunol.*, 20, 651–68, 2020.
84. Tang, L., Zheng, Y., Melo, M.B., Mabardi, L., Castano, A.P., Xie, Y.Q., *et al.*, Enhancing T cell therapy through TCR signaling-responsive nanoparticle drug delivery. *Nat. Biotechnol.*, 36, 707–16, 2018.

85. Xuan, N., Shumilina, E., Nasir, O., Bobbala, D., Götz, F., Lang, F., Stimulation of Mouse Dendritic Cells by Gum Arabic. *Cell. Physiol. Biochem.*, 25, 641–8, 2010.
86. Strobel, S. and Ferguson, A., Induction of oral tolerance, in mice, to gum arabic. *Food Addit. Contam.*, 3, 1, 43–6, 1986.
87. Ouyang H.Q., Liu, L., Chen, Z., Luo, J.M., Yu, E.X., Effects of Qingyi Huaji decoction on serum levels of interleukin-6, interleukin-8 and tumor necrosis factor-alpha in nude mice bearing pancreatic tumors. *Zhong Xi Yi Jie He Xue Bao*, 8, 7, 655–61, 2010.
88. Tanaka, T., Immunomodulatory action of citrus auraptene on macrophage functions and cytokine production of lymphocytes in female BALB/c mice. *Carcinogenesis.*, 20, 1471–6, 1999.
89. Bray, F., Ferlay, J., Soerjomataram, I., Siegel, R.L., Torre, L.A., Jemal, A., Global cancer statistics 2018: GLOBOCAN estimates of incidence and mortality worldwide for 36 cancers in 185 countries. *CA Cancer J. Clin.*, 68, 394–424, 2018.
90. Talib, W.H. and AbuKhader, M.M., Combinatorial Effects of Thymoquinone on the Anticancer Activity and Hepatotoxicity of the Prodrug CB 1954. *Sci. Pharm.*, 81, 519–30, 2013.
91. Dias, D.A., Urban, S., Roessner, U., A Historical Overview of Natural Products in Drug Discovery. *Metabolites.*, 2, 303–36, 2012.
92. Wright, G.D., Opportunities for natural products in 21st century antibiotic discovery. *Nat. Prod. Rep.*, 34, 7, 694–701, 2017.
93. Rayan, A., Raiyn, J., Falah, M., Nature is the best source of anticancer drugs: Indexing natural products for their anticancer bioactivity. *PLoS One.*, 9,12, 11, e0187925, 2017.
94. Abulateefeh, S.R., Spain, S.G., Aylott, J.W., Chan, W.C., Garnett, M.C., Alexander, C., Thermoresponsive polymer colloids for drug delivery and cancer therapy. *Macromol. Biosci.*, 11, 12, 1722–34, 2011.
95. Nagai, T. and Machida, Y., Buccal delivery systems using hydrogels. *Adv. Drug Deliv. Rev.*, 11, 179–91, 1993.
96. Madhav, N.V.S., Shakya, A.K., Shakya, P., Singh, K., Orotransmucosal drug delivery systems: a review. *J. Control. Release*, 140, 1, 2–11, 2009.
97. Sudhakar, Y.N., Kuotsu, K., Bandyopadhyay, A.K., Buccal bioadhesive drug delivery–a promising option for orally less efficient drugs. *J. Control. Release*, 114, 1, 15–40, 2006.
98. Donnelly, R.F., McCarron, P.A., Tunney, M.M., Woolfson, A.D., Potential of photodynamic therapy in treatment of fungal infections of the mouth. Design and characterisation of a mucoadhesive patch containing toluidine blue O. *J. Photochem. Photobiol. B*, 86, 1, 59–69, 2007.

99. Barclay, T.G., Day, C.M., Petrovsky, N., Garg, S., Review of polysaccharide particle-based functional drug delivery. *Carbohydr. Polym.*, 221, 94–112, 2019.
100. Bhardwaj, T.R., Kanwar, M., Lal, R., Gupta, A., Natural Gums and Modified Natural Gums as Sustained-Release Carriers. *Drug Dev. Ind. Pharm.*, 26, 1025–38, 2000.
101. Dinarello, C.A., The paradox of pro-inflammatory cytokines in cancer. *Cancer Metastasis Rev.,* 25, 307–13, 2006.
102. Aka, J.A., Mazumdar, M., Lin, S.X., Reductive 17$β$-hydroxysteroid dehydrogenases in the sulfatase pathway: Critical in the cell proliferation of breast cancer. *Mol. Cell. Endocrinol.*, 301, 183–90, 2009.
103. Lai, J., Thompson, J.R., Sandhu, D.S., Roberts, L.R., Heparin-degrading sulfatases in hepatocellular carcinoma: roles in pathogenesis and therapy targets. *Future Oncol.*, 4, 6, 803–14, 2008.
104. Orlowski, R.Z. and Kuhn, D.J., Proteasome Inhibitors in Cancer Therapy: Lessons from the First Decade. *Clin. Cancer Res.*, 14, 1649–57, 2008.
105. Deaglio, S., Aydin, S., Vaisitti, T., Bergui, L., Malavasi, F., CD38 at the junction between prognostic marker and therapeutic target. *Trends Mol. Med.*, 14, 5, 210–8, 2008.
106. Jin, T., Fantus, I.G., Sun, J., Wnt and beyond Wnt: multiple mechanisms control the transcriptional property of beta-catenin. *Cell. Signal.*, 20, 10, 1697–704, 2008.
107. Kim, Y.S. and Milner, J.A., Dietary modulation of colon cancer risk. *J. Nutr.*, 137, 11 Sup, 2576S–2579S, 2007.
108. Aldawsari, H.M., Singh, S., Alhakamy, N.A., Bakhaidar, R.B., Halwani, A.A., Badr-Eldin, S.M., Gum Acacia Functionalized Colloidal Gold Nanoparticles of Letrozole as Biocompatible Drug Delivery Carrier for Treatment of Breast Cancer. *Pharm.*, 13, 1554, 2021.
109. Pal, K., Roy, S., Parida, P.K., Dutta, A., Bardhan, S., Das, S., *et al.*, Corrigendum to "Folic acid conjugated curcumin loaded biopolymeric gum acacia microsphere for triple negative breast cancer therapy in *in vitro* and *in vivo* model". *Mater. Sci. Eng. C Mater. Biol. Appl.,* 111, 110866, 2020.
110. Sun, H., Jia, J., Jiang, C., Zhai, S., Gold Nanoparticle-Induced Cell Death and Potential Applications in Nanomedicine. *Int. J. Mol. Sci.*, 19, 3, 754, 2018.
111. Venkatesan, J., Hur, W., Gupta, P., Son, S.E., Lee, H.B., Lee, S.J., *et al.*, Gum Arabic-mediated liquid exfoliation of transition metal dichalcogenides as photothermic anti-breast cancer candidates. *Int. J. Biol. Macromol.*, 244, 124982, 2023.

112. Aliabbasi, N., Fathi, M., Emam-Djomeh, Z., Gum arabic-based nanocarriers for drug and bioactive compounds delivery. *Micro- Nanoeng. Gum-Based Biomater. Drug Deliv. Biomed. Appl.*, 13, 333–345, 2022
113. De, A.K., Nayak, A.K., Kundu, A., Das, B., Samanta, A., Gum arabic-based nanomaterials in drug delivery and biomedical applications, 7, 165–182, 2021.
114. Hasanin, M.S., Taha, N.F., Abdou, A.R., Emara, L.H., Green decoration of graphene oxide Nano sheets with gelatin and gum Arabic for targeted delivery of doxorubicin. *Biotechnol. Rep.*, 34, e00722, 2022.
115. Molaei, M.J., Two-dimensional (2D) materials beyond graphene in cancer drug delivery, photothermal and photodynamic therapy, recent advances and challenges ahead: A review. *J. Drug Deliv. Sci. Technol.*, 61, 101830, 2020.
116. Murugan, C., Sharma, V., Murugan, R.K., Malaimegu, G., Sundaramurthy, A., Two-dimensional cancer theranostic nanomaterials: Synthesis, surface functionalization and applications in photothermal therapy. *J. Control. Release.*, 299, 1–20, 2019
117. Lee, H.B., Son, S.E., Gupta, P., Venkatesan, J., Hur, W., Park, J., *et al.*, Mesoporous platinum nanozyme-based competitive immunoassay for sensitive detection of 25-hydroxyvitamin D. *Mater. Lett.*, 330, 133286, 2023.
118. Mostafavi, E., Zarepour, A., Barabadi, H., Zarrabi, A., Truong, L.B., Medina-Cruz, D., Antineoplastic activity of biogenic silver and gold nanoparticles to combat leukemia: Beginning a new era in cancer theragnostic. *Biotechnol. Rep.*, 26, 34, e00714, 2022.
119. Paulino, A.T., Guilherme, M.R., Mattoso, L.H.C., Tambourgi, E.B., Smart Hydrogels Based on Modified Gum Arabic as a Potential Device for Magnetic Biomaterial. *Macromol. Chem. Phys.*, 211, 1196–205, 2010.
120. Tiwari, A., Gum Arabic-Graft-Polyaniline: An Electrically Active Redox Biomaterial for Sensor Applications. *J. Macromol. Sci. Part A.*, 44, 7, 735–45, 2007.
121. Zhang, L., Yu, F., Cole, A.J., Chertok, B., David, A.E., Wang, J., *et al.*, Gum Arabic-Coated Magnetic Nanoparticles for Potential Application in Simultaneous Magnetic Targeting and Tumor Imaging. *AAPS J.*, 11, 693–9, 2009.
122. Williams, D., Gold, K., Holoman, T., Ehrman, S., Wilson, O., Surface Modification of Magnetic Nanoparticles Using Gum Arabic. *J. Nanopart. Res.*, 8, 749–53, 2006.
123. Kattumuri, V., Katti, K.K., Bhaskaran, S., Boote, E.J., Casteel, S.W., Fent, G.M., *et al.*, Gum arabic as a phytochemical construct for the stabilization of gold nanoparticles: *in vivo* pharmacokinetics and X-ray-contrast-imaging studies. *Small.*, 3, 2, 333–41, 2007.

124. Zhang, H., Shan, G., Liu, H., Xing, J., Surface modification of $γ$-Al2O3 nano-particles with gum arabic and its applications in adsorption and biodesulfurization. *Surf. Coat. Technol.*, 201, 6917–21, 2007.
125. Roque, A.C.A. and Wilson, O.C., Adsorption of gum Arabic on bioceramic nanoparticles. *Mater. Sci. Eng. C.*, 28, 3, 443–7, 2008.
126. Yadav, M., Yadav, A., Yadav, J.P., *In vitro* antioxidant activity and total phenolic content of endophytic fungi isolated from Eugenia jambolana Lam. *Asian Pac. J. Trop. Med.*, 7, S256–61, 2014.
127. Singh, S., Gill, A.A.S., Nlooto, M., Karpoormath, R., Prostate cancer biomarkers detection using nanoparticles based electrochemical biosensors. *Biosens. Bioelectron.*, 137, 213–21, 2019.
128. Singh, S., Numan, A., Somaily, H.H., Gorain, B., Ranjan, S., Rilla, K., *et al.*, Nano-enabled strategies to combat methicillin-resistant Staphylococcus aureus. *Mater. Sci. Eng. C.*, 129, 112384, 2021.
129. Bayda, S., Hadla, M., Palazzolo, S., Riello, P., Corona, G., Toffoli, G., *et al.*, Inorganic Nanoparticles for Cancer Therapy: A Transition from Lab to Clinic. *Curr. Med. Chem.* 25, 34, 4269–303, 2017.
130. Bobo, D., Robinson, K.J., Islam, J., Thurecht, K.J., Corrie, S.R., Nanoparticle-Based Medicines: A Review of FDA-Approved Materials and Clinical Trials to Date. *Pharm. Res.*, 33, 2373–87, 2016.
131. Ventola, C.L., Progress in Nanomedicine: Approved and Investigational Nanodrugs. *P T Peer-Reviewed J. Formul. Manag.*, 42, 12, 742–55, 2017.
132. Lombardo, D., Kiselev, M., Caccamo, M.T., Smart Nanoparticles for Drug Delivery Application: Development of Versatile Nanocarrier Platforms in Biotechnology and Nanomedicine. *J. Nanomater.*, 26, 702518, 2019.
133. Kato, R.B., Roy, B., de Oliveira, F.S., Ferraz, E.P., de Oliveira, P.T., Kemper, A.G., *et al.*, Nanotopography Directs Mesenchymal Stem Cells to Osteoblast Lineage Through Regulation of microRNA-SMAD-BMP-2 Circuit. *J. Cell. Physiol.*, 11, 25482, 2014.
134. Zhang, X., Li, Y., Dong, X., Wang, H., Chen, B., Li, R., *et al.*, 3D-printed bioactive ceramic scaffolds with MoSe2 nanocrystals as photothermal agents for bone tumor therapy. *RSC Adv.*, 12, 30588–97, 2022
135. Gao, J., Mao, Y., Xiang, C., Cao, M., Ren, G., Wang, K., *et al.*, Preparation of $β$-lactoglobulin/gum arabic complex nanoparticles for encapsulation and controlled release of EGCG in simulated gastrointestinal digestion model. *Food Chem.*, 354, 129516, 2021.
136. Song, X., Chen, Y., Sun, H., Liu, X., Leng, X.J., Physicochemical stability and functional properties of selenium nanoparticles stabilized by chitosan, carrageenan, and gum Arabic. *Carbohydr. Polym.*, 255, 117379, 2020.
137. Lei, Z., Zhu, W., Xu, S., Ding, J., Wan, J., Wu, P., Hydrophilic MoSe2 Nanosheets as Effective Photothermal Therapy Agents and Their Application in Smart Devices. *ACS Appl. Mater. Interfaces.*, 832, 20900–8, 2016.

138. Feng, X., Wang, X., Xing, W., Zhou, K., Song, L., Hu, Y., Liquid-exfoliated MoS2 by chitosan and enhanced mechanical and thermal properties of chitosan/MoS2 composites. *Compos. Sci. Technol.*, 93, 76–82, 2014.
139. Ansari, M.J., Jasim, S.A., Taban, T.Z., Bokov, D.O., Shalaby, M.N., Al-Gazally, M.E., *et al.*, Anticancer Drug-Loading Capacity of Green Synthesized Porous Magnetic Iron Nanocarrier and Cytotoxic Effects Against Human Cancer Cell Line. *J. Cluster Sci.*, 34, 467–77, 2022.
140. Sarika, P.R. and Nirmala, R.J., Curcumin loaded gum arabic aldehyde-gelatin nanogels for breast cancer therapy. *Mater. Sci. Eng. C Mater. Biol. Appl.*, 65, 331–7, 2016.
141. Udompornmongkol, P. and Chiang, B.H., Curcumin-loaded polymeric nanoparticles for enhanced anti-colorectal cancer applications. *J. Biomater. Appl.*, 30, 537–46, 2015.
142. Shahgholian, N. and Rajabzadeh, G., Fabrication and characterization of curcumin-loaded albumin/gum arabic coacervate. *Food Hydrocolloids.*, 59, 17–25, 2016.

6

Cyclodextrins: Inclusion Complexes and Drug Delivery in Cancer Therapy

Mohd Hafizur Rehman Ansari[1,2*], Mohan Lal[2,3] and Ravindra K. Rawal[3,4†]

[1]*Department of Pharmacy, School of Healthcare and Allied Sciences, G.D. Goenka University, Gurugram, Haryana, India*
[2]*Agrotechnology and Rural Development Division, CSIR-Northeast Institute of Science and Technology, Jorhat, Assam, India*
[3]*Academy of Scientific and Innovative Research (AcSIR), Ghaziabad, Uttar Pradesh, India*
[4]*Natural Product Chemistry, Chemical Sciences and Technology Division, CSIR-North East Institute of Science and Technology, Jorhat, Assam, India*

Abstract
Natural oligosaccharides generated from starch called cyclodextrins (CDs) have become critical cyclic compounds with comprehensive uses because of their special structural and chemical characteristics. As drug delivery vehicles, CDs are very useful in the pharmaceutical sector because they make it easier for hydrophobic medications to be included in complexes, improving the solubility, stability, and bioavailability of these medications. This chapter explores the introductory chemistry of CDs, including their structures, solubility profiles, dissolution features, and the way host–guest compounds are formed. Additionally, it investigates the biological compatibility of CDs and their strategic use as nanostructured carriers in creating anticancer drugs. In the context of targeted therapy for solid tumors, in the case of breast, stomach, esophagus, liver, colon, and prostate, the dual role of CDs is highlighted. The topic of inclusion of various genes and phytochemicals into CD-based delivery systems is covered, along with the difficulties of solubility, bioavailability, and biodistribution. Through the use of CDs, these innovative compounds derived from natural sources have the unsung caliber to surmount the drawbacks of traditional radiation and chemotherapies, offering a

**Corresponding author*: rehman.ansari1988@gmail.com
†*Corresponding author*: rawal.ravindra@gmail.com; drrkrawal@neist.res.in

Luqman Jameel Rather, Showkat Ali Ganie and Mohammed A. Assiri (eds.) Polysaccharide Biomaterials in Cancer Research and Therapy: From Lab to Life, (149–192) © 2026 Scrivener Publishing LLC

strong substitute for treating second primary neoplasms in cancer survivors. This book chapter will emphasize how CDs may improve the effectiveness of tailored cancer treatments and point to possible future research areas in this cutting-edge area.

Keywords: Cyclodextrins, formulations, solubility, drug molecules, host–guest complexes, targeted drug delivery, nanostructures carriers in anticancer drug development therapy

6.1 Introduction

Cyclodextrins' (CDs') basic interactions were first discovered by Villars and Schardinger over 100 years ago. The first CD document-based patent was recorded in terms of chemistry and their complexes in 1953 [1]. Generally speaking, oligosaccharides (cyclic form), mainly CDs, are mostly manufactured industrially by cyclomaltodextrin glucanotransferase, which breaks down starch enzymatically. They are devising D-glucopyranose units linked by α-(1-4) glucosidic linkages [2]. Currently, alpha-cyclodextrin (α-CD), beta-cyclodextrin (β-CD), and gamma-cyclodextrin (γ-CD) are the three primary pharmaceutical product categories that use CDs, with corresponding glucopyranose units of 6, 7, and 8 (Figure 6.1) [3]. Additionally, the amount of glucose units, specific cavity sizes, solubility, and molecular weight all affect CDs; each factor is represented by a Greek letter based on the quantity of units [3]. During the last three decades, certain biotechnological advances have resulted in case surplus use of CDs in favor of numerous therapies for cancer and other complex biological disorders. Therefore, the overall turnover of CDs has naturally increased but significantly decreased the overall cost. Despite this, accessibility

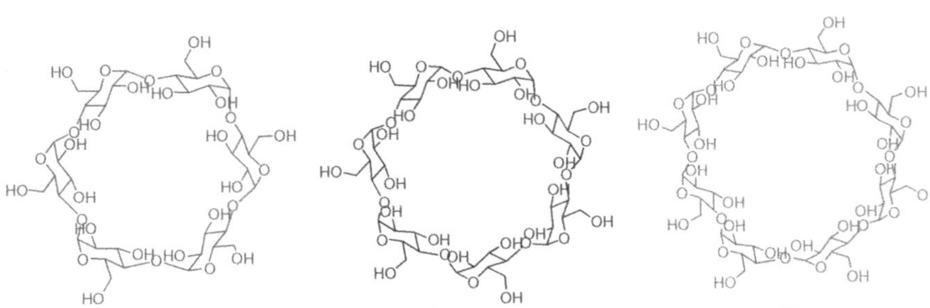

Figure 6.1 The general structure of CDs and their derivatives.

also increased in terms of purity and vast applicability with ameliorating patient compliance using other derivative products such as hydroxypropyl-CD, heptakis-2,6-dimethyl-β-CD, heptakis-2,3,6-trimethyl-β-CD, methylated-β-CD, etc. [1].

6.1.1 Structures and Properties of CDs

A type of cyclic oligosaccharides known as CDs—also called α-, β-, and γ-CD—is created when enzymes break down starch and present six, seven, or eight glucose units connected by α-1,4 glycosidic linkages (Figure 6.1) [4, 5]. CDs have a hollow-shaped, truncated cone structure or torus. This is having a hydrophobic cavity and an external hydrophilic surface due to the chair structure of the glucopyranose groups. Because of this structural configuration, hydrophobic medications can be encapsulated in CD cavities for use in host–guest complexes without the need for complex chemical interactions [6]. Furthermore, the CDs and diverse guest molecules generally form the complexes (Figure 6.2), which is advantageous for loading drugs and their absorption, release, taste, or odor masking; controlling drug-releasing profiles; improving drug permeability and biodistribution; and lowering undesirable side effects at the desired site or biological barriers [7]. Therefore, CDs' physical and chemical properties offer some important benefits across biomedical, pharmaceutical, and other applications nowadays. Moreover, the dual properties of CDs to improve

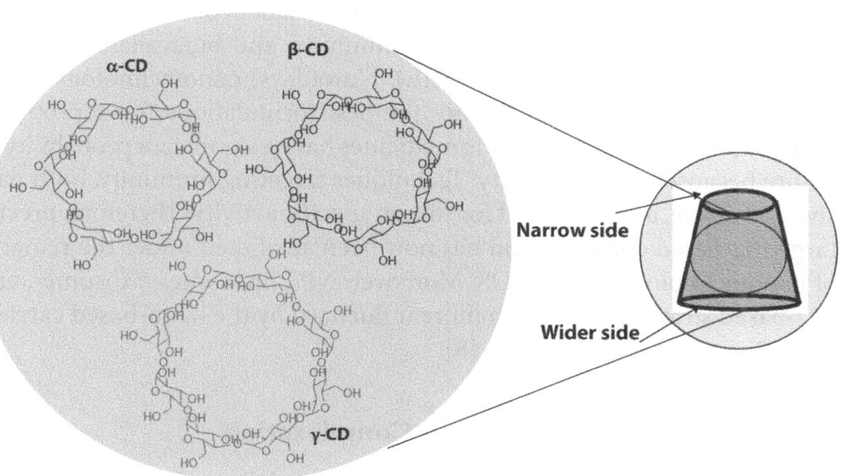

Figure 6.2 The keen derivatives of CD (α, β, and γ, respectively) molecules in formulations concern.

the well-known pharmaceutical features such as inclusion capability, solubility, controlled drug delivery (DD) strategy, and toxicities have been synthesized [5, 7]. Similarly, the major objectives are often realized because of CDs' ability to form complexes with host cavities and guest molecules [3, 5].

6.1.2 Derivatives of CDs

Enzymes, nucleic acids, photosensitizers, chemotherapeutic drugs, nanoparticles (NPs), and various interactions among metal and its oxides, polymers, liposomes, and micelles have all been positively laden onto native CDs and their derivatives. Moreover, CDs' exceptional chemical diversity allows for the co-delivery of many biomolecules to construct a biocompatible that combines the advantages of multiple therapeutic approaches to provide synergistic effects [5].

6.2 Impact of CDs on Properties of Formulations

CDs have several applications in pharmaceutical formulations and are functional dual-hatted excipients for targeted drug delivery consideration for many anticancer medications. This, including the well-known paclitaxel (PTX), docetaxel, cisplatin, and methotrexate drugs, can readily be amalgamated with CD to increase their steering and diverse special effects. Broadly, chemotherapeutic drugs have many chances of failure due to their toxicity, efficacy, active and passive immunity, and bioavailability across the tumor microenvironment (TME). Nowadays, nanotechnology-based drug delivery systems (DDSs) are the best formulations for appropriate targeting [8]. Chemotherapeutic medicines have a significant probability of failure because of their toxicity. Techniques targeting immunity, both passive and active, are developed for tumor-specific activity. Therefore, precise targeting-based consideration has now been attributed under the remarks of nanotechnology-based DDS. Moreover, NP-, liposome-, exosome-, and CD-based strategies are much more influenced by the nano-based carriers for DD in numerous therapies [8].

6.2.1 Mechanism of Inclusion Complexation

CDs are generally produced by enzymatic degradation of starch molecules, where the glucose residues are linked together by glycosidic bonds (α-1,4-form). CDs are categorized into three valuable parts, i.e., derivatives as per the number of basic subunits of glucose 6, 7, and 8 form, correspondingly. The basic uniqueness of structure and properties of CDs are already mentioned in the above section. Moreover, these types of things are amalgamated to form inclusion complexes for further consideration of numerous characteristics of drug properties. Therefore, this marvelous approach improves solubility, dissolution, half-life, and aqueous stability of poor drug bioavailability. The two similar sulfobutylether β-CD (SBE) and hydroxypropyl β-CD (HP) derivatives have both been recently classified by the Food and Drug Administration (FDA) as inactive pharmaceutical ingredients, because both derivatives were used as parenteral formulation for a more extended period with less cytotoxic effects than β-CDs [9]. The primary aim of the mechanisms of the inclusion complexation procedure depends upon three important properties: firstly, the inclusion of complexes with CDs and their *in vivo* and *in vitro* biological investigations; secondly, assessing and contrasting the bioactive effectiveness of compounds that are complex with those that are not; lastly, inclusion complexes were

Table 6.1 Characteristic features of CDs and their derivatives [13].

S. no.	CD derivatives	Solubility (mg/mL)	Molecular weight (Dalton)
Natural CDs			
1	α-CD	145	972
2	β-CD	18.5	1135
3	γ-CD	232	1297
Polymerized CDs			
1	Epichlorohydrin-β-CD	>500	112000
2	Carboxymethyl epichlorohydrin-β-CD	>200	2000000-15000000
Chemically modified CDs			
1	Hydroxypropyl-β-CD	≥600	1400
2	Sulfobutyl ether-β-CD	≥500	2163
3	Hydroxypropyl-γ-CD	≥500	1576
4	Randomly methylated-β-CD	≥500	1312

put through chemical and biological performance tests, i.e., the interface area of sciences to create novel pharmaceuticals [10]. Therefore, CD and its derivatives play a significant role in designing and developing mechanistic insight-based inclusion agents and ameliorate the chemical and biological behavior and further improve the solubility and aqueous stability of weak bioavailable drugs (Table 6.1) [11, 12].

6.2.2 Types of Complexes

CD-based simple inclusion complexes can increase only the aqueous solubility and actual stability of drugs without unwanted toxic effects. However, in the case of biology, specific receptors are overexpressed on the surface of tumor cells, while in the case of normal cells, their expression is significantly lower, such as glucose, biotin, and folate receptors. Subsequently, ligands such as CDs, using numerous complex-based approaches, have been further optimized in terms of physicochemical parameters to better target DD concerns. Furthermore, the nanotechnology (as per desired particle sizes of 50–200 nm) of numerous drugs with CDs is a fruitful remark of absorption *via* enhanced permeability and retention rate in numerous biological experiments using nanovesicles, nanomicelles, and liposome procedures. Due to these procedures, good therapeutic efficacy was achieved across the tumor cells or the microenvironment with minute side effects of drugs on the human body to a certain level [14]. Furthermore, the entire ligand–complex-based system was modified to meet modern requirements for a variety of biological illnesses using the best pharmatech process method.

6.2.3 Host–Guest Complexes

CDs are also called cycloamylases; these all are cyclic sugars made up of joined d-glucopyranose units α-(1-4-form) and created *via* employing CD glucosyltransferases to break down starch enzymatically. These agents participated in reaction mixtures, including n-octanol firstly with α-CD, secondly β-CD by toluene, and finally, cyclohexadec-8-en-1-one/cyclohexadecenol for γ-CDs to isolate each derivative. The absence of the precipitation agents led to the subsequent separation of other oligomers using chromatographic techniques. However, the bigger CD molecule is made up of 26 glucose units. Therefore, 95% of all pharmacological formulations use all three derivatives—α-, β-, and γ-CDs—among others in case of numerous health implications [15]. From numerous resources, the well-known report reveals that some natural and synthetic substances have been showcased as complex with CDs and their derivatives [10] in terms of

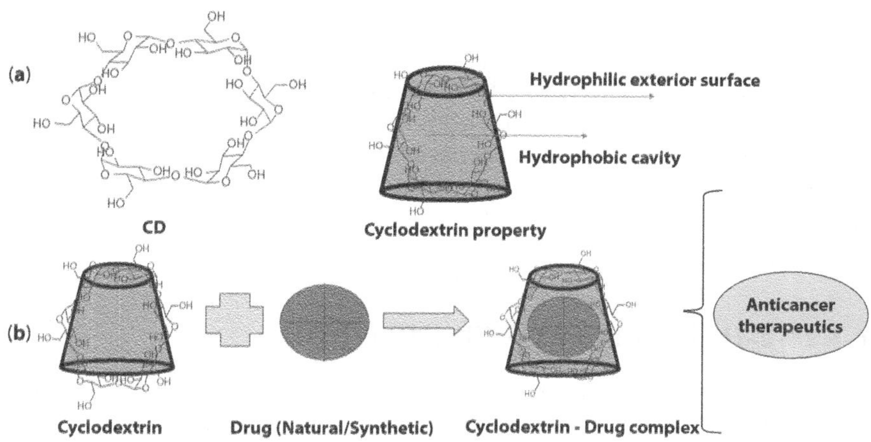

Figure 6.3 (a) Basic architecture of CD molecules. (b) Diagrammatic representation of association of the CD and drug to form drug–CD complex.

understanding numerous therapeutic properties such as anticancer activities (Figures 6.3a and b) [16]. Despite this, some well-known studies of CDs are given below with some significant points across health implications.

This present report shows some recent trends of progress of CD-based optimized DD concerns for the assessment of anticancer consideration using *in vivo* murine models. Despite this, some evidence as per the *in vitro–in vivo* concerns has been enlisted with some natural products and other agents either in single or in combinatorial form (Table 6.2) [10]. Therefore, numerous *in vivo* studies of drugs with remarkable characteristics of CDs have addressed further setbacks of conventional anticancer medications.

6.3 Application of CDs

6.3.1 Methylated-β-CD

CDs and other probable derivatives majorly form complexes with several guest molecules, generally hydrophobic ones. These molecules get transformed into cell membrane constituents like cholesterol and phospholipids resulting from the hemolysis of humans. Similarly, methylated CDs are more hydrophobic than parent CDs as per their affinity across the constituents of cell membranes. The mechanism of death attributed to methylated β-CDs is apoptosis resulting from the breakdown of cholesterol across the cellular membranes [16]. In cholesterol extraction in the cell membrane, the methylated β-CDs marked apoptotic cellular death in squamous carcinoma M213 cells. Therefore, there is a progressive relationship between the CD-based hemolytic property with the uneven caliber to solubilize the cholesterol across the cellular barriers. Moreover, methylated β-CDs are considerably more hazardous than parent β-CDs. Methylated β-CDs must first be thoroughly toxicologically examined before being developed as a cancer treatment [16].

6.3.2 2-Hydroxy Propyl-β-CD (HP-β-CD)

Another study revealed that the accumulation of cholesterol in terms of dysbiosis further leads to numerous malignancies in the case of cancer. There, HP-β-CD already revealed that the reduction of cholesterol intracellularly further leukemic growth through the G2/M cell-cycle arrest and apoptosis. Furthermore, at higher doses of 50 and 150 mM, respectively, HP-β-CD intraperitoneal injection treatment significantly extended the lifetime in leukemic mice xenografted with BV173 and Ba/F3 BCR-ABLWT while also inhibiting the development of leukemic cells. However, this derivative showed limited toxicity as well as tolerability after IP administration for 5 consecutive days with a predefined dose of 2086.5 mg/kg. Another study documented that the dose at optimal 10,000 mg/kg IP of HP-β-CD is well abided.

Therefore, the CD dose is generally required to be higher for inhibiting the tumor growth. In the case of parenteral usage, CDs are mainly required at lower doses with the safest approach. Furthermore, HP-β-CD is comparatively more promising than methylated β-CDs. Therefore, nowadays, HP-β-CD is most widely used in animals and humans as parenterally without any single adverse effects [16].

6.3.3 CD Complexation with Anticancer Drugs

To enhance solubility and stability, boost bioavailability and bio-dissolution, lessen toxicity, and alter physicochemical properties, some anticancer medications have been amalgamated among CDs and their derivatives [13, 16]. Some important examples of the complexation of diverse anticancer medications with CDs and further derivatives are listed in Table 6.2. After developing CD-based polyrotaxanes or pseudopolyrotaxanes (CDPRs), the Caruso group was used as a degradable linker, i.e., cystamine, to crosslink CDPRs. Clickable PEG moieties were then added and further functionalized. Doxorubicin (Dox) was conjugated to the hydroxyl moieties

Table 6.2 Some promising anticancer activities of CD inclusion complexes with host–guest interaction strategy [10].

CD type	Complex substance	Dose	Animal	Activity	Improved characteristics	Ref.
β-CD	Curcumin	100 mg/kg	Mice	Anticancer	Curcumin–CD complexes enhanced	[17]
β-CD	Ricobendazole and Albendaz ole	30 mg/kg	BALB/c mice 8 weeks old	Anticancer	Solubility was highest when β-CD was used as a carrier. This increase in solubility was higher for albendazole, indicating the formation of a more stable complex than with ricobendazole. *In vivo* studies showed that the ABZ:β-CD complex produced a reduction in the tumor growth kinetics on mice with no signs of toxicity	[18]

(Continued)

Table 6.2 Some promising anticancer activities of CD inclusion complexes with host–guest interaction strategy [10]. (*Continued*)

CD type	Complex substance	Dose	Animal	Activity	Improved characteristics	Ref.
β-CD	Pumbagin	Subcutaneous (subq.) 5 mg/kg	Male/female C57BL/6J mice	Anticancer	Plumbagin–β-CD complex in niosomes is a potential tool for the effective delivery of plumbagin and could enhance its antitumor property in skin cancer	[19]
β-CD	3-(4′-geranylox y3 methoxyphenyl)-2-transpropenoic acid (GOFA) and auraptene (AUR).	Oral (p.o.) 100 and 500 ppm	Male Crj: CD-1(ICR) mice	Anticancer	GOFA/β-CD and AUR/β-CD are effective in inhibiting colon cancer development in a two-stage colitis-related mouse colon carcinogenesis model through modulation of inflammation, proliferation, and expression of several proinflammatory cytokines	[20]

(*Continued*)

Table 6.2 Some promising anticancer activities of CD inclusion complexes with host–guest interaction strategy [10]. (*Continued*)

CD type	Complex substance	Dose	Animal	Activity	Improved characteristics	Ref.
B-Cyclodextrin (β-CD) and 2-hydroxypropyl-β-cyclodextrin (HPβ-CD)	Paclitaxel	Oral (p.o.) 125 mg/kg	C57BL/6 J mice	Anticancer	Paclitaxel by encapsulation in poly(anhydride) NPs containing CDs and poly(ethylene glycol) possessed significant antitumor effect in a syngenic tumor model of carcinoma in mice	[21]
β-Cyclodextrin	Paclitaxel	10.0 mg/kg PTX	Female BALB/c nude mice	Anticancer	Anticancer efficacy, cell proliferation inhibition, apoptosis rate (30.0%), PTX accumulation in resistant cells	[22]
α, β-Cyclodextrin (CD) and 2-hydroxypropylβ-CD	LGK974	Oral (p.o.) 10 mg/kg	Nude (Nu/Nu088) mice	Anticancer	In a mouse lung cancer allograft model, CD: LGK 974 complexes induced potent Wnt signaling inhibition with reduced intestinal toxicity	[23]

(*Continued*)

Table 6.2 Some promising anticancer activities of CD inclusion complexes with host–guest interaction strategy [10]. (*Continued*)

CD type	Complex substance	Dose	Animal	Activity	Improved characteristics	Ref.
β-CD	Camptothecin	12.9 and 25.8 mg/kg (CPT)	BALB/c nude female mice	Anticancer	↓Tumor volume ↑Tumor growth delay (13 days of difference)	[24]
β-CD	Doxorubicin	6.0 mg/kg DOX	Male NCRNU nude mice	Anticancer	Tumor volume [9] (9.4-, 9.1-,and 7.7-fold) ↑Tumor necrosis ↑ Cytotoxicity rate ↓ Cell viability rate [10]: (5.5-, 4.6-, and 2.9-fold)	[25]
β-CD	Methotrexate	5 mg/kg	BALB/c mice (20–25 g)	Anticancer	Increase in solubility and dissolution rate, enhancement of bioavailability and antitumor activity	[26]

of the treaded α-CDs to form Dox-loaded capsules. The disulfide bonds within the capsules were cleaved by glutathione, which resulted in the conjugation of α-CDs-Dox through dethreading. According to this study, click chemistry for post-functionalization, in conjunction with tunable CDPRs, allows the formation of capsules that can be precisely regulated in terms of their composition and functionality. Therefore, this makes CDPR-based biomaterials even more promising for targeted DDS [27].

Other antitumor drugs, such as PTX, have demonstrated great promise when used to treat STs using polypropylene glycol (PPG) complexed with the β-CD-N3 group. Wu and Jiang›s group recently synthesized the CDPR. Approximately 11-β-CDs were locked on one axle, and a succinate-based PTX was covalently joined to the hydroxyl groups in the case of a CDPR-based hydrophilic spacer. The ideal drug loading level of approximately 29% was demonstrated by the supermolecular CDPR–PTX conjugates, and esterase catalysis can speed up the release of PTX. Later, human neuroblastoma (SH-SY5Y) cells may easily internalize the CDPR–PTX conjugates and preserve the scientific investigation of the pharmacological activity of PTX [28, 29]. Gamma scintillation counting yielded a half-life of 5.8 hours for the 99mTc-labeled CDPRs in blood circulation, which is significantly longer than the 18.8 ± 1.5 min reported for Taxol. Antitumor assessment of CDPRs was assessed by an s.c. hepatic H22 tumor-transplanted mice model. The results demonstrated that, at an equivalent dosage of PTX, the resulting CDPRs had a promising antitumoral impact when compared with the standard drug Taxol. The results investigated the 78.7% tumor growth inhibition by CDPRs as compared to 30.7% for Taxol (15th day). Consequently, the life span of median survival time for tumor-transplanted mice was significantly longer as compared to all the formulation treatment groups. Overall, the findings showed how promising these CDPRs are in clinical settings [28, 29]. According to a different study report, host–guest interaction was used to load PTX layer by layer in the wall. The integrated anticancer medication was progressively increased with biological settings, and capsules held their stability. Competitive CD added to the exterior surfaces can stimulate the release of PTX. When breast cancer–based cells were incubated by the capsules, further results revealed that the cells only adhered to capsules because the CD44 receptor overexpressed HA. The PTX-loaded capsules were ultimately investigated to dramatically lower the breast cancer cell viability during their cultivation process. Collectively, these findings demonstrate the promise of these capsules containing HA and CD in case of anticancer therapy [30, 31].

6.4 DD Approaches

The major concern of DDS is to carry the exact quantity of drug molecules specifically bound to the different sites in an accurate manner (Figure 6.4). The unwanted side effects can be restrained by the evolution of the new strategy, i.e., the DD approach. Therefore, nowadays, CDs are one of the most promising candidates for fully utilizing guest molecule due to their unsung properties in addressing numerous complex biological disorders. Therefore, CDs, through complexation procedures, have the potential to amplify or ameliorate numerous characteristics, including solubility, dissolution, bioavailability, and biodistribution. Similarly, prostaglandins E2 has gained significant attention in the market due to improvements in terms of its solubility, stability, and bioavailability. However, CD molecules are naturally less hydrophilic, posing challenges related to the use of organic solvents and their derivatives [32].

6.4.1 Oral Route

As with the traditional concerns of pharmaceutical formulations, i.e., conventional tablets, they are economical, offer good patient compliance, and are easy to produce. Therefore, in this case, drug administration orally is the rate-limiting step for preferred DD for solid oral dosage formulations [33]. These biopharmaceutical-type formulations have immediate release

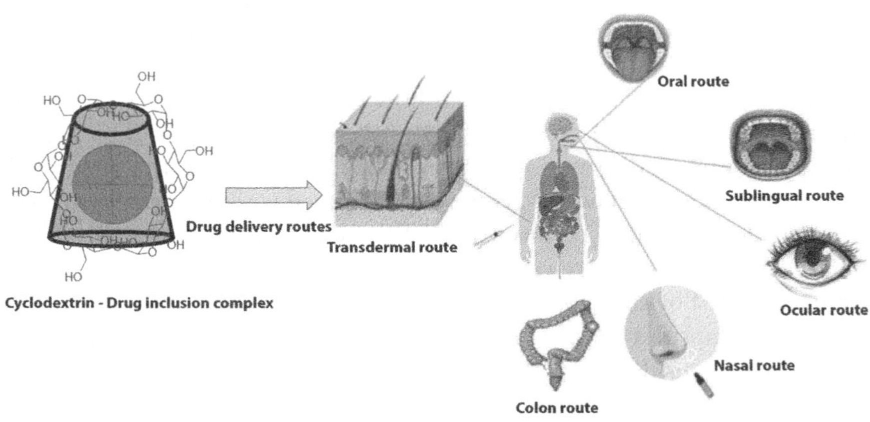

Figure 6.4 Schematic depiction of DDS pathways with CD–drug inclusion complex considerations.

of tablets with numerous series of processes such as tablet disintegration, release rate, particle size, dissolution, permeation of the molecules across the biological barriers, partition coefficient, and others. Generally, the hydrophilicity of a drug is slow in certain cases if the values are below 0.1–0.05 mg/Ml, and the rate is limited also. Therefore, the partition coefficient strategy (aqueous exterior to lipophilic mucosa) improvises the rate-limiting steps of the less absorption and dissolution-based drugs [34]. Furthermore, numerous formulation techniques have been developed to overcome critical points in the case of DD by oral route. Therefore, a general CD and its other derivatives nowadays are much more significant in terms of pharmaceutical applications and documented excellent reviews for readers from the last two decades [34].

In the case of oral dosage forms intended for quick release, the highest permissible dose to the solubility D/S ratio must be maintained under 250 ml and within the suitable pH range of 1–7.5 as per the biopharmaceutical classification system. Likewise, medications exhibiting aqueous solubility exceeding 0.1–0.05 mg/ml will have demonstrated a dissolving rate that limits absorption when incorporated into a traditional immediate-release tablet. Therefore, the conventional oral tablet size is 800 mg, which is particularly fixed for the upper size limit. In case of excipient requirements, 700 mg of the complex can be fixed for immediate tablets. Despite this, certain measures of CDs for drugs are applied at an average potency of 0.1–1 mg/kg. Therefore, CD-based oral dosage forms particularly follow two basic guidelines [35]. The aqueous solubility of phenytoin is 24 μg/mL, with a log K(octanol/water) value of 2.5 and a D:S ratio of around 2000 mL. Phenytoin's oral bioavailability, or its sodium counterpart, is approximately 90%, but it varies depending on the conditions, likely because of its poor lipophilicity. Despite this, the bioavailability of phenytoin by the oral route is significantly increased through the CD-based complexation approach [35]. The water solubility of spironolactone is 28 μg/mL; its log K(octanol/water) value is 2.8 with a D:S ratio of 10,000 mL and oral bioavailability of 25%. Oral bioavailability was increased by approximately 2.4 times when spironolactone was formulated as a CD inclusion complex [35]. Acyclovir is a class III medication, and its membrane permeability is what slows down the drug's rate of absorption from the gastrointestinal system. Adding CD to an oral formulation has little influence on the medication's oral bioavailability because this type of DD enhancer works solely through the water diffusion barrier [36].

6.4.2 Sublingual DD

This is the most effective behavior to pass by the pre-systemic metabolism across the hepatic system. Drugs are generally transported systemically by thawing the mucosal barriers in this DDS. Hydrophilic drugs complexed with CDs have been numerously documented to raise solubility, absorption, and bioavailability properties. 17β-Estradiol, androstenediol, clomipramine, and danazol have significantly increased the bioavailability using the formulation with 2-hydroxy propyl-β-CD. This process is particularly governed by the rate-limiting step of the process of absorption for lipophilic compounds [35]. Another study looked into the Δ9-tetrahydrocannabinol (Δ9-THC) complexed with methyl-β-CD and 2-hydroxy-propyl-β-CD to achieve a sublingual formulation. The findings demonstrated that the dose of 400 mg of 2-hydroxy-propyl-β-CD and the dose of 1 mg THC 1 mg may create a complex, i.e., water-soluble; however, the dose of 400 mg is thought to be the maximum amount for sublingual delivery in a bulk formulation. Likewise, a soluble complex formulation containing THC (1 mg) and methylated-β-CD (25 mg) might be formed. Thus, when compared to oral delivery, the bioavailability of THC is increased by a formulation including random methylated-β-CD [37].

6.4.3 Ocular DD

Medicine is quality-assured, safe, economical, and self-applicable whenever effective therapy and good patient compliance are required. Topical eye-drop-type formulations are unique if they are generally prepared based on the traditionally mentioned requirements. In the last two decades, several research groups have revealed scientific documents with improved ocular DDS. Therefore, selected APIs were typically dissolved and complexed with the aqueous solution of CDs, estimated to get promising therapeutic concern with increased residence time with mucoadhesive polymers [38]. Albino rabbits were used as test subjects for the standardized and optimized NPs' potential as ocular medication delivery systems. Subsequent *in vivo* investigations demonstrated that the produced mucoadhesive NPs were more adept than the ECO solution at maintaining the antifungal action of ECO. Thus, chitosan/SBE-β-CD NPs were developed to offer a viable vehicle for the regulated administration of medication to the ocular cavity [39]. Phase solubility analysis and PXRD techniques were both utilized to develop the procedure of inclusion behavior with the usage of the modified CD to address the issues related to azithromycin (AZM). Clarity, pH, gelling, drug release pattern by *in vitro*, eye irritability property, drug content, and antibacterial activity of the developed and optimized formulation F4, including the composition of polymers, were assessed. Ultimately, it was determined that *in situ* gel AZM: SBE-β-CD was a viable formulation for effective ocular intervention attributed to its increased antibacterial efficacy and longer residence time [40].

A different study found that thiolation of HP-β-CD was accomplished, along with a two-fold rise in viscosity and residence time of corneal tissues. Following instillation, HP-β-CD with the thiol group increased the time of precorneal residence and area under the curve of eye drops of dexamethasone by 4 and 11.7 times, respectively. Additionally, between 30 and 150 minutes after injection, a consistent raised level of targeted drug achieved in humor was seen in the occurrence of polymer-targeted based consideration. The results revealed that HP-β-CD with the thiol group is a great excipient to use as ocular formulations of weakly soluble medications to raise their bioavailability with residence time in the ocular site [41]. Other marketed pharmaceutical products that contain HP-β-CD and HP-γ-CD as solubilizing agents are indomethacin (Indocid) and diclofenac sodium (Voltranen-Ophtha). Ocular drops (aqueous) containing cyclosporin A-CD-based NPs have been further used in rabbits for *in vivo* toxicologic research. Despite this, pluronic with sodium alginate was complexed with HP-β-CD-voriconazole (an antifungal ocular formulation) through cold gelation process to facilitate its production synthesis [42].

6.4.4 Nasal DD

Regarding the nasal DD method, studies have investigated the use of diverse polymers, including complexes with chitosan and other materials, to treat various neurodegenerative diseases [43]. Di Gioia *et al.* (2015) documented the intranasal targeting of the striatum using NPs composed of a drug complexed with glycol, polyanion, and various linking candidates [44]. Furthermore, compared to oral or IM injections, intranasal administration of carfentanil-DM-β-CD results in higher bioavailability and faster absorption, according to pharmacokinetic studies [45]. In another study, sheep mucosa's drug permeability was enhanced using an *in situ* polymeric drug approach, i.e., pH triggered [46]. Similarly, quick nasal absorption was documented following the *in situ* gel delivery of the CD-mediated atypical antipsychotic drug asenapine [47]. To increase targeting efficiency and enhance bioavailability, CD-based microparticles and emulsions have been developed and synthesized for intranasal administration [42]. The EMA states that HP-β-CD and SBE-β-CD are well tolerated by the nasal mucosa up to 10% of HP-β-CD in solution form and are fully compatible with nasal delivery. In addition, RM-β-CD and DM-β-CD can also be used in solutions up to 10% and work directly to increase nasal permeability. Because of its poor water solubility, β-CD can only be utilized in solutions up to 1.5%; nevertheless, it can be successfully used in solid products in the form of dry powders [48].

Two of more than 80 pharmaceutical medicines with CDs on the market were given approval for nasal administration by the FDA and EMA in 2019. BaqsimiTM, i.e., dry-powder formulation especially for nasal, is intended for use to treat hypoglycemia. Alternatively, for hormone replacement therapy, Aerodiol® is the most widely consumed [49]. Nasal midazolam (with 90% bioavailability) that was produced and included a complex with RM-β-CD seemed to be particularly effective for systemic drug absorption. The drug's absorption rate was able to be increased by the addition of chitosan to the formulations [50]. To target carnosic acid in the brain and increase endogenous neurotrophin levels, a nasal formulation was created. This will help prevent and treat neurodegenerative illnesses. The solubility of carnosic acid in water was improved when HP-β-CD was present. Rats were given aqueous solutions of this combination *via* the nasal route and subcutaneously with chitosan. It seems that the chitosan-containing nasal formulations could maximize the rat brain's synthesis of neurotrophins [51]. In a different investigation, ribavirin composed of α-CD microparticles, i.e., spray dried, was found to raise the drug accumulation in multiple brain regions when administered *via* the nasal route as opposed to ribavirin, which was micronized without excipients. Furthermore, compared to intravenous ribavirin administration, this was capable of significantly raising the ribavirin across the brain by more than ~5 times [52].

An effective anti-Alzheimer drug called timosaponin BII was created in a nasal formulation by an *in situ* hydrogel approach. Other gums, like gellan, were procured to form the gel while HP-β-CD was present. Mice were given this formulation intravenously for 38 days, which resulted in high therapeutic efficacy by brain-targeting of timosaponin BII compared to an Alzheimer's disease model [53]. Disulfiram with HP-β-CD was advocated as a treatment for glioblastoma. Moreover, with this complex appropriately applied nasally together with copper ions, it demonstrated effective therapeutic benefits against male rats that were harboring cerebral gliomas. Robust targeting of the brain for the transportation of nasal-brain medication administration was verified by Cy5.5/HP-β-CD dye in terms of a fluorescence signal [54].

6.4.5 Transdermal DD

The application of HP-β-CD to hairless mouse skin for up to four hours improves transdermal penetration. HP-β-CD was removed, and solutions containing corticosteroids were applied. Two model medicines were then used, and their transdermal flux and skin accumulation were examined. The results imply that this host–guest interaction-based strategy does not eliminate lipids through the dermis but rather increases transdermal penetration by improving the drug's apparent solubility in the formulation [55]. An *in vitro* study examined the skin penetration of captopril (CP) from β-CD *via* hairless mouse skin, suggesting additional features of β-CD. CP was used as a model drug in this investigation. As the concentration dependence of β-CD grew, the stability of β-CD was reduced, and vice versa, as the concentration of CP increased. The parameters that determine the stability of β-CD were shown to be more stable in β-CD with greater yield stress levels, according to the data. However, CP's skin permeability could be increased by employing β-CD with the oil phase, and free CP concentration in β-CD determined the CP flux in the aqueous phase [56]. Due to its higher stability compared to the β-CD complex, the complex containing HP-β-CD allowed for higher encapsulation percentages and resulted in more stable MLV systems. Due to CDs' solubilizing action, permeation studies were executed, and the results revealed no significant impact of the CD-based drug-permeation rate. The rhodamine–CD complex was used as a fluorescent marker in confocal laser scanning microscopy investigations. These findings provided support by demonstrating that the label penetrated rat skin layers more deeply with the solution than it did when it was encapsulated in liposomes [57]. Due to its increased stability over pure curcumin (CMN), HP-β-CD demonstrated optimal transdermal flow, suggesting improved penetration through CMN-2-hydroxypropyl-β-CDs (HP-β-CD). The action of CDs has a better effect on the rate of drug permeation, as demonstrated by studies, complexation, and various enhancers across the skin of rats. This contrasts with pure drug's erratic, inadequate skin penetration [58].

Loftsson *et al.* examined the impact of a glycerol monoether extract with HP-β-CD on the transport of testosterone from o/w cream in a hairless mice model. Firstly, an approximate 60% rise in the testosterone flow was noted with the addition of the host complex to the ointment. Secondly, a similar 40% raise was noted when the sample was passed through it. Thirdly, the flux was noted to increase to 80% in case both agents were mixed. When prostaglandin E1 was delivered transdermally using a guest molecule and CM-β-CD, similar results were obtained. However, in this instance, CM-β-CD also functioned as a penetration enhancer in the case of the dermal delivery of HPE-101 [59]. Another study revealed that the ACADFE-β-CD inclusion complex enters the skin through both transcellular and follicular pathways using confocal scanning laser microscopy [60]. Carvedilol (CAR)-CD complexes were prepared using *in situ* methods. Among the formulations tested, Soluplus 20% + α-CD (5–10%) and Solutol poly(pseudo)rotaxanes exhibited higher G' and G" as well as more rapid release of CAR. This difference in PEG chain position between the two amphiphilic polymers can be explained. The outcomes demonstrated how adaptable the formulations were of their spontaneous flow behavior and release patterns for transdermal CAR delivery [61]. Another feature that best characterized the formulations that were created was their ability to permeate through the skin of excised rabbit ears. In particular, Me-β-CD microemulsions, which were later selected for *in vivo* biological studies, revealed the significant permeation across the membrane of excised rabbit ears [62].

6.4.6 Colonic DD

The colon contains a complex and large microbial flora, composed of both permanent and sporadic members. The *Bacteroides* genus contains most of the colon's polysaccharide-degrading bacteria. The primary polysaccharidases are amylase, pectinase, and xylanase, as well as primary glycosidases found in the colonic microbiota. These enzymes are in charge of breaking down the undigested carbohydrates, including CDs. CD-based prodrug solubility and linkage type influence the drug release. Alpha-amylase in the colon hydrolyzes CD conjugates into tiny saccharide conjugates, such as maltose conjugates. By enzymatically breaking down to release the medication, these conjugates reduce steric hindrance for subsequent attacks [63]. A study revealed that α- and γ-CD with ester-based prodrugs, particularly those with drug conjugates, reached the intestines. Similarly, α- and γ-CD with amide-based prodrugs were further hydrolyzed and released the conjugates of glucose into the intestine but without rheological characteristics [28]. However, due to the limited hydrophilicity of β-CD, neither β-CD ester nor amide prodrugs were able to release the drug effectively [63]. A series of conjugates of scutellarin-β-CD (SCU-CD) exhibited greater solubility in water compared to the freely formed medication. Cytotoxicity studies on HCT116, SW480, and HT-29 colon cells indicated that SCU-CD conjugates showed better anticancer activities than scutellarin [64]. In a different investigation using artesunate-β-CD conjugates, similar results were also seen [65]. Diclofenac–β-CD combination was used to study the impact of feeding status on the release of drugs in Wistar rats with 4 different meal timings. The pH and mass of the gut were also evaluated, and prodrug metabolism was examined. The feeding schedule was discovered to have an impact on the pace at which diclofenac–β-CD hydrolyzes. Fasting causes the most rapid breakdown of diclofenac–β-CD because there is less competition for microbial enzymatic activity (absence of food) [63].

6.5 CDs-Based Nanostructures in Cancer Therapy

Different medications have been used to treat cancer, with varying degrees of success. Even with encouraging anti-cancer qualities, conventional medications frequently do not have the necessary physicochemical characteristics to be effective treatments for the illness. It is difficult for the compounds to reach the intended site at an optimal quantity in a way that is harmless or safe for the tissues because of their specific characteristics, which include insolubility in water, instabilities, poor permeability, short period of drug cycle, and lesser biocompatibility. Therefore, the development of DD systems that deliver anticancer drugs to tumor cells with increased effectiveness became essential. Nowadays, a diversity of materials has sparked

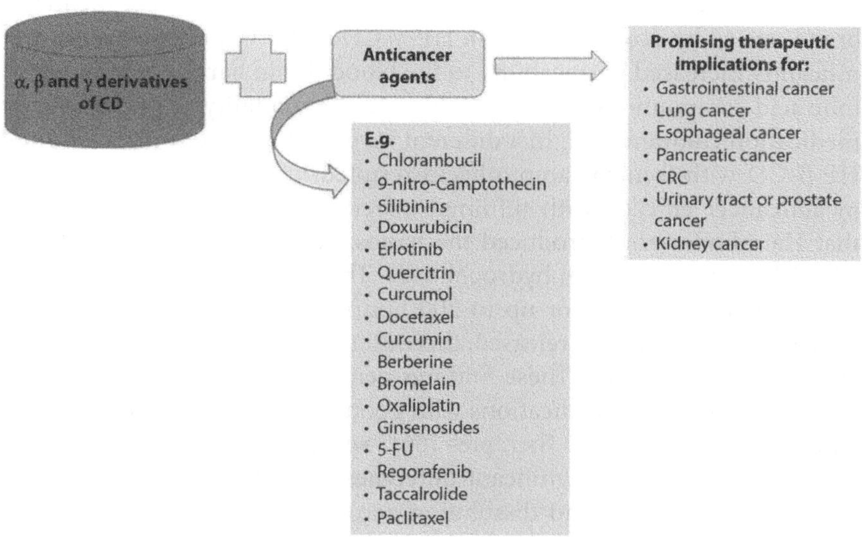

Figure 6.5 Overviews of substantial possibilities of CDs for DD in case of anticancer drug developments.

current scientific interest in the development of personalized nanocarriers (NCs) as biocompatible and stable for anticancer drug development [5]. CDs are a particularly interesting choice for encapsulating anticancer medicines. These substances are naturally occurring cyclic oligomers that have shown promise in medication administration. Enzymatic hydrolysis of starch yields CDs, which are easily modified chemically. The low immunogenicity, biocompatibility, safety, and commercial accessibility of CDs make them a valuable addition to pharmaceutical formulations required for cancer treatment (Figure 6.5). Researchers used CDs to create a variety of cutting-edge anticancer DDS with these benefits in mind. In this regard, we provide a brief explanation of the characteristics of CDs that enable the creation of effective NCs and go over the recently developed CD-based anticancer pharmaceutical products [5, 66].

6.6 CDs as Carriers of the Anticancer Drug Development

The development of inclusion complexes with nontoxic substances enhances the drug's physicochemical characteristics. Nowadays, to improve the process of solubility and dissolution stability, raise bioavailability, decrease toxicity, and change the rheological parameters, anticancer medicines have been complexed with CDs and other agents. The breakdown of the membrane caused by doxorubicin with HP-γ-CD and γ-CD complexation significantly increased permeability to the blood–brain barrier. Similarly, the folic acid compound β-CD-PEG enhanced the solubility of the anticancer medication chlorambucil. In a different investigation, the complexation of HP-β-CD with 9-nitro camptothecin resulted in a notable improvement in anticancer efficacy with minimal toxicity [13]. Another study found that Haimhoffer *et al.* produced the nanospheres using chitosan bonded with CD and doxorubicin hydrochloride. The medication was continually delivered through NPs for up to 200 hours; within the initial 24 hours, approx. 18% of drugs get released; thereafter, the release rate decreases and eventually reaches 40%. These findings demonstrate that chitosan can be used to manufacture medications with good solubility for prolonged drug administration in cancer therapies [66]. Some of the CDs as carriers of anticancer drugs have significant outcomes in terms of improvement of absorption, solubility, and dissolution across the biological barrier with several examples [13].

6.6.1 Gastrointestinal Cancer

Using the entrapment method, phytochemicals with nanostructured biocompatible polymers have been effectively used to improve cancer treatment. To assess silibinin's antioxidant and apoptotic impact on cancer cell lines such as HT-29 and stomach, i.e., AGS, the compound was added to the Zein–β-CD complex. The results were investigated in that it reduced the effects on AGS and normal cell lines. Furthermore, it showed considerable antioxidant potential by a developed carrier as well as surprising anticancer effects on HT-29, i.e., colon-specific cancer cell lines [67]. Designing DDS with nanotechnology is a possible new direction in the treatment of cancer. Nowadays, Lawson, a nonpolar phytochemical with anticancer properties, was ensnared in β-CD to assess its targeted cytotoxicity against several cancer cell lines. A powerful ultrasound-mediated homogenization approach was used to create the Lawson-loaded β-CD nanocarriers (LB-NCs). The results showed that by upregulating caspase 3, 8, and 9 proteins in MCF-7 cells, the artificially created negatively charged (−23.8 mV) NPs with the desired size demonstrated significant apoptotic properties. Additionally, when LB-NCs were compared to normal HUVEC cells, they demonstrated a notable promising antiproliferative activity on cancer cell lines [68]. Introducing a poly-6-cationic-CD-heptakis[6-(2-amino-ethylthio)-6-deoxy-2-O- octylsulfanylpropyl] into 45-epithelial cells (Caco-2) that are both undifferentiated and differentiated, the β-CD-hepta-N-trifluoroacetate strategy has been examined, resulting in elevated expression levels of reporter genes. CD-based NPs coated *via* siRNA were delivered rectally for targeted distribution to macrophages. Clinical benefits have been observed in a colitis-based murine model [69].

Delivery vehicles based on CD offer desired physicochemical and pharmacokinetic features without sacrificing consumer safety. CD derivatives have been reported to be an effective carrier for anticancer medications, helping to conceal the undesirable aspects of chemotherapeutics, increasing drug bioavailability, and overcoming their poor water solubility and instability. Consequently, extending the life of healthy and regenerative cells while improving therapeutic effects against different types of cancer cells becomes possible when employing CD-based oral delivery nanoformulations [70, 71]. The α-, ß-, and γ-CDs and New Zealand propolis were complexed and further showed potent antiproliferative effects on four cell lines of gastrointestinal cancer, including gastric carcinoma cells. Additionally, it has been found that this administration method has strong antioxidant and anti-inflammatory properties for lipids. The bulk of the benefits were associated not only with the components of propolis but also with the CDs that were dually combined and worked in concert [71]. Chitosan and CDs have distinct intrinsic features that make them promising candidates for gastrointestinal-specific DDD design. Chitosan's preferential protonation and solubilization in acidic environments, high zeta potential, and ability to open tight junctions between epithelial cells can enhance chemotherapeutic uptake. CD-based inclusion complexes can be degraded by pH changes or heat/enzymes, resulting in α-1,4 link cleavages between glucose units. Using CDs in medication formulations can selectively target tumor cells due to their high glucose consumption [71].

6.6.2 Lung Cancer

The greatest morbidity and death rates are associated with lung cancer, a major hazard to human health. Despite this, the majority of cancer-related deaths each year are caused by metastatic lung cancer. This study reported the use of RGD-functionalized-CD metal-organic framework (CDF) based NPs for co-delivering and doxorubicin (DOX) and heparin for cancer treatment, with regard to lung-targeting features. After intravenous treatment, RGD-CDF-LMWH NPs are effectively targeted for lung tumors; the accumulation of RCLD is 5.8 times more than that in the liver. Additionally, in B16F10 and A549 lung cancer transplanted-based murine models, respectively, RCLD dramatically reduces the tumor nodule count and area of dissemination of the lung and usually blocks the cancer extravasation–intravasation process across *in vitro–in vivo* mechanism [72].

The primary goal was to create an inhalable treatment that would use sulfobutylether-β-CD complexation to ameliorate water solubility and stability of resveratrol (RES). The stability of RES was significantly improved following host–guest complexation, as evidenced by a significantly extended half-life in stability experiments conducted in plasma and at pH 7.4. For effective deposition and pulmonary administration, CD-RES and the percentage mass median aerodynamic diameter were significantly increased [73]. Using poly(lactic-co-glycolic) (50:50, 25–35 kDa) nanoformulations is a technique for preventing and mitigating non-small cell lung cancer (NSCLC) that has developed erlotinib resistance. The findings showed that Erlo-CD-loaded NPs, with a size of 210 ± 8 nm, had a sustained release characteristic of around 5% loading efficiency and a 3-fold greater entrapment. The NPs showed markedly enhanced therapeutic efficiency against NSCLC cells, as evidenced by low IC50 values, decreased cancer cell colony formation, elevated apoptosis, and inhibition of autophagy. Remarkably, a 3D spheroid investigation showed that Erlo-CD NPs had superior antitumor efficacy compared to erlotinib alone. Despite this, research has demonstrated that modifying nanoErlo formulations can increase treatment efficacy against lung cancer that is resistant to erlotinib [74].

Another study demonstrated the creation of a CD-based nano-sponge (CD-NS) for quercitrin loading (QCT). The 2-hydroxypropyl-β-CD (2-HPβCD) and β-CD were cross-linked using diphenyl carbonate. Entrapment efficiency was generally found in the QCT-loaded CD-NS, ranging from 94.17 to 99.03%, with particle sizes from 97.10 to 325.90 nm. The findings, which hold biological importance, demonstrated unequivocally that the QCT IC50 values on human A549 cells and SARS-CoV-2 increased by 1.57- to 5.35-fold and 5.95- to 26.95-fold, respectively [75]. Paduraru *et al.* developed and unveiled that a permethyl-β-CD-camptothecin prodrug, a water-soluble adamantane–porphyrin complex, hyaluronic acid joined by triphenylphosphine, and β-CD through host–guest interaction properties are all present in CD prodrug supramolecular NPs. The porphyrin component of the well-designed system allows it to be readily occupied by the mitochondria of A549 cancer cells, which in turn releases active anticancer agents *in situ* and generates ROS when exposed to light. Furthermore, this study investigated the use of nanoassemblies, which showed synergistic chemo-photodynamic effects and offered a major and effective strategy against lung cancer [5].

According to Leclercq *et al.*, the porcupine inhibitor, or LGK974, is a new orally accessible cancer treatment currently undergoing clinical testing, complexed with CDs. This strategy made it possible to administer LGK974 more safely and repeatedly by mouth or intravenously, improving both its solubility and bioavailability process and lowering its toxicity in the Wnt signaling homeostasis process [76]. Another study examines how inclusion complexes with CDs can improve the solubility of Zn (DDC)2. The inclusion complexes were made with two types of beta-CDs: SBE-CD and HP-CD. After assessing phase solubility diagrams, the solutions were freeze-dried for further characterization by DSC, TGA, XRD, and FTIR. The MTT assay was used to assess the cytotoxicity of the generated inclusion complexes on human lung cancer cells. Adding beta-CDs considerably enhanced the solubility of Zn (DDC)2, reaching around 4 mg/mL in 20% w/w CD solutions. The Higuchi and Connors model indicated that Zn (DDC)2 has an Ap-type phase solubility diagram. Characterization tests revealed the presence of the amorphous drug in CD-Zn (DDC)2 complexes. The inclusion complexes significantly increased the cytotoxicity of Zn (DDC)2 by a factor of ten compared to the free drug. CD-Zn (DDC)2 inclusion complexes have the potential to treat lung cancer [77].

6.6.3 Esophageal Cancer

The curcumol–β-CD inclusion complex (CβC) was applied to EC cell lines, and its radiosensitizing activity was analyzed using targeted experimental procedures. A synergistic insight-based study of CβC and irradiation clearly demonstrated antiproliferative effects, decreased cellular colony formation, and increased apoptotic behavior compared to either compound alone, which counteracts the hypoxia-mediated radioresistance symptoms of EC cells. Under hypoxic conditions, the sensitization enhancement ratios (SERs) for TE-1 and ECA109 were 1.39 and 1.48, respectively. Under normoxia, the SERs for TE-1 and ECA109 were 1.25 and 1.32, respectively. When compared to either treatment alone, CβC and irradiation limited tumor growth to a maximum level [78]. Another study demonstrated that the cellular absorption of NPs was improved by CD-based polymers with hydrophobic arms and an acrylate group. At the optimal pH of 6, the groups can typically be protonated, which allows them to transfer the NPs from vesicles and use them as a platform for nanochemotherapeutics by releasing drugs intracellularly. Gadade *et al.* reviewed the possible impacts of CDs on the distribution of drugs across cellular membranes. By reducing the targeted drug's efflux, docetaxel/SBE-β-CD/CS NPs showed a considerable improvement in small intestine absorption and bioavailability profile [79].

In another instance, CDs were further used to transport siRNA to target tumor cells using an NP system composed of CD, polyethylene glycol, and transferrin as a targeting ligand. CDs function as polycations in the creation of NP for siRNA delivery, which additionally enables the assembly of nucleic acids of various sizes and types through electrostatic interactions. The primary purpose of nano-assembly production is to increase resistance against nuclease degradation. Findings from a phase 1 clinical study using this targeted treatment in the case of STs showed that there was a decrease in both protein RRM2 (M2 subunit of ribonucleotide reductase) and specific messenger RNA [80, 81]. One of the most promising natural products, curcumin, has been further developed into a water-soluble complex using HP-γ-CD encapsulated within CS NPs. According to the findings, this not only improves passive-targeting but also increases drug release and drug efficacy in the case of cancer cells. In another study, Hattori revealed the targeted CDs that had been altered with folic acid. Similarly, utilizing the folate receptor protein and Caco-2 cell layer model, the anticancer medication doxorubicin was used to demonstrate the targeting efficacy of CDs treated with folic acid. Erdogar *et al.* examined the use of CDs to target NPs [82]. An excellent investigation was conducted on the supramolecular assembly that uses sulfonato-β-CD-based polysaccharides (controlling technique) at different physiological pHs with balanced delivery of berberine. The sulfonato-β-CD-based carrier containing the natural compound berberine exhibits stability in the gastric environment and permits drug release at intestinal pH [83]. These previously mentioned recent results demonstrate how CD derivatives can be used to treat a variety of illnesses. A β-CD-based NP composition called CRLX 101 has been observed to be effective in treating a class of cancers, such as esophageal cancer [83]. Deng *et al.* developed a T7 peptide-modified pH-responsive nanosystem loaded with curcumin and docetaxel to treat esophageal cancer. This nanocarrier transports drugs in a pH-responsive way, improves cellular absorption, and inhibits growth in a KYSE150 esophageal cancer model. Additionally, the combination therapy demonstrated a synergistic anticancer effect, highlighting its potential for treating esophageal cancer [84].

6.6.4 Pancreatic Cancer

Pancreatic ductal adenocarcinoma (PDAC) is among the most frequent types of cancer, killing more people every year than lung and colorectal cancers. It is attributed to only 3% of all new cancer instances in the US, but it also causes more than 7% of all fatalities, with a survival rate after 5 years of less than 5% [85]. In pancreatic cancer, CD-based preparations have been documented for both oral and intravenous administration to facilitate the absorption and bioavailability of the targeted drug and prevent presystemic metabolism [71]. To improve the systemic distribution of new cancer therapy chemicals, such as derivatives of CD, many formulations have been created. Additionally, the CDF-β-CD inclusion complex (1:2) (CD-F-CD) formulation and characterization have been established. It was evident from the data that CDF-β-CD reduced the growth inhibitory effects by 50%, when analyzed across several human cancer cell lines. The pancreas was the site of preferential accumulation where animals exhibited levels of CDF-β-CD ten times higher than those found in serum [86]. As an additional illustration, bromelain is known to break down the extracellular matrix in malignant tissues and cells. However, the medication has a brief half-life in blood and little tissue accumulation. To address this, "PEGylation Retaining Activity for Self-assembly" was employed. In this method, adamantane-modified bromelain with multi-substituted-PEGylated β-CDs (β-CyDs) comprising 2 or 20 kDa PEG chains was combined with water to create the SPRA's more recent method using bromelain. Accumulation of fluorescein isothiocyanate (FITC)-dextran (2 MDa) in tumors was enhanced by the results, which also demonstrated high *in vitro* gelatin-degrading activity. Furthermore, intravenous administration of doxorubicin encapsulated in PEGylated liposomes (DOXIL) after tumor-bearing mice was shown to have antitumor activities *in vivo*. According to the findings, SPRA-bromelain may prove promising for distributing additional drugs to patients with pancreatic cancer [87].

Due to curcumin's low solubility in water, limited absorption, and poor biodistribution, its clinical relevance for treating PDAC is restricted. Significant progress has been made with the development of a difluorinated curcumin (CDF) derivative, which specifically accumulates in the pancreas and suppresses PDAC growth in both *in vitro* and *in vivo* models. Thus, the 2-hydroxy-propyl-β-CD (HCD) helps it to pass through biological barriers with greater hydrolytic stability and water solubility. Additionally, in PDAC cell lines, CDF and CDFHCD increased cell cycle and apoptosis and prevented colony and spheroid formation. According to the findings, CDFHCD self-assembly is a successful strategy for improving solubility and anticancer therapeutic efficacy, and it is being used to help PDAC patients reach a clinical proof of concept [88]. The carcinogenic effects of well-known CDs have been assessed in multiple mouse models using the oral route of β-CD and HP-β-CD. When mice were given doses (500–5,000 mg/kg/day of HP-β-CD orally) through diet, there was no discernible evidence of the drug's ability to cause cancer. On the other hand, in rat-based models, exocrine acinar cell neoplasia was found to significantly increase at 500, 2,000, and 5,000 mg/kg. In spite of this, there was also a little rise in large intestine neoplasms at 5,000 mg/kg. However, after a dose-dependent method of osmotically active foods, there was a major achievement of adaptive hypertrophy of the large intestines. Furthermore, after receiving HP-β-CD orally, rats' pancreas underwent notable changes that started off as exocrine pancreatic hyperplasia at 12 months and progressed to neoplasia by 24 months. The findings unequivocally demonstrated that in rat-based murine models, cholecystokinin (CCK) selectively induces hyperplasia in pancreatic acinar cells [89]. In another research, a CD-conjugated-α-bisabolol complex (CD-BSB) was shown to alter cytomorphological changes and cause apoptosis in pancreatic cancer cells. CD-BSB inhibited phosphorylation of focal adhesion kinase. CD-BSB inhibited pFAK 397 in cancer cells in a concentration-dependent manner. In subcutaneous xenograft models, CD-BSB groups showed decreased tumor volumes compared to controls. The CD-BSB-treated group showed fewer Ki67-positive cells than the GEM-treated group. In conclusion, these findings clarify the efficiency of CD [90].

6.6.5 Colorectal Cancer (CRC)

CRC is the second-leading cause of cancer-related deaths and the third most common type of cancer. Generally, it is considered a life-threatening type of illness. To improve health outcomes of CRC patients, it is imperative to enhance disease prevention or mitigation, identification, and therapy [71]. A β-CD-based composite was proposed and produced by Altoom *et al.* to administer the medication oxaliplatin. This study demonstrated a significant increase in the cytotoxic potential, showing significant cytotoxicity effects against HCT-116 cancer cells, and a targeted rheological behavior for chemotherapeutics as a healthier one and compared to normal CRC cells [91]. A supramolecular system based on poly(β-CD) has been created by Zhang *et al.* to deliver the prodrug Pt(IV)-ADA2. The results investigated the issues with nanocarrier DD, including prolonged blood circulation, tumor-specific accumulation, an effective therapeutic substance in case of cellular uptake of CT-26 cells, cell cycle arrest specificity procedures, and no other harmful effects [92]. Sun *et al.*'s research has also outlined several crucial steps in the use of delivery methods that target folate. More specifically, the authors created folate-targeted amphiphilic CD NPs modified by polyethylene glycol (PEG) and co-encapsulated the two promising natural compounds, quercetin and ginsenoside Rg3 (Rg3) (Figure 6.4). Thus, in a well-planned orthotopic CRC mouse model, the optimized and developed nanoformulation demonstrated notable effects in terms of better tumor targeting and prolonged blood circulation duration. Therefore, when combined with PD-L1 inhibitors, the treatment further prolonged the survival of mice, which clearly demonstrated the promise of this suggested DD method for the treatment of CRC [93]. Fai *et al.* suggested using a medication with a natural basis of tetrahydrocurcumin (THC) encapsulated within β-CD and further loaded into chitosan particles, i.e., inclusion complex (IC), to generate a new DD vehicle (THC IC-laden CPs). Furthermore, the THC IC-loaded CPs revealed an instantaneous cellular uptake and dose-dependent cytotoxic behavior when tested on Caco-2 cells [94].

In another investigation, Akkin *et al.* reported that 5-fluorouracil and interleukin-2 (IL-2) may be carried by a CD nanoplex that was created based on a charge interaction. When evaluated on CT-26 colorectal cancer cells, nanoplex-based drug loading clearly demonstrated profoundly better permeability and promising anticancer effects than a free form of the drug, displaying more than 80% in 12 hours. The study concluded that the delivery system's design and development represent a viable option for the advancement of cancer treatment since they provide a synergistic approach. In the event that there are health consequences from CRC, this additional co-transport of immunotherapeutic compounds and chemotherapeutic medications will protect healthy tissues from unintended harm [95]. In a different case study, Zou and colleagues suggested a folate-targeted delivery method. They have produced amphiphilic cationic CD-based NPs customized with PEGylated folate loaded with small interfering RNA (siRNA) and docetaxel. Subsequently, this dual-delivery system provided both gene therapy and chemotherapeutic activity specifically targeted to CRC cells. As a result, the design and created nanoformulation improved the drug's encapsulating apoptotic impact by expressing RelA. As a result, the previously noted effect of this nanosystem may considerably impede the growth of tumors without endangering healthy cells [96]. Regorafenib and γ-CD modified NPs with mannose have been reported by Bai *et al.* Furthermore, this has contributed to TME modulation and targeting. Nevertheless, by targeting macrophages, the NPs were able to reduce inflammatory pathways and prevent tumor-associated factors. Despite the potentiation of suppression of enzymatic kinases, this enhanced the anticancer activity of the included medication and shows potential as a focused and effective treatment for CRC [97].

In another research, an Oxa(IV) prodrug with anti-inflammatory effects (desmethyl naproxe, DN) and GSH-depleting CD pseudo-polyrotaxane carriers was synthesized and self-assembled into micellar NPs (DNPt@PPRI). The release of DN from DNPt@PPRI can reduce PGE2 levels, inhibiting inflammation and tumor spreading by decreasing COX-2 protein, and can also synergize with Oxa to inhibit tumor. More critically, GSH depletion can impair Oxa detoxification and thereby increase chemotherapy-induced apoptosis. DNPt@PPRI has a good GSH depletion ability to increase Oxa sensitivity, indicating a possibility for synergistic chemotherapy and chemosensitization of colorectal cancer [98]. Silibinin-loaded Zeinβ CD nanocarriers (SZBCNCs) were produced using progressive ultrasound homogenization and analyzed for zeta potential, DLS, FESEM, and FTIR. Finally, the selective toxicity of SZBCNCs and the mechanism of cellular death induction were investigated in HT29 and AGS cancer cells by assessing cell survival and apoptotic gene (Caspase 3, 9), which were confirmed by DAPI staining. Furthermore, the significant decrease in the IC50 concentrations of SZBCNCs among the HT29 and AGS cancer cell lines demonstrated their selective cytotoxicity. The enhanced apoptotic and downregulated necrotic (NFKB) gene expressions following SZBCNCs treatment dosages showed SZBCNCs' apoptotic activity, which was confirmed by the increased apoptotic morphology of DAPI-stained HT29 cancer cells. SZBCNCs are an effective anticolon cancer nanodelivery method due to their antioxidant and apoptotic properties. These strategies have the potential to be a safe and effective treatment for colon cancer. Additional research, particularly *in vivo* tests with animal cancer models, is needed [67].

6.6.6 Urinary Tract or Prostate Cancer (PC)

The most promising medications for healthy and adult patients with specific STs are those that target microtubules. Taccalonolide AJ (AJ) alleviates tubulin polymerization by adhering to protein covalently. This property makes it an important therapy tool for malignancies. By inducing cell cycle arrest, apoptosis, and blocking tumor cell invasion and migration process, the taccalonolide AJ-hydroxypropyl-β-CD (AJ-HP-β-CD) demonstrated selective activity toward the ccRCC cells 786-O compared to noncancerous hepatic cell lines, as demonstrated by the scientific investigation. The maximum tolerated dose of the targeted drug during acute toxicity testing was determined to be 10.71 mg/kg, which is approximately 20 times more than the selected single dose alone [99]. In the case of murine models, Wistar rats injected with 1,000 ppm of N-ethyl-N- hydroxyethyl nitrosamine (EHEN) showed a substantial increase in the number of renal cell tumors upon subcutaneous (s.c.) injection of β-CD. The results concluded that, after a 32-week trial, 50% of the rats treated with 1,000 ppm EHEN for two weeks and 100% of the rats treated with 1,000 ppm EHEN for two weeks, followed by daily subcutaneous injections of β-C for one week, developed kidney tumors. According to these findings, in a mouse model, β-C stimulates renal tubular cell carcinogenesis produced by EHEN [100].

TNFa and KC levels were reversed at both local and systemic levels by HP-β-CD in the poloxamer formulation. Histological analysis clearly demonstrated the infiltration of mononuclear cells into the lamina propria and urothelium, made possible by the poloxamer-HP-β-CD combination. In an orthotopic mouse bladder cancer model, the tumor burden in mice treated with R-837 was significantly lower than those in animals treated with vehicle or not treated at all [101]. Two CD-conjugated compounds, N,N′-Bis(6A-deoxy-γ-CD-6A-yl)succinamide (66γCD2su) and N,N′-bis(6A-deoxy-γ-CD-6A-yl)urea (66γCD2ur), were developed to effectively prevent the deprivation of curcumin. The findings showed that 66γCD2su and 66γCD2ur have the potential to be highly effective intracellular curcumin delivery agents for cancer cells. The curcumin–66γCD2su complex also effectively maintained the dose-dependent antiproliferative activity of curcumin in human PC (PC-3) cells. When comparing curcumin complexed with either 66γCD2su or 66γCD2ur to curcumin alone, we also found similar patterns of gene regulation in PC-3 cells. However, curcumin provided by either 66γCD2su or 66γCD2ur induces a somewhat higher upregulation of heme oxygenase-1 [102]. The primary challenge for the synthesis of complexes based on CD and medicinal preparations is the host–guest complexation, given the distinct structural features of CD. Sun's silicic acid-bound CD/CSF-1R siRNA supermolecule NPs are useful in the treatment of PC because they can specifically target siglec-1 (CD169), which is overexpressed by M2 macrophages. This targets the upregulated CSF-1/CSF-1R signaling pathway, which is linked to a poor prognosis for cancer patients [103].

The recent research reported a unique technique to treating prostate cancer using a nanocarrier consisting of folic acid (FA), β-cyclodextrin (β-CD), and magnetic graphene oxide (MGO) as a theranostic. The carrier is intended to boost curcumin's solubility and bioavailability as a potential prostate cancer treatment. Folic acid receptors overexpressed on the surfaces of solid tumors, including prostate cancer, may allow for targeted medication delivery to tumor cells while avoiding nonspecific effects on healthy tissues. Folic acid-curcumin@β-CD-MGO's anticancer activity was tested *in vitro* on LNCaP (androgen-dependent) and PC3 (androgen-independent) prostate cancer cells. The relaxivity of NPs in MRI images was also examined as a diagnostic parameter. The results revealed a concentration-dependent inhibitory effect on cell growth, oxidative damage, and apoptosis. Furthermore, resultant data suggest a prospective theranostic agent for improving curcumin administration and traceability while also increasing its therapeutic potential in the treatment of prostate cancer [104]. This study reports the development of a multivalent DD and targeting system using β-cyclodextrin perfunctionalized with dipeptide-like urea arms, a well-established mimic of a selective ligand against PSMA. Initially, fluorescein was utilized to validate the method on cells that express high amounts of PSMA (prostate tumoral cells, LNCap) or extremely low levels of PSMA (non-tumoral cells, Hek293T). The antineoplastic drug doxorubicin complexed with β-cyclodextrin functionalized with PSMA-like ligand induces cytotoxicity on LNCap cells faster than doxorubicin alone. This could be a promising DD strategy for selectively targeting prostate cancer cells [105].

6.6.7 Kidney Cancer

The most frequent type of primary kidney cancer is called hepatocellular carcinoma (HCC), which is also one of the deadliest cancers worldwide. Although chemotherapy remains the mainstay of cancer treatment, there are comparatively few licensed chemotherapeutic medicines for head and neck cancer. For this reason, it is vital to address developing and urgent therapies. According to Li *et al.* [106], the study found that the folate receptor (FR) is significantly expressed on the membrane of hepatic cancer cells. The FA-targeted PEGylated CD NP was utilized in this investigation to administer Melarsopol (MEL) to HCC in an optimal manner. Thus, in contrast to its non-targeted form (CD.MEL.PEG), the targeted nanoformulation (specifically CD.MEL.PEG-FA) achieved substantially promising cellular uptake, cell migration inhibition, cytotoxicity effects, and apoptotic cell death, thereby enabling the HCC-specific delivery of MEL *via* FR. When given intravenously to orthotopic HCC mice, the new medication dramatically slowed the growth of the tumors and extended the animals' lives without having any negative side effects [106]. In a separate investigation, Janssen's modified CD, HP-β-CD, and the polyanionic, variably substituted sulfobutyl ether of β-CD, SBE-β-CD (Captisol), were found to be non-nephrotoxic derivatives. The study showed that the complexes including SBE-β-CD and HP-β-CD with different medications rapidly dissociate following parenteral drug administration, do not cause any negative effects following intramuscular injection, and improve the bioavailability of oral weakly water-soluble pharmaceuticals. Some typical pharmacokinetics, biodistribution, and cellular effects of drugs have already been studied. Therefore, human experience with CD derivatives, in particular SBE-β-CD and HP-β-CD, shows that these two CDs, when administered orally or intravenously, are well tolerated and do not negatively affect the kidneys or other organs [89].

The capacity of PTX-modified solid lipid NPs (SLNs) with 2-hydroxypropyl-β-CD (HPCD) to improve medication absorption and lessen nephrotoxic effects when administered intravenously was examined. By heating and sonicating, PTX-loaded SLNs (PS) and PTX-loaded SLNs modified with HPCD (PSC) were created. The enhanced cellular uptake and anticancer activity in MCF-7 cells were demonstrated by the results. Furthermore, PSC was more bioavailable in rats than PTX solution following intravenous treatment; nevertheless, there were no appreciable variations in kidney damage [107]. In an additional investigation, a suitable quaterrylene bisimide derivative (QDI-CD) was developed through modification using permethyl-β-CD. QDI-CD, a biocompatible molecule, may be successfully excreted with a renal clearance efficiency of (67.00 ± 2.37)% after 24 hours as per the administration by tail-vein immunization. As a result, following metabolism, the QDI-CD remains unchanged in the case of urine. Moreover, QDI-CD demonstrated the effective PTT in a mouse-based model and, as a powerful photoacoustic-thermal candidate, could be efficiently enhanced in a tumor tissue-based model. This study examined a strong agent for renal clearance from the body and further use for potential clinical considerations [108]. Another study used 786-O cells to create xenografted mice to test the antitumor activity of AJ-hydroxypropyl-β-cyclodextrin (AJ-HP-β-CD) *in vivo*. Results showed that AJ-HP-β-CD outperformed docetaxel and sunitinib in terms of tumor growth and weight. These findings demonstrated that adding CD significantly enhanced AJ's antitumor therapeutic window. This work suggests that the AJ-HP-β-CD complex could be a promising tubulin stabilizer for treating clear-cell renal-cell carcinoma. Furthermore, this medication delivery technology has the potential to widen the scope of translational research into other chemotherapeutic medicines [99]. Despite the fact that a number of CD-based medications have been shown to be successful in treating cancer, their uses have been restricted due to their physicochemical characteristics, which include toxicity, poor water solubility, photolability, and an unpleasant smell. Numerous investigations on various CD-based chemotherapy drug carrier systems and their effects on human health are presented in this study.

6.7 Future Perspective/Direction

The potential features of CDs to form inclusion complexes with a variety of medications have reinforced efforts to develop more effective anticancer chemotherapeutic approaches. Consequently, a great deal of research has looked into the introduction of bioactive traditional medications into various cavities and examined their possible impacts against different cancer cell lines, either as *in vitro* or *in vivo* therapeutic options in numerous murine models. A variety of bioactive substances, including chemotherapeutic medications that have already been discussed in the study, have been loaded into CDs and their derivatives using various combinations of polymers. Additionally, the flexibility of CDs allows for the co-delivery of many biomolecules, with the goal of developing platform-based techniques that work synergistically across a wide range of therapeutic implications. Furthermore, functionalization with the host-to-guest molecules has enabled the designed nanocarriers to fix the appropriate dose at the targeted site with amelioration of the physical--chemical and as well as biopharmaceutical properties. The gap between DDD is growing larger by the day, as the quest for innovative medicinal chemicals becomes more time-consuming and much crucial due to the increase of chemical space. Artificial intelligence (AI) in medicinal chemistry has recently sparked widespread interest as a potential means of transforming the pharmaceutical industry. AI approaches, such as machine learning and natural language processing, have the potential to speed up and improve the medicine development process across numerous phases from zero to finished pharmaceutical products. AI-based technologies aid in drug development by identifying and validating drug targets, modeling medications, and improving druggability. Creating patient-centered clinical trials enhances decision-making processes.

Many drugs have been discovered to fail often in clinical trials. Every day, fewer drugs are released into the market. Certain drug products excel in clinical trials but face several challenges when they reach the market. As a result, a particular digital platform must be developed to handle these issues. While AI has numerous applications, there are currently no empirical data to justify its use in clinical research. AI plays a significant role in clinical research.

- It is influencing the parameters such as drug product success and failure rates.
- Reduced overall product development expenses.
- Shorter time for drug product to reach the market.
- Product recalls have decreased significantly.

6.8 Conclusion

CDs and their derivatives have already been used as pharmaceutical necessities for the last two to three decades. Broadly, these all are supramolecular assemblies used in a biomedical application. Nowadays, nanostructure-based strategies of CDs as a carrier used with pharmaceutical applications are majorly applied in terms of amelioration of physicochemical- to biopharmaceutical-based properties of bioactive natural molecules. Moreover, this is most widely accepted for DD in the case of numerous classes of tumors targeting consideration. As an interface of chemistry to biology, these CDs and their derivatives are most widely accepted to develop as self-assembly-based concerns with nanocarriers, such as NPs and others, to attach with host–guest interactions. This CD-based nanosized system further improves the drug release across biological barriers, pharmacokinetics, and bio-distribution in case of targeted DD across cancer. Despite this, systemic toxicity and mechanism of elimination must be required and further validated for candidate products. Recently, the production of CDs and their yield-based purity have become much more pronounced for the further development of the specified DD in the case of targeted cancer. Therefore, with these aforementioned challenges, the CD-based nanocarriers with reference to bioactive molecules in the case of controlled DD are still promising for designing and developing new pharmaceutical products.

Acknowledgments

The authors would like to thank Dr. Virendra M. Tiwari, director of the Council of Scientific and Industrial Research, Northeast Institute of Science and Technology (CSIR-NEIST), Jorhat, 785006, Assam, India, for his immense help, co-operation, fortitude, and sincere counsel to complete the manuscript. Without his healthy criticism and lively discussions, this work would not have emerged in the present form.

AI disclosure statement: The author acknowledges the use of AI-based tools for minor language editing or grammatical correction. However, all intellectual contributions, analyses, and conclusions presented in this chapter are entirely the author's own.

References

1. Gandhi, S.R., Quintans, J.D.S.S., *et al.*, The use of cyclodextrin inclusion complexes to improve anticancer drug profiles: a systematic review. *Expert Opin. Drug Deliv.*, 17, 1069–1080, 2020.
2. Kurkov, S.V. and Loftsson, T., Cyclodextrins. *Int. J. Pharm.*, 453, 167–180, 2013.
3. Santos, A.C., Costa, D., *et al.*, Cyclodextrin-based delivery systems for *in vivo*-tested anticancer therapies. *Drug Deliv. Transl. Res.*, 11, 49–71, 2021.
4. Merisko-Liversidge, E., Liversidge, G.G., *et al.*, Nanosizing: a formulation approach for poorly-water-soluble compounds. *Eur. J. Pharm. Sci.*, 18, 113–120, 2003.
5. Paduraru, D.N., Niculescu, A.G., *et al.*, An Updated Overview of Cyclodextrin-Based Drug Delivery Systems for Cancer Therapy. *Pharmaceutics*, 14, 1748, 2022.
6. Brewster, M.E. and Loftsson, T., Cyclodextrins as pharmaceutical solubilizers. *Adv. Drug Deliv. Rev.*, 59, 645–666, 2007.
7. Erdoğar, N. and Bilensoy, E., Cyclodextrin-Based Nanosystems in Targeted Cancer Therapy. in: *Cyclodextrin Applications in Medicine, Food, Environment and Liquid Crystals*. S. Fourmentin, G. Crini, E. Lichtfouse, (Eds),

Environmental Chemistry for a Sustainable World, vol. 17, pp. 59–80, Springer, Cham, 2018, doi: 10.1007/978-3-319-76162-6_3.
8. Vyas, K., Rathod, M., Patel, M.M., Insight on nano drug delivery systems with targeted therapy in treatment of oral cancer. *Nanomedicine*, 49, 102662, 2023.
9. Said Suliman, A., Khoder, A., *et al.*, Cyclodextrin Diethyldithiocarbamate Copper II Inclusion Complexes: A Promising Chemotherapeutic Delivery System against Chemoresistant Triple Negative Breast Cancer Cell Lines. *Pharmaceutics*, 13, 84, 2021.
10. Carneiro, S., Duarte, C., *et al.*, Cyclodextrin–Drug Inclusion Complexes: *In Vivo* and *In Vitro* Approaches. *Int. J. Mol. Sci.*, 20, 642, 2019.
11. Conceicao, J., Adeoye, O., *et al.*, Cyclodextrins as Drug Carriers in Pharmaceutical Technology: The State of the Art. *Curr. Pharm. Des.*, 24, 1405–1433, 2018.
12. Davis, M.E. and Brewster, M.E., Cyclodextrin-based pharmaceutics: past, present and future. *Nat. Rev. Drug Discov.*, 3, 1023–1035, 2004.
13. Gidwani, B. and Vyas, A.A., Comprehensive Review on Cyclodextrin-Based Carriers for Delivery of Chemotherapeutic Cytotoxic Anticancer Drugs. *Biomed Res. Int.*, 2015, 1–15, 2015.
14. Zhang, D., Lv, P., *et al.*, Cyclodextrin-based delivery systems for cancer treatment. *Mater. Sci. Eng.: C*, 96, 872–886, 2019.
15. Sanku, R.K.K., Karakus, O.O., *et al.*, Inclusion Complexes in Drug Delivery and Drug Targeting: Formation, Characterization, and Biological Applications. in: *Targeted Nanosystems for Therapeutic Applications: New Concepts, Dynamic Properties, Efficiency, and Toxicity.* Chapter 9, K. Sakurai, M.A. Ilies, (eds), pp. 187–221, ACS Publications, 2019, doi: 10.1021/bk-2019-1309.ch009.
16. Qiu, N., Li, X., Liu, J., Application of cyclodextrins in cancer treatment. *J. Incl. Phenom. Macrocycl. Chem.*, 89, 229–246, 2017.
17. Zhang, L., Man, S., *et al.*, Curcumin-cyclodextrin complexes enhanced the anti-cancer effects of curcumin. *Environ. Toxicol. Pharmacol.*, 48, 31–38, 2016.
18. Wang, L., Jiang, X., *et al.*, Complexation of tanshinone IIA with 2- hydroxypropyl-β-cyclodextrin: Effect on aqueous solubility, dissolution rate, and intestinal absorption behavior in rats. *Int. J. Pharm.*, 341, 58–67, 2007.
19. Oommen, E., Shenoy, B.D., *et al.*, Antitumour Efficacy of Cyclodextrin-complexed and Niosome-encapsulated Plumbagin in Mice Bearing Melanoma B16F1. *Pharm. Pharmacol. Commun.*, 5, 281–285, 1999.
20. Tanaka, T., De Azevedo, M.B.M., *et al.*, Colorectal cancer chemoprevention by 2 β-cyclodextrin inclusion compounds of auraptene and 4′-geranyloxyferulic acid. *Int. J. Cancer*, 126, 830–840, 2010.
21. Calleja, P., Espuelas, S., *et al.*, Pharmacokinetics and Antitumor Efficacy of Paclitaxel–Cyclodextrin Complexes Loaded in Mucus-Penetrating Nanoparticles for Oral Administration. *Nanomedicine*, 9, 2109–2121, 2014.

22. Shen, Q., Shen, Y., *et al.*, Paclitaxel/hydroxypropyl-β-cyclodextrin complex-loaded liposomes for overcoming multidrug resistance in cancer chemotherapy. *J. Liposome Res.*, 30, 12–20, 2020.
23. Guimaraes, P.P.G., Tan, M., *et al.*, Potent *in vivo* lung cancer Wnt signaling inhibition *via* cyclodextrin-LGK974 inclusion complexes. *J. Control. Release*, 290, 75–87, 2018.
24. Gaur, S., Chen, L., *et al.*, Preclinical study of the cyclodextrin-polymer conjugate of camptothecin CRLX101 for the treatment of gastric cancer. *Nanomedicine*, 8, 721–730, 2012.
25. Hyun, H., Lee, S., *et al.*, Engineered beta-cyclodextrin-based carrier for targeted doxorubicin delivery in breast cancer therapy *in vivo*. *J. Ind. Eng. Chem.*, 70, 145–151, 2019.
26. Ray, S., Roy, N., *et al.*, Synthesis and Characterization of an Inclusion Complex of dl- Aminoglutethimide with β-Cyclodextrin and Its Innovative Application in a Biological System: Computational and Experimental Investigations. *ACS Omega*, 7, 11208–11216, 2022.
27. Dam, H.H. and Caruso, F., Modular Click Assembly of Degradable Capsules Using Polyrotaxanes. *ACS Nano*, 6, 4686–4693, 2012.
28. Irie, T. and Uekama, K., Pharmaceutical Applications of Cyclodextrins. III, Toxicological Issues and Safety Evaluation. *J. Pharm. Sci.*, 86, 147–162, 1997.
29. Wei, H. and Yu, C., Cyclodextrin-functionalized polymers as drug carriers for cancer therapy. *Biomater. Sci.*, 3, 1050–1060, 2015.
30. Velhal, K., Barage, S., *et al.*, A Promising Review on Cyclodextrin Conjugated Paclitaxel Nanoparticles for Cancer Treatment. *Polymers (Basel)*, 14, 3162, 2022.
31. Tong, F., Zhou, Y., *et al.*, Supramolecular nanomedicines based on host–guest interactions of cyclodextrins. *Exploration*, 3, 20210111, 2023.
32. Singh, J., Dhamija, I., *et al.*, Chronicle updates in cyclodextrin-based carriers for drug delivery. *Bull. Natl. Res. Cent.*, 46, 202, 2022.
33. Golhen, K., Buettcher, M., *et al.*, Meeting Challenges of Pediatric Drug Delivery: The Potential of Orally Fast Disintegrating Tablets for Infants and Children. *Pharmaceutics*, 15, 1033, 2023.
34. Comoglu, T. and Dilek Ozyilmaz, E., Orally disintegrating tablets and orally disintegrating mini tablets – novel dosage forms for pediatric use. *Pharm. Dev. Technol.*, 24, 902–914, 2019.
35. Rasheed, A., Cyclodextrins as Drug Carrier Molecule: A Review. *Sci. Pharm.*, 76, 567–598, 2008.
36. Shin, S., Kim, T.H., *et al.*, Development of a gastroretentive delivery system for acyclovir by 3D printing technology and its *in vivo* pharmacokinetic evaluation in Beagle dogs. *PLoS One*, 14, e0216875, 2019.
37. Godge, G.R., Hiremath, S., *et al.*, Pharmaceutical Advances in Cyclodextrin Inclusion Complexes for Improved Bioavailability of Poorly-Soluble Drugs. *Int. J. Pharm. Sci. Nanotechnol.*, 8, 2894–2905, 2015.

38. Biro, T. and Aigner, Z., Current Approaches to Use Cyclodextrins and Mucoadhesive Polymers in Ocular Drug Delivery—A Mini-Review. *Sci. Pharm.*, 87, 15, 2019.
39. Mahmoud, A.A., El-Feky, G.S., *et al.*, Chitosan/sulfobutylether- β-cyclodextrin nanoparticles as a potential approach for ocular drug delivery. *Int. J. Pharm.*, 413, 229–236, 2011.
40. Thakur, A., Jain, S., *et al.*, Cyclodextrin Derivative Enhances the Ophthalmic Delivery of Poorly Soluble Azithromycin. *ACS Omega*, 7, 23050–23060, 2022.
41. Grassiri, B., Knoll, P., *et al.*, Thiolated Hydroxypropyl-β-cyclodextrin: A Potential Multifunctional Excipient for Ocular Drug Delivery. *Int. J. Mol. Sci.*, 23, 2612, 2022.
42. Jacob, S. and Nair, A.B., Cyclodextrin complexes: Perspective from drug delivery and formulation. *Drug Dev. Res.*, 79, 201–217, 2018.
43. Gavini, E., Rassu, G., *et al.*, Mucoadhesive microspheres for nasal administration of cyclodextrins. *J. Drug Target.*, 17, 168–179, 2009.
44. Di Gioia, S., Trapani, A., *et al.*, Intranasal delivery of dopamine to the striatum using glycol chitosan/sulfobutylether-β-cyclodextrin based nanoparticles. *Eur. J. Pharm. Biopharm.*, 94, 180–193, 2015.
45. Yang, P., Li, Y., *et al.*, Preparation and evaluation of carfentanil nasal spray employing cyclodextrin inclusion technology. *Drug Dev. Ind. Pharm.*, 44, 953–960, 2018.
46. Sherje, A.P. and Londhe, V., Development and Evaluation of pH-Responsive Cyclodextrin-Based *in situ* Gel of Paliperidone for Intranasal Delivery. *AAPS PharmSciTech*, 19, 384–394, 2018.
47. Kulkarni, J.A. and Avachat, A.M., Pharmacodynamic and pharmacokinetic investigation of cyclodextrin-mediated asenapine maleate *in situ* nasal gel for improved bioavailability. *Drug Dev. Ind. Pharm.*, 43, 234–245, 2017.
48. Rassu, G., Sorrenti, M., *et al.*, Versatile Nasal Application of Cyclodextrins: Excipients and/or Actives. *Pharmaceutics*, 13, 1180, 2021.
49. Jambhekar, S.S. and Breen, P., Cyclodextrins in pharmaceutical formulations I: structure and physicochemical properties, formation of complexes, and types of complex. *Drug Discov. Today*, 21, 356–362, 2016.
50. Haschke, M., Suter, K., *et al.*, Pharmacokinetics and pharmacodynamics of nasally delivered midazolam. *Br. J. Clin. Pharmacol.*, 69, 607–616, 2010.
51. Vaka, S.R.K., Murthy, S.N., *et al.*, Upregulation of Endogenous Neurotrophin Levels in the Brain by Intranasal Administration of Carnosic Acid. *J. Pharm. Sci.*, 100, 3139–3145, 2011.
52. Giuliani, A., Balducci, A.G., *et al.*, *In vivo* nose-to-brain delivery of the hydrophilic antiviral ribavirin by microparticle agglomerates. *Drug Deliv.*, 25, 376–387, 2018.
53. Chen, W., Li, R., *et al.*, Nasal timosaponin BII dually sensitive *in situ* hydrogels for the prevention of Alzheimer's disease induced by lipopolysaccharides. *Int. J. Pharm.*, 578, 119115, 2020.

54. Qu, Y., Sun, X., *et al.*, Therapeutic effect of disulfiram inclusion complex embedded in hydroxypropyl-β-cyclodextrin on intracranial glioma-bearing male rats *via* intranasal route. *Eur. J. Pharm. Sci.*, 156, 105590, 2021.
55. Kear, C.L., Yang, J., *et al.*, Investigation into the Mechanism by Which Cyclodextrins Influence Transdermal Drug Delivery. *Drug Dev. Ind. Pharm.*, 34, 692–697, 2008.
56. Taguchi, H., Tanaka, H., *et al.*, Application of Pickering Emulsion with Cyclodextrin as an Emulsifier to a Transdermal Drug Delivery Vehicle. *Biol. Pharm. Bull.*, 42, 116–122, 2019.
57. Maestrelli, F., González-Rodríguez, M.L., *et al.*, Preparation and characterisation of liposomes encapsulating ketoprofen–cyclodextrin complexes for transdermal drug delivery. *Int. J. Pharm.*, 298, 55–67, 2005.
58. Ghanghoria, R., Kesharwani, P., *et al.*, Transdermal delivery of cyclodextrin-solubilized curcumin. *Drug Deliv. Transl. Res.*, 3, 272–285, 2013.
59. Loftsson, T. and Masson, M., Cyclodextrins in topical drug formulations: theory and practice. *Int. J. Pharm.*, 225, 15–30, 2001.
60. Ding, Z., Wu, M., *et al.*, Encapsulation of a Flavonoid-rich Allium cepa L. var. *agrogatum* Don Extract in β-Cyclodextrin for Transdermal Drug Delivery. *J. Agric. Food Chem.*, 61, 4914–4920, 2013.
61. Taveira, S.F., Varela-Garcia, A., *et al.*, Cyclodextrin-based poly(pseudo) rotaxanes for transdermal delivery of carvedilol. *Carbohydr. Polym.*, 200, 278–288, 2018.
62. Mura, P., Bragagni, M., *et al.*, Development of liposomal and microemulsion formulations for transdermal delivery of clonazepam: Effect of randomly methylated β-cyclodextrin. *Int. J. Pharm.*, 475, 306–314, 2014.
63. Shahiwala, A., Cyclodextrin conjugates for colon drug delivery. *J. Drug Deliv. Sci. Technol.*, 55, 101448, 2020.
64. Yang, B., Zhao, Y.L., *et al.*, Scutellarin-cyclodextrin conjugates: Synthesis, characterization and anticancer activity. *Carbohydr. Polym.*, 92, 1308–1314, 2013.
65. Jiang, R., Zhao, Y., *et al.*, Synthesis, characterization, and *in vitro* evaluation of artesunate-β- cyclodextrin conjugates as novel anti-cancer prodrugs. *Carbohydr. Res.*, 400, 19–25, 2014.
66. Haimhoffer, A., Rusznyak, A., *et al.*, Cyclodextrins in Drug Delivery Systems and Their Effects on Biological Barriers. *Sci. Pharm.*, 87, 33, 2019.
67. Al Alabdullah, M.A.A., Goodarzi, M.T., *et al.*, The silibinin-loaded Zein-β cyclodextrin nano-carriers (SZBC-NCs) as a novel selective cancer cell drug delivery system in HT-29 cell line. *Sci. Rep.*, 14, 14769, 2024.
68. Alboabdullah, A.K.A., Goodarzi, M.T., *et al.*, The Lawson-loaded β-cyclodextrin nanocarriers (LB-NCs) a novel targeted cancer cell in stomach and breast cancer as a drug delivery system. *Naunyn Schmiedebergs Arch. Pharmacol.*, 397, 6623–6631, 2024, doi: 10.1007/s00210-024-03042-6.
69. Simões, S.M.N., Rey-Rico, A., *et al.*, Supramolecular cyclodextrin-based drug nanocarriers. *Chem. Commun.*, 51, 6275–6289, 2015.

70. Adeoye, O. and Cabral-Marques, H., Cyclodextrin nanosystems in oral drug delivery: A mini review. *Int. J. Pharm.*, 531, 521–531, 2017.
71. Najm, A., Niculescu, A.G., *et al.*, Chitosan and Cyclodextrins—Versatile Materials Used to Create Drug Delivery Systems for Gastrointestinal Cancers. *Pharmaceutics*, 16, 43, 2023.
72. He, Y., Xiong, S., *et al.*, Pulmonary Targeting Crosslinked Cyclodextrin Metal–Organic Frameworks for Lung Cancer Therapy. *Adv. Funct. Mater.*, 31, 2004550, 2021.
73. Wang, X., Parvathaneni, V., *et al.*, Cyclodextrin Complexation for Enhanced Stability and Non-invasive Pulmonary Delivery of Resveratrol—Applications in Non-small Cell Lung Cancer Treatment. *AAPS PharmSciTech*, 21, 183, 2020.
74. Vaidya, B., Parvathaneni, V., *et al.*, Cyclodextrin modified erlotinib loaded PLGA nanoparticles for improved therapeutic efficacy against non-small cell lung cancer. *Int. J. Biol. Macromol.*, 122, 338–347, 2019.
75. Abou Taleb, S., Moatasim, Y., *et al.*, Quercitrin loaded cyclodextrin based nanosponge as a promising approach for management of lung cancer and COVID-19. *J. Drug Deliv. Sci. Technol.*, 77, 103921, 2022.
76. Leclercq, L., Interactions between cyclodextrins and cellular components: Towards greener medical applications. *Beilstein J. Org. Chem.*, 12, 2644–2662, 2016.
77. Kaya, A., Arafat, B., *et al.*, Preparation and characterisation of zinc diethyldithiocarbamate–Cyclodextrin inclusion complexes for potential lung cancer treatment. *Pharmaceutics*, 16, 1–14, 2024.
78. Su, M., Ren, X., *et al.*, Curcumol β-cyclodextrin inclusion complex enhances radiosensitivity of esophageal cancer under hypoxic and normoxic condition. *Jpn. J. Radiol.*, 41, 1275–1289, 2023.
79. Gadade, D.D. and Pekamwar, S.S., Cyclodextrin Based Nanoparticles for Drug Delivery and Theranostics. *Adv. Pharm. Bull.*, 10, 166–183, 2020.
80. Davis, M.E., Zuckerman, J.E., *et al.*, Evidence of RNAi in humans from systemically administered siRNA *via* targeted nanoparticles. *Nature*, 464, 1067–1070, 2010.
81. Davis, M.E., The First Targeted Delivery of siRNA in Humans *via* a Self-Assembling, Cyclodextrin Polymer-Based Nanoparticle: From Concept to Clinic. *Mol. Pharm.*, 6, 659–668, 2009.
82. Erdogar, N., Varan, G., *et al.*, Cyclodextrin-based polymeric nanosystems, in: *Drug Targeting and Stimuli Sensitive Drug Delivery Systems*, pp. 715–748, 2018.
83. Chen, X.M., Chen, Y., *et al.*, Sulfonato-β-Cyclodextrin Mediated Supramolecular Nanoparticle for Controlled Release of Berberine. *ACS Appl. Mater. Interfaces*, 10, 24987–24992, 2018.
84. Deng, L., Zhu, X., *et al.*, Novel T7-Modified pH-Responsive Targeted Nanosystem for Co-Delivery of Docetaxel and Curcumin in the Treatment of Esophageal Cancer. *Int. J. Nanomed.*, 15, 7745–7762, 2020.

85. Iacobazzi, R.M., Cutringnelli, A., *et al.*, Hydroxy-Propil-β-Cyclodextrin Inclusion Complexes of two Biphenylnicotinamide Derivatives: Formulation and Anti-Proliferative Activity Evaluation in Pancreatic Cancer Cell Models. *Int. J. Mol. Sci.*, 21, 6545, 2020.
86. Dandawate, P.R., Vyas, A., *et al.*, Inclusion Complex of Novel Curcumin Analogue CDF and β- Cyclodextrin (1:2) and Its Enhanced *In Vivo* Anticancer Activity Against Pancreatic Cancer. *Pharm. Res.*, 29, 1775–1786, 2012.
87. Higashi, T., Kogo, T., *et al.*, Efficient Anticancer Drug Delivery for Pancreatic Cancer Treatment Utilizing Supramolecular Polyethylene-Glycosylated Bromelain. *ACS Appl. Bio Mater.*, 3, 3005–3014, 2020.
88. Bhattacharyya, S., Ghosh, H., *et al.*, Anticancer Activity of Novel Difluorinated Curcumin Analog and Its Inclusion Complex with 2-Hydroxypropyl-β-Cyclodextrin against Pancreatic Cancer. *Int. J. Mol. Sci.*, 24, 6336, 2023.
89. Stella, V.J. and He, Q., Cyclodextrins. *Toxicol. Pathol.*, 36, 30–42, 2008.
90. Kano, M.T., Kokuryo, T., *et al.*, Cyclodextrin conjugated α-Bisabolol suppresses FAK phosphorylation and induces apoptosis in pancreatic cancer. *Anticancer Res.*, 43, 1009–1016, 2023.
91. Altoom, N., Ibrahim, H.M., *et al.*, Characterization of β-cyclodextrin/phillipsite (β-CD/Ph) composite as a potential carrier for oxaliplatin as therapy for colorectal cancer; loading, release, and cytotoxicity. *Colloids Surf. A Physicochem. Eng. Asp.*, 648, 129144, 2022.
92. Zhang, R., You, X., *et al.*, Poly(β-cyclodextrin)/platinum prodrug supramolecular nano system for enhanced cancer therapy: Synthesis and *in vivo* study. *Carbohydr. Polym.*, 292, 119695, 2022.
93. Sun, D., Zou, L., *et al.*, A cyclodextrin-based nanoformulation achieves co-delivery of ginsenoside Rg3 and quercetin for chemo-immunotherapy in colorectal cancer. *Acta Pharm. Sin. B*, 12, 378–393, 2022.
94. Fai, T.K., Yee, G.H., *et al.*, Preparation of Chitosan Particles as a Delivery System for Tetrahydrocurcumin: β-cyclodextrin Inclusive Compound for Colorectal Carcinoma. *Curr. Drug Ther.*, 16, 430–438, 2021.
95. Akkın, S., Varan, G., *et al.*, A different approach to immunochemotherapy for colon Cancer: Development of nanoplexes of cyclodextrins and Interleukin-2 loaded with 5-FU. *Int. J. Pharm.*, 623, 121940, 2022.
96. Zou, Y., Xiao, F., *et al.*, A folate-targeted PEGylated cyclodextrin-based nanoformulation achieves co-delivery of docetaxel and siRNA for colorectal cancer. *Int. J. Pharm.*, 606, 120888, 2021.
97. Bai, H., Wang, J., *et al.*, Cyclodextrin-based host-guest complexes loaded with regorafenib for colorectal cancer treatment. *Nat. Commun.*, 12, 759, 2021.
98. Wang, W., He, X., *et al.*, Glutathione-depleted cyclodextrin pseudo-polyrotaxane nanoparticles for anti-inflammatory oxaliplatin (IV) prodrug delivery and enhanced colorectal cancer therapy. *Chin. Chem. Lett.*, 35, 108656, 2024.

99. Han, J., Zhang, S., *et al.*, Development of Taccalonolide AJ-Hydroxypropyl-β-Cyclodextrin Inclusion Complexes for Treatment of Clear Cell Renal-Cell Carcinoma. *Molecules*, 25, 5586, 2020.
100. Hiyasa, Y., Ohshima, M., *et al.*, β-Cyclodextrin: Promoting Effect on the Development of Renal Tubular Cell Tumors in Rats Treated With N-Ethyl-N-hydroxyethylnitrosamine. *JNCI: J. Natl. Cancer Inst.*, 4, 963–967, 1982.
101. Hayashi, T., Crain, B., *et al.*, Intravesical Toll-like receptor 7 agonist R-837: Optimization of its formulation in an orthotopic mouse model of bladder cancer. *Int. J. Urol.*, 17, 483–490, 2010.
102. Harada, T., Giorgio, L., *et al.*, Diamide Linked γ-Cyclodextrin Dimers as Molecular-Scale Delivery Systems for the Medicinal Pigment Curcumin to Prostate Cancer Cells. *Mol. Pharm.*, 10, 4481–4490, 2013.
103. Wei, X., Yu, C.Y., *et al.*, Application of Cyclodextrin for Cancer Immunotherapy. *Molecules*, 28, 5610, 2023.
104. Einafshar, E., Javid, H., *et al.*, Curcumin loaded β-cyclodextrin-magnetic graphene oxide nanoparticles decorated with folic acid receptors as a new theranostic agent to improve prostate cancer treatment. *Carbohydr. Polym.*, 340, 122328, 2024.
105. Imperio, D., Grolla, A.A., *et al.*, Functionalization of β-cyclodextrin with a urea-based PSMA ligand and preliminary studies on targeting prostate cancer cells. *Bioorg. Med. Chem. Lett.*, 73, 128890, 2022.
106. Li, Y.N., Li, X., *et al.*, Delivery of melarsoprol using folate-targeted PEGylated cyclodextrin- based nanoparticles for hepatocellular carcinoma. *Int. J. Pharm.*, 636, 122791, 2023.
107. Cho, C.W., Baek, J.S., *et al.*, Modification of paclitaxel-loaded solid lipid nanoparticles with 2-hydroxypropyl-β-cyclodextrin enhances absorption and reduces nephrotoxicity associated with intravenous injection. *Int. J. Nanomed.*, 10, 5397–5405, 2015.
108. Luo, Y.L., Rong, R.X., *et al.*, Effective Renal Clearance and Photothermal Therapy of a Cyclodextrin- Modified Quaterrylene Derivative. *ACS Appl. Bio Mater.*, 3, 3390–3400, 2020.

7

Hyaluronic Acid: Targeted Delivery Strategies for Anticancer Agents

Atharva Anand Mahajan[1†], Gauri Panzade[1†], Souhardya Bandyopadhyay[2] and Subhrojyoti Ghosh[3*]

[1]*Advance Centre for Treatment Research and Education in Cancer, Navi Mumbai, India*
[2]*School of Biosciences and Bioengineering, Indian Institute of Technology Mandi, Himachal Pradesh, India*
[3]*Infection Biology Group, Centre for Cellular and Molecular Biology, Hyderabad, Telangana, India*

Abstract

Hyaluronic acid (HA) has garnered significant interest as a multifaceted biomaterial for the targeted delivery of anticancer agents, attributed to its unique characteristics and the frequent overexpression of its receptors in various cancer cells. This chapter delves into recent advancements and potential applications of HA-based delivery platforms in oncology. HA, a naturally occurring polysaccharide in the extracellular matrix, offers several benefits that render it an optimal drug delivery carrier. Its high biocompatibility, biodegradability, and non-immunogenic nature make it suitable for numerous biomedical uses. HA can specifically bind to CD44 receptors, commonly overexpressed on cancer cell surfaces, facilitating targeted delivery of therapeutic agents to tumors and minimizing off-target impacts. A notable advantage of HA-based systems is their capacity to enhance the solubility and stability of hydrophobic anticancer drugs. By conjugating hydrophobic drugs with HA, HA–drug complexes have been developed to protect and encapsulate the drugs, thus improving their bioavailability and pharmacokinetics. Additionally, HA provides a versatile framework for delivering various anticancer agents, including small molecule drugs, nucleic acids (such as siRNA and miRNA), and nanoparticles (like liposomes and polymeric nanoparticles). The targeting mechanisms of HA-based delivery systems

**Corresponding author*: subhrojyotighosh8@gmail.com
†First two authors have equal contribution

Luqman Jameel Rather, Showkat Ali Ganie and Mohammed A. Assiri (eds.) Polysaccharide Biomaterials in Cancer Research and Therapy: From Lab to Life, (193–222) © 2026 Scrivener Publishing LLC

are intricate. Through binding to CD44 receptors on cancer cells, HA triggers receptor-mediated endocytosis, allowing intracellular drug release and subsequent cytotoxic effects. Moreover, HA exploits tumor-specific features, including heightened vascular permeability and inadequate lymphatic drainage, to accumulate in tumors *via* the enhanced permeability and retention effect. HA-based nanoparticles can be further functionalized with targeting ligands or imaging agents to enhance tumor specificity and facilitate real-time tracking of drug delivery and therapeutic outcomes. Preclinical research has demonstrated that HA-based delivery systems can augment the therapeutic efficacy of anticancer agents while reducing toxicity. Clinical trials with HA-based drugs have yielded promising outcomes, indicating their potential for clinical use. Nonetheless, challenges persist in optimizing the pharmacokinetics, biodistribution, tumor penetration, and cellular uptake, as well as addressing immunogenicity and clearance concerns. In summary, HA-based delivery systems hold substantial promise for revolutionizing cancer treatment by enabling more precise therapies. By harnessing HA's properties and its interactions with the tumor microenvironment, researchers can innovate drug delivery systems that enhance efficacy, minimize side effects, and ultimately improve patient outcomes in cancer therapy.

***Keywords*:** Hyaluronic acid, anticancer agents, targeted drug delivery, CD44 receptors, tumor targeting, nanoparticles

7.1 Introduction

7.1.1 Overview of Cancer and the Need for Targeted Therapies

Cancer is a group of diseases marked by the unregulated growth of cells, which can invade other areas of the body, making it one of the most challenging and deadly health issues globally. In 2020, around 19.3 million new cases of cancer were reported, with nearly 10 million deaths resulting from the disease globally [1]. These striking numbers underscore the persistent public health challenge that cancer represents, emphasizing the critical need for improved treatment strategies. The conventional approaches to cancer treatment—surgery, chemotherapy, and radiation—are often limited by their non-specific nature, which can lead to significant side effects and damage to healthy tissues. Chemotherapy involves the systemic use of cytotoxic drugs that target rapidly dividing cells, affecting both cancerous and healthy ones. This non-selective action diminishes its therapeutic effectiveness and causes significant side effects, including immunosuppression, organ damage, and severe gastrointestinal issues [2]. Moreover, the development of drug resistance, tumor heterogeneity, and poor drug penetration into tumor tissues further complicates treatment outcomes with traditional therapies. Given these limitations, targeted therapies have emerged as a promising alternative in the treatment of cancer. Targeted therapies are designed to specifically identify and attack cancer cells while sparing normal, healthy cells, thereby reducing systemic toxicity [3]. These treatments typically target molecular markers or pathways that are distinctly altered or overexpressed in cancer cells, such as certain proteins, receptors, or genes associated with tumor development and progression. For instance, therapies aimed at the human epidermal growth factor receptor 2 (HER2) have been highly effective in treating HER2-positive breast cancer by specifically blocking the growth of cancer cells that have an overabundance of this receptor [4]. Targeted drug delivery, in particular, has gained significant traction as it enhances the precision of drug delivery by exploiting unique features of the tumor microenvironment or cancer-specific markers. Nanocarrier systems, including liposomes, nanoparticles, and micelles, are developed to transport therapeutic agents directly to tumor cells, typically utilizing receptor-mediated pathways or passive targeting through the enhanced permeability and retention (EPR) effect [5]. These can encapsulate various types of drugs—chemotherapeutics, immunotherapies, or gene therapies—providing controlled release and minimizing off-target effects.

7.1.2 The Importance of Targeted Drug Delivery in Reducing Side Effects and Improving Treatment Efficiency

One of the significant limitations of conventional cancer therapies, particularly chemotherapy, is their lack of selectivity, which results in substantial damage to healthy cells alongside cancer cells [6]. Traditional chemotherapy drugs are designed to target rapidly dividing cells, a hallmark of cancer. However, they also affect other healthy tissues that divide quickly, such as the bone marrow, gastrointestinal tract, and hair follicles. This lack of specificity results in significant side effects, including immunosuppression, nausea, hair loss, and organ damage, which not only diminish the patient's quality of life but also restrict the safe dosage of these drugs. Targeted drug delivery systems (DDS) aim to address these obstacles by directing therapeutic agents specifically to cancer cells, reducing harm to healthy tissues. This precise targeting is accomplished through various mechanisms, such as receptor-mediated endocytosis, which delivers drugs to cells with an abundance of certain receptors, or passive targeting, which leverages the EPR effect in tumors. The EPR effect describes the accumulation of nanoparticles in tumor tissues due to their leaky blood vessels and inadequate lymphatic drainage, enabling localized drug delivery [7]. Targeted delivery systems enhance the effectiveness of anticancer drugs by concentrating them at the tumor site. This approach allows for higher drug concentrations at the intended location, boosting the drug's capacity to destroy cancer cells while minimizing the exposure of healthy tissues to harmful substances. This strategy is especially critical for drugs with narrow therapeutic windows, where the margin between a beneficial dose and a toxic one is very slim. For example, liposomal formulations of doxorubicin (such as Doxil) have demonstrated improved efficacy and reduced cardiotoxicity compared to conventional doxorubicin due to the ability of the liposomes to selectively accumulate in tumors *via* the EPR effect [8].

Targeted DDS reduce side effects while boosting therapeutic efficacy by optimizing the pharmacokinetics and bioavailability of medications. Numerous anticancer drugs encounter obstacles such as low solubility, quick elimination from the bloodstream, or instability in biological environments. Nanocarrier-based systems, such as liposomes, nanoparticles, and micelles, protect drugs from premature breakdown, prolong their circulation in the body, and facilitate controlled, sustained release at tumor sites, thereby preserving the drug's activity over an extended duration [9, 10]. Moreover, targeted delivery can help mitigate the development of drug resistance, which is a significant challenge in cancer treatment. Resistance often develops when drug concentrations at the tumor site are insufficient, allowing some cancer cells to survive and adapt to the therapy. By ensuring higher drug concentrations are delivered directly to the tumor, targeted systems can decrease the chances of resistant cells emerging, thereby enhancing overall treatment efficacy.

7.1.3 Introduction to Hyaluronic Acid as a Biocompatible and Versatile Polymer for Drug Delivery

Hyaluronic acid (HA) is a naturally occurring linear polysaccharide composed of repeating disaccharide units of D-glucuronic acid and N-acetyl-D-glucosamine [11]. HA is a key component of the extracellular matrix (ECM) in connective tissues, playing a crucial role in maintaining tissue hydration, elasticity, and structural integrity. Its distinctive physicochemical and biological properties have made HA a highly regarded biocompatible and versatile polymer for use in DDS [12]. One of the main benefits of HA in drug delivery is its outstanding biocompatibility. Being a naturally occurring component in the human body, HA is non-immunogenic, non-toxic, and biodegradable, making it an excellent vehicle for therapeutic agents.

When administered, HA is broken down by hyaluronidases or through free radical-induced degradation, ensuring it is safely cleared from the body without causing harmful immune reactions [12]. These qualities make HA especially ideal for repeated or extended therapeutic applications. HA's high water-binding capacity enables it to form hydrogels and other structures that can encapsulate a diverse range of drugs, including small-molecule chemotherapeutics, proteins, peptides, and nucleic acids [13]. This versatility in drug loading has led to the development of various HA-based DDS, such as nanoparticles, micelles, liposomes, and hydrogels, which can be designed to deliver drugs in a controlled, sustained, and targeted manner [14].

A critical feature of HA in cancer therapy is its ability to target cancer cells through its interaction with the CD44 receptor, which is overexpressed on the surface of many tumor cells, including those in breast, ovarian, lung, and colon cancers [15]. This receptor-mediated targeting allows HA-based DDS to accumulate in tumor tissues, enhancing drug delivery specificity and reducing off-target effects. In addition to CD44, HA can also bind to other receptors, such as RHAMM (receptor for hyaluronan-mediated

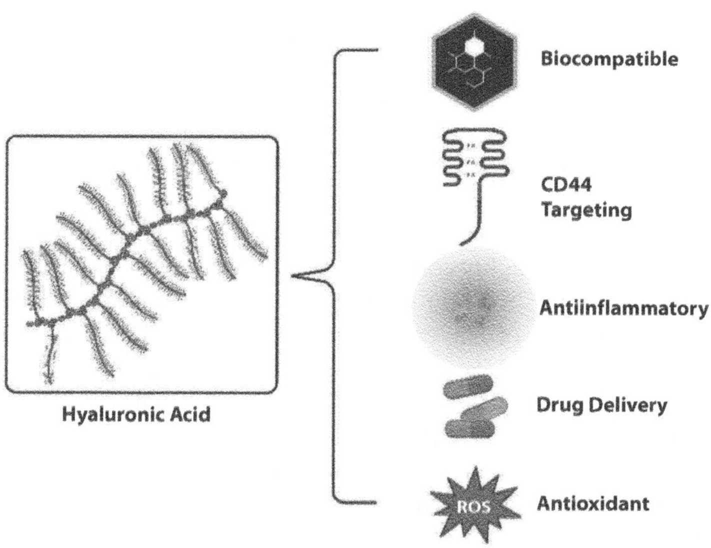

Figure 7.1 HA possesses antioxidant and anti-inflammatory properties. It is biocompatible and can target CD44 receptors. these characteristics make it a valuable tool for drug delivery applications.

motility), expanding its potential for targeted delivery across various cancer types. Moreover, HA can be chemically modified to enhance its functionality as a drug carrier. By introducing functional groups or conjugating HA with other polymers or targeting ligands, researchers can improve its stability, drug-loading capacity, and targeting efficiency [16]. For example, HA-functionalized nanoparticles and liposomes have been shown to enhance the cellular uptake of anticancer drugs and improve their therapeutic efficacy in preclinical models. Figure 7.1 illustrates the different properties of HA.

7.2 HA: Structure and Biological Role

HA is a naturally occurring glycosaminoglycan present in the ECM of various tissues. Its distinctive biophysical and biochemical properties make it a crucial molecule in tissue hydration, repair, and cancer progression. Structurally, HA is a simple yet versatile polymer composed of repeating disaccharide units. Biologically, HA plays a range of roles, from providing structural support to mediating cellular signaling. In cancer, HA interacts with various cell surface receptors, such as CD44, RHAMM, and LYVE-1, promoting tumor growth and metastasis. These characteristics have made HA a vital target in DDS, especially in cancer treatment [17].

7.2.1 Chemical Structure of HA

HA is a linear polysaccharide composed of repeating disaccharide units made up of D-glucuronic acid and N-acetyl-D-glucosamine. These disaccharides are linked by alternating β-(1→3) and β-(1→4) glycosidic bonds [18]. This structure is highly conserved across species and is synthesized in the plasma membrane by hyaluronan synthases (HAS1, HAS2, and HAS3). The molecular weight of HA can range from several thousand to several million Daltons, with its size influencing its biological function [19]. High-molecular-weight HA is known for its anti-inflammatory effects, while lower-molecular-weight HA fragments can promote inflammation and angiogenesis. Due to its structure, HA is highly hydrophilic, allowing it to absorb and retain water, forming thick gels. This property is crucial for HA's function in maintaining tissue hydration and providing lubrication. Additionally, the carboxyl groups on D-glucuronic acid confer a polyanionic character, allowing HA to interact with various proteins and cations within the ECM. HA's chemical simplicity belies its multifunctionality in biological systems, especially in maintaining the structural and functional integrity of tissues [17, 20].

7.2.2 Biological Functions of HA in the Human Body

- **Role in the ECM:** In the ECM, HA provides a scaffold that supports cellular organization and tissue architecture. HA binds to water molecules, forming a hydrated, gel-like matrix that supports the diffusion of nutrients and signaling molecules. It interacts with proteoglycans and other ECM components, enhancing the structural integrity of tissues like cartilage and skin. HA is especially prevalent in connective tissues, where it plays a crucial role in regulating cell migration, proliferation, and differentiation [12, 17].
- **Tissue Hydration:** HA's hydrophilic nature allows it to bind up to 1,000 times its molecular weight in water, making it crucial for tissue hydration. This property is essential in the skin, where HA maintains moisture and elasticity. In synovial joints, HA serves as a lubricant, reducing friction between articular cartilage surfaces during movement. It also plays a role in maintaining the viscoelasticity of the vitreous body in the eye and the integrity of the intervertebral discs [17].
- **Tissue Repair and Wound Healing:** HA is actively involved in tissue repair and regeneration. During the early stages of wound healing, HA levels in the ECM increase significantly, creating a provisional matrix that supports cell migration and tissue remodeling. HA interacts with fibroblasts, keratinocytes, and immune cells to regulate inflammation, angiogenesis, and collagen deposition, which are critical for effective wound healing. Low-molecular-weight HA fragments can stimulate the production of pro-inflammatory cytokines and promote the recruitment of immune cells, while high-molecular-weight HA is associated with anti-inflammatory effects [21].

7.2.3 Interaction with CD44 and Other HA Receptors Overexpressed in Cancer Cells

HA interacts with several cell surface receptors that mediate its biological functions. The most well-known HA receptor is CD44, a transmembrane glycoprotein widely expressed on various cell types, including cancer cells [22]. CD44 mediates cell adhesion, migration, and proliferation, and its interaction with HA is implicated in cancer progression. In many tumors, including breast, ovarian, and colon cancers, CD44 is overexpressed, promoting tumor growth, invasion, and resistance to apoptosis [23]. The interaction between HA and CD44 activates key downstream signaling pathways, such as the Ras-MAPK and PI3K-Akt pathways, which play vital roles in cancer cell survival and metastasis. In addition to CD44, HA also binds to other receptors, including RHAMM and LYVE-1 (lymphatic vessel endothelial hyaluronan receptor-1). RHAMM is involved in regulating cell motility and is often overexpressed in aggressive cancer phenotypes, promoting metastasis by enhancing cellular migration and invasion [11]. LYVE-1, primarily expressed in lymphatic endothelial cells, is involved in lymphangiogenesis and lymphatic metastasis, facilitating the spread of cancer cells through the lymphatic system. The overexpression of these HA receptors in cancer cells has provided a target for HA-based DDS. HA-conjugated nanoparticles, micelles, and hydrogels have been designed to exploit the natural affinity of HA for CD44 and RHAMM, enhancing the selective delivery of anticancer agents to tumor tissues while minimizing off-target effects.

7.3 Mechanism of Targeting *Via* HA

7.3.1 HA's Role in Receptor-Mediated Endocytosis

HA is essential in receptor-mediated endocytosis, primarily through its interactions with cell surface receptors like CD44 and RHAMM. Receptor-mediated endocytosis is a specific cellular process where molecules, such as HA, bind to cell surface receptors, triggering the formation of vesicles that internalize the molecule into the cell [19]. In the case of HA, this mechanism is highly relevant in cancer biology, where it facilitates the cellular uptake of HA-conjugated drug carriers, leading to targeted intracellular drug delivery. The endocytic uptake of HA–drug conjugates primarily occurs through the CD44 receptor, which binds to the HA chains on the cell surface, triggering clathrin-mediated endocytosis. Once internalized, these HA–drug complexes are trafficked through endosomal compartments and may eventually reach the lysosomes for degradation or the cytoplasm for drug release, depending on the design of the DDS. This receptor-mediated endocytosis mechanism not only allows for the selective delivery of therapeutic agents but also enhances the cellular uptake and accumulation of HA-based nanoparticles. The overexpression of CD44 in many types of cancer cells, such as breast, ovarian, and lung cancers, makes this a valuable pathway for the delivery of chemotherapy drugs, nucleic acids, or imaging agents [24].

7.3.2 Binding to CD44 and RHAMM Receptors, Which are Often Upregulated in Cancer Cells

The interaction between HA and its primary receptors, CD44 and RHAMM, is central to both normal cellular processes and cancer progression. However, exploiting these interactions in the heterogeneous tumor microenvironment presents several challenges. Tumor heterogeneity can lead to variable expression of CD44 and RHAMM among different cancer types and even within different regions of the same tumor, potentially impacting the efficacy of HA-based therapeutic strategies. This variability necessitates the development of more sophisticated delivery systems that can adapt to or overcome these heterogeneities to ensure consistent targeting and treatment outcomes. CD44, a cell surface glycoprotein, and RHAMM, an intracellular and extracellular receptor, are frequently overexpressed in various cancer types, including breast, colon, and pancreatic cancers [22]. These receptors mediate several key processes in tumor biology, such as cell proliferation, migration, and invasion [15].

- **CD44**: CD44 is the most widely studied HA receptor. It mediates cellular responses by binding to HA, which triggers downstream signaling pathways such as Ras, PI3K/Akt, and MAPK [25]. These pathways regulate cancer cell survival, proliferation, and metastasis. Overexpression of CD44 is a hallmark of many aggressive cancer phenotypes and is associated with poor prognosis. CD44's role in HA-mediated signaling makes it a prime target for HA-based DDS. When HA is conjugated to therapeutic agents, it selectively binds to CD44 on the surface of cancer cells, enhancing the uptake and retention of the drugs. Compared to other biomaterials such as liposomes, dendrimers, and synthetic polymers, HA offers the advantage of biocompatibility and natural targeting capabilities due to its affinity for CD44. However, the susceptibility of HA to enzymatic degradation and potential variations in its binding efficiency pose challenges that must be overcome for its successful clinical application.

- **RHAMM**: RHAMM plays a complementary role to CD44, particularly in promoting cell motility and metastasis. Unlike CD44, RHAMM can localize intracellularly and in the ECM, contributing to cytoskeletal dynamics and migration. It is often upregulated in metastatic tumors and is implicated in the progression of aggressive cancers. However, targeting RHAMM in heterogeneous tumor environments presents specific challenges, such as variable expression levels and the potential for compensatory pathways that may reduce therapeutic efficacy. RHAMM interacts with HA to regulate the mitotic spindle, motility, and cellular invasion [22].

The simultaneous targeting of both CD44 and RHAMM with HA-based DDS provides a dual advantage, as both receptors are involved in tumorigenic signaling and are upregulated in many cancers. This makes them highly effective for the selective accumulation of HA–drug conjugates in cancerous tissues.

7.3.3 Selective Accumulation of HA-Based Drug Carriers at Tumor Sites

One of the most significant advantages of using HA-based DDS in cancer therapy is the selective accumulation of these carriers at tumor sites [25]. This selective accumulation occurs through two primary mechanisms: receptor-mediated endocytosis *via* HA-binding receptors (such as CD44 and RHAMM) and the EPR effect observed in tumors. Tumor tissues often exhibit abnormal vascular architecture, with leaky blood vessels and poor lymphatic drainage. This abnormality allows nanoparticles, such as HA–drug conjugates, to preferentially accumulate in the tumor microenvironment through the EPR effect. When HA is incorporated into drug carriers, its high affinity for overexpressed CD44 and RHAMM receptors in cancer cells further enhances this selective targeting. As a result, HA-based nanoparticles, micelles, or hydrogels can effectively localize at the tumor site, where they are internalized by cancer cells through receptor-mediated endocytosis [26]. HA's biocompatibility and its ability to interact specifically with cancer-associated receptors make it an ideal candidate for delivering chemotherapeutic agents, nucleic acids, and immune modulators directly to tumors. HA-based drug carriers have been shown to reduce off-target toxicity and improve the therapeutic index of various anticancer drugs, including doxorubicin, paclitaxel, and siRNA-based therapies.

7.4 HA-Driven DDS

7.4.1 Nanoparticles: Formulation, Advantages, and Examples of Anticancer Agents Delivered *Via* HA-Coated Nanoparticles

Nanoparticles have become a promising system for drug delivery due to their small size, capacity to encapsulate various therapeutic agents, and potential for controlled release. HA-coated nanoparticles, a significant category in this system, are specifically designed for targeted cancer treatment. These nanoparticles are generally made from materials such as lipids, polymers, or inorganic compounds and are coated with HA to enhance their specificity for cancer cells. The HA coating promotes selective uptake by cancer cells that overexpress HA receptors like CD44 and RHAMM. The process of creating HA-coated nanoparticles usually involves conjugating HA to the nanoparticle surface during or after their synthesis, which enhances their biocompatibility and stability in the bloodstream [27]. HA-coated nanoparticles offer several advantages: enhanced tumor targeting, increased circulation time, reduced systemic toxicity, and efficient cellular uptake. Additionally, these nanoparticles can be loaded with a wide range of anticancer agents, including chemotherapeutic drugs (e.g., paclitaxel, doxorubicin), nucleic acids (e.g., siRNA, mRNA), and imaging agents [27]. Examples of HA-coated nanoparticles used in cancer therapy include the use of HA-coated polymeric nanoparticles for paclitaxel delivery in ovarian cancer and HA-coated liposomal nanoparticles for doxorubicin delivery in breast cancer [28]. These HA-coated formulations significantly improve drug accumulation in tumors, leading to enhanced therapeutic efficacy with minimal side effects [29].

7.4.2 Micelles: Self-Assembling HA-Based Micelles for Hydrophobic Drug Loading

Micelles are nanoscale colloidal carriers formed by the self-assembly of amphiphilic molecules in water. HA-based micelles have gained interest as DDS, particularly for hydrophobic drugs, because they can encapsulate poorly soluble compounds within their hydrophobic core, improving their solubility and stability. These micelles are typically created by linking HA to hydrophobic segments, like fatty acids, to produce amphiphilic copolymers. When exposed to water, these copolymers spontaneously form micelles with a hydrophilic outer shell and a hydrophobic core, ideal for solubilizing lipophilic drugs [30]. This self-assembly is advantageous because it allows for a simple, solvent-free formulation process, and the HA shell ensures that the micelles have enhanced biocompatibility, prolonged circulation time, and tumor targeting *via* HA-receptor binding. The use of HA-based micelles for anticancer drug delivery has been demonstrated in multiple studies, such as the incorporation of hydrophobic paclitaxel, doxorubicin, and curcumin. These micelles have shown enhanced therapeutic efficacy in cancer models by increasing drug accumulation at tumor sites, improving the solubility of hydrophobic drugs, and minimizing systemic toxicity [27].

7.4.3 Liposomes: HA-Functionalized Liposomes for Improved Delivery and Targeting

Liposomes are lipid-based vesicles capable of encapsulating both hydrophobic and hydrophilic drugs, making them versatile carriers for a wide range of therapeutic agents [10]. Liposomes are commonly used in DDS because of their biocompatibility, ability to carry various therapeutic agents, and potential to improve drug pharmacokinetics. HA-functionalized liposomes are a specialized type of liposome where the surface is coated with HA, enabling tumor-specific targeting and enhancing the delivery of drugs to cancerous tissues [31]. HA-functionalized liposomes offer several advantages: (1) enhanced stability and circulation time in the bloodstream due to the HA coating, (2) preferential uptake by tumor cells *via* receptor-mediated endocytosis, and (3) controlled release of encapsulated drugs, improving their therapeutic efficacy. HA functionalization of liposomes has been demonstrated to significantly enhance drug accumulation at tumor sites, particularly in cancers that overexpress CD44 or RHAMM. For instance, HA-functionalized liposomes have been used to deliver doxorubicin, paclitaxel, and siRNA to cancer cells. Research indicates that these HA-coated liposomes improve the therapeutic efficacy of these drugs and reduce the side effects commonly associated with traditional chemotherapy [32].

7.4.4 Hydrogels: Injectable HA Hydrogels for Localized Drug Release in Tumors

Hydrogels are three-dimensional, cross-linked polymer networks that can absorb large amounts of water, providing a soft and biocompatible environment for drug delivery. HA-based injectable hydrogels have gained attention for their potential in targeted cancer therapy. These hydrogels can be injected directly into tumors or their surrounding microenvironments, where they solidify in place, allowing for the sustained release of therapeutic agents. HA-based hydrogels offer several advantages, including biocompatibility, localized drug delivery, and the flexibility to be combined with various treatment modalities, such as chemotherapy, gene therapy, and immunotherapy [33]. The hydrogels can be designed to release drugs gradually over an extended period, ensuring sustained therapeutic action at the tumor site while minimizing off-target effects and reducing systemic toxicity. For instance, HA-based hydrogels have been utilized for the

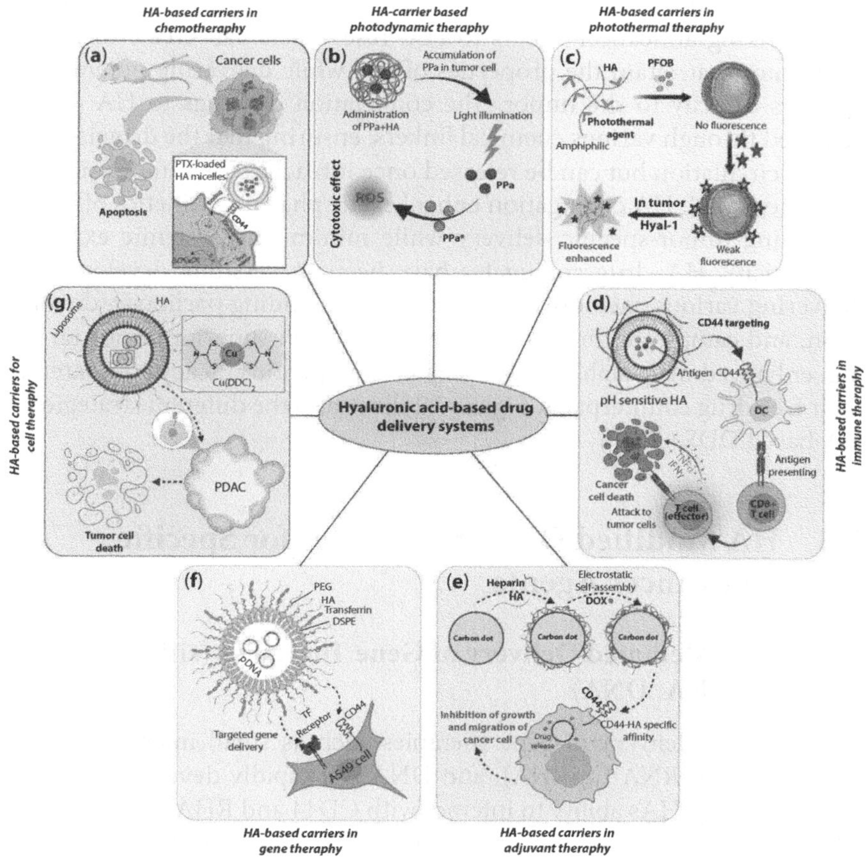

Figure 7.2 HA-based DDS are versatile and have found applications across various therapeutic modalities, including chemotherapy, photothermal therapy, photodynamic therapy, cell therapy, adjuvant therapy, immune therapy, and gene therapy. These systems utilize the unique properties of HA to target specific cells, enhance therapeutic efficacy, and reduce side effects, making them suitable for a wide range of treatments.

localized delivery of chemotherapeutic drugs like doxorubicin and protein therapeutics such as antibodies. These systems are particularly advantageous for treating solid tumors, as they enable direct drug delivery to the tumor site, enhancing the treatment's efficacy and limiting the adverse effects on healthy tissues.

7.4.5 Conjugates: Direct Conjugation of Anticancer Drugs with HA for Enhanced Stability and Targeting

Direct conjugation of anticancer drugs to HA molecules is a strategy aimed at enhancing the stability, solubility, and targeting of the drugs. By covalently linking anticancer agents to HA, researchers can create drug–HA conjugates that retain the properties of HA while delivering potent therapeutics directly to the tumor. The conjugation of drugs to HA can be achieved through various chemical linkers, ensuring that the drug is stable during circulation but can be released once it reaches the tumor microenvironment [34]. HA conjugation enhances the pharmacokinetics of drugs, improving tumor-specific delivery while minimizing systemic exposure and toxicity. HA–drug conjugates have been successfully developed for delivering various chemotherapeutic agents, including paclitaxel, doxorubicin, and camptothecin. These conjugates exhibit superior tumor targeting, enhanced drug stability, and greater therapeutic efficacy compared to their free drug counterparts. Figure 7.2 illustrates the different strategies of HA-based DDS.

7.5 HA Modified Delivery Vehicles for Specific Anticancer Agents

7.5.1 HA-Mediated Delivery of Gene Therapies (siRNA, MiRNA, DNA)

HA-mediated delivery of gene therapies such as small interfering RNA (siRNA), microRNA (miRNA), and DNA is a rapidly developing area in cancer therapy. HA's ability to interact with CD44 and RHAMM receptors, which are overexpressed on many cancer cells, makes it an ideal carrier for gene-based therapies. By conjugating or encapsulating gene therapies within HA-based nanoparticles or hydrogels, researchers can achieve targeted and efficient delivery of genetic material to tumor cells, thereby improving therapeutic outcomes [35]. In particular, HA is utilized in the delivery of siRNA and miRNA to suppress oncogenic gene expression or restore the function of tumor suppressors. This approach is especially beneficial for silencing genes that contribute to cancer progression, resistance to chemotherapy, or metastasis. For example, HA-based nanoparticles have been used to deliver siRNA targeting genes such as Bcl-2 and KRAS in various cancer models, demonstrating significant gene silencing effects and tumor growth inhibition [36]. Similarly, DNA delivery using HA nanoparticles has shown promising results in gene therapy for cancer. HA-modified vectors, such as plasmid DNA or viral vectors, can be targeted to cancer cells, improving transfection efficiency and minimizing systemic toxicity. Several studies have demonstrated the effectiveness of HA in facilitating the *in vivo* delivery of plasmid DNA encoding for immune-stimulating factors, such as cytokines or tumor-associated antigens, to enhance anticancer immunity [37].

7.5.2 Immunotherapy Agents and HA-Targeted Delivery (Antibodies, Checkpoint Inhibitors)

Immunotherapy has transformed cancer treatment, with HA-based DDS gaining attention for the targeted administration of immunotherapeutic agents. These agents, including monoclonal antibodies, immune checkpoint inhibitors, and cytokines, have demonstrated potential in activating the immune system to combat cancer cells. HA functionalization improves the targeting of these agents to tumor tissues, minimizing off-target effects and enhancing therapeutic effectiveness. Monoclonal antibodies, such as trastuzumab (anti-HER2) and rituximab (anti-CD20), are commonly used to treat cancers like breast cancer and lymphoma, respectively [38]. HA-coated nanoparticles improve the delivery of antibodies to cancer cells, boosting their ability to efficiently bind to target receptors such as HER2 or CD20. Likewise, immune checkpoint inhibitors like pembrolizumab (anti-PD-1) and ipilimumab (anti-CTLA-4) can be delivered *via* HA-based nanocarriers, enhancing tumor targeting while minimizing systemic immune-related side effects [39]. HA-based systems have been utilized for the targeted delivery of cytokines, such as interleukin-2 (IL-2) and granulocyte-macrophage colony-stimulating factor (GM-CSF), to strengthen anti-tumor immune responses. Studies suggest that HA-functionalized immunotherapeutic agents not only increase the concentration of these therapies at the tumor site but also activate immune cells, including T-cells and macrophages, to effectively target and destroy cancer cells [40].

7.5.3 Combination Therapies (HA in Delivering Multiple Drugs or Drugs with Imaging Agents)

Combination therapies, where two or more therapeutic agents are used together, are gaining traction in oncology [41]. The use of HA-based delivery systems to deliver multiple drugs simultaneously, or to co-deliver drugs along with imaging agents, offers a promising strategy for improving treatment outcomes and monitoring therapeutic responses in real time. HA can be used to encapsulate or conjugate various therapeutic agents, including chemotherapy drugs, targeted therapies, gene therapies, and imaging agents, allowing for their synergistic delivery to the tumor. HA-based nanoparticles can be engineered to release different drugs at controlled rates, thereby achieving the desired therapeutic effect without excessive systemic toxicity [42]. For example, studies have demonstrated the co-delivery of doxorubicin (a chemotherapeutic agent) and paclitaxel (another chemotherapy drug) using HA-coated nanoparticles [43]. These formulations show improved anticancer effectiveness when compared to administering each drug individually, as the drugs work together to more effectively block cancer cell growth and spread. Beyond chemotherapy, HA-based nanoparticles can also facilitate the simultaneous delivery of immunotherapies and imaging agents. For example, HA-coated liposomes have been utilized to deliver both immune checkpoint inhibitors and fluorescence-based imaging agents to cancer cells [44]. This approach not only enhances the therapeutic effect of the drugs but also provides a non-invasive means to monitor drug distribution and tumor response *in vivo* using imaging techniques like fluorescence or magnetic resonance imaging [42].

7.6 Challenges in HA-Based Targeted Delivery

7.6.1 Optimization of Molecular Weight for Targeting Efficacy

The molecular weight of HA plays a crucial role in its effectiveness for targeted drug delivery, particularly in cancer treatment. HA interacts with CD44 and RHAMM receptors, which are frequently overexpressed on cancer cells, and its molecular weight affects the affinity and efficiency of this binding. Higher-molecular-weight HA tends to have stronger interactions with these receptors, improving targeting and enhancing therapeutic outcomes. HA with a lower-molecular-weight offers better solubility and can diffuse more readily through tissues. In contrast, HA with a higher molecular weight has a stronger binding affinity for these receptors, which could lead to more efficient targeting of cancer cells [45]. Optimization of HA's molecular weight is essential to balance its targeting ability, tissue penetration, and bioavailability. Several studies have demonstrated that HA derivatives with intermediate molecular weights (50–200 kDa) tend to show the best combination of receptor targeting and cellular uptake. For instance, HA nanoparticles composed of high-molecular-weight HA were found to exhibit enhanced binding to tumor cells overexpressing CD44, whereas lower-molecular-weight HA (less than 10 kDa) can exhibit better tissue penetration due to reduced viscosity and higher diffusivity [46]. Moreover, the modulation of HA's molecular weight has been shown to affect its clearance rate from the body. High-molecular-weight HA tends to build up in the liver and spleen because of its larger size, while low-molecular-weight HA is eliminated more quickly by the kidneys. Therefore, the optimal molecular weight is essential for achieving prolonged circulation time while minimizing systemic side effects.

7.6.2 Overcoming Drug Resistance and Tumor Heterogeneity

Tumor heterogeneity and the development of drug resistance are major challenges in cancer treatment. HA-based DDS have shown promise in overcoming these obstacles. Tumor heterogeneity, characterized by the presence of various cell types within a tumor, complicates the effectiveness of conventional therapies by limiting their ability to target and treat all cancerous cells effectively. HA-based systems offer the potential to specifically target diverse tumor cells, improving therapeutic outcomes and reducing the chances of resistance [29]. HA-based systems can be engineered to respond to the dynamic conditions of the tumor microenvironment by incorporating stimuli-responsive components, such as pH-sensitive or temperature-sensitive polymers, which release the drug specifically at the tumor site. Additionally, HA's ability to bind to CD44 and RHAMM receptors, commonly overexpressed on cancer stem cells (CSCs), helps address the challenge of drug resistance. CSCs are key contributors to drug resistance due to their self-renewal capacity and resistance to apoptosis. By using HA-based nanoparticles that specifically target these CSC populations, drug resistance can be minimized, thereby improving the overall therapeutic efficacy [47]. Furthermore, HA-based carriers can be combined with chemotherapeutic agents or targeted therapies to overcome multi-drug resistance (MDR). For example, HA-functionalized nanoparticles have been used to deliver MDR modulators (verapamil) to cancer cells, thereby enhancing the efficacy of standard chemotherapy drugs by reversing MDR mechanisms [48].

7.6.3 Controlling Drug Release Rates and Bioavailability

The controlled release of drugs from HA-based delivery systems is essential for enhancing therapeutic efficacy while minimizing side effects. By modifying the physicochemical properties of HA, such as its molecular weight, crosslinking density, and incorporating stimuli-responsive elements, drug release can be tailored to respond specifically to the conditions of the tumor microenvironment, ensuring that the drug is released at the right time and location. This approach optimizes treatment outcomes and reduces off-target effects [27]. For example, HA can be conjugated to pH-sensitive groups, allowing for the release of the drug in the acidic tumor microenvironment, which is characteristic of many solid tumors. In addition, HA-based DDS can be designed to provide sustained and localized drug release over prolonged periods. This can be accomplished by encapsulating the drug within nanoparticles, micelles, liposomes, or hydrogels derived from HA. These systems can be further enhanced by modifying them with targeting ligands, which improve specificity toward tumor cells and minimize off-target effects, ensuring more efficient and precise treatment [49]. HA is essential in these systems as it facilitates the targeted delivery of therapeutic agents to the tumor site, improving bioavailability and boosting treatment efficacy. Moreover, the integration of

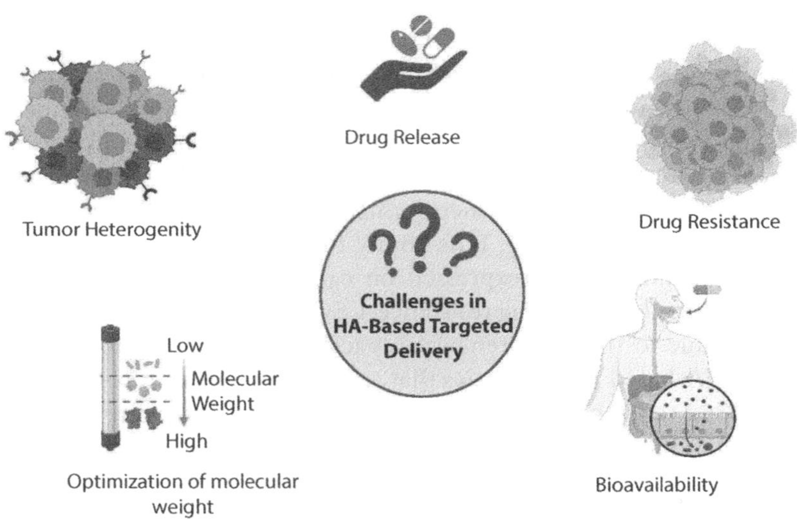

Figure 7.3 Challenges in HA-based targeted delivery. Challenges such as tumor heterogeneity, drug release, drug resistance, optimization of molecular weight, and bioavailability must be encountered.

imaging agents into HA-based DDS enables *in vivo* monitoring of drug release. By using HA-functionalized nanoparticles with embedded contrast agents, real-time tracking of drug distribution and release becomes feasible, providing valuable insights into the pharmacokinetics and overall effectiveness of the treatment [50]. Figure 7.3 illustrates the different challenges in HA-based targeted delivery.

7.7 Clinical Applications and Current Advances

7.7.1 Preclinical and Clinical Trials of HA-Based DDS

HA-based DDS have undergone extensive preclinical and clinical investigations, focusing on their use in targeted cancer therapies. Preclinical studies have demonstrated the ability of HA-coated nanoparticles, liposomes, micelles, and hydrogels to effectively deliver anticancer agents to tumors, thereby improving drug solubility, stability, and bioavailability [44]. In these studies, HA-functionalized drug carriers exhibited enhanced tumor accumulation due to receptor-mediated endocytosis *via* CD44 and RHAMM receptors, which are overexpressed on cancer cells. Several clinical trials have translated these promising preclinical results into human testing [51]. For example, HA-coated liposomes containing paclitaxel have shown favorable pharmacokinetics and enhanced tumor targeting in phase I/II trials for breast and ovarian cancer patients. Other research has explored the use of HA-based micelles to deliver hydrophobic anticancer drugs such as doxorubicin, demonstrating improved therapeutic outcomes and fewer side effects compared to traditional formulations [52]. Additionally, HA-functionalized nanoparticles have been used to deliver RNA-based therapies such as siRNA, demonstrating significant potential in treating resistant cancers and gene therapy applications. While the clinical application of HA-based DDS is still in the early stages, ongoing trials have shown promising results. However, challenges such as scaling up production, obtaining regulatory approval, and fully understanding the long-term safety profiles of these systems still need to be addressed [53].

7.7.2 Success Stories of HA-Targeted Therapies in Specific Cancers

HA-based targeted therapies have shown considerable potential in treating different cancers, especially breast and ovarian cancers, by exploiting

HA's ability to target CD44, which is overexpressed on tumor cells. In breast cancer, nanoparticles functionalized with HA have been utilized to deliver paclitaxel and other chemotherapy drugs directly to the tumor site, minimizing systemic toxicity and improving treatment effectiveness [54]. These formulations have shown increased tumor accumulation, improved drug retention within the tumor microenvironment, and better clinical outcomes in preclinical models. In ovarian cancer, clinical trials have investigated HA-modified liposomes loaded with paclitaxel, demonstrating improved pharmacokinetics, extended circulation time, and enhanced tumor targeting. These therapies are designed to minimize the side effects of conventional chemotherapy while increasing the bioavailability of the drug at the tumor site, leading to more effective treatment outcomes [55]. Furthermore, HA-targeted therapies have demonstrated effectiveness in treating various cancers, including lung, colon, and pancreatic cancer. HA-functionalized carriers are employed to deliver a broad spectrum of therapeutic agents, such as small molecules, nucleic acids, and immunotherapeutic agents. The success of these therapies highlights the promising potential of HA-based DDS in advancing personalized cancer treatments [56].

7.7.3 Recent Innovations in HA-Based Delivery Systems, Including Smart Drug Delivery Technologies

Recent advancements in HA-based DDS have led to several innovations designed to improve the targeting and effectiveness of anticancer treatments. A major advancement is the development of "smart" DDS that respond to specific stimuli in the tumor microenvironment, such as variations in pH, temperature, or enzyme activity. These systems enable the controlled release of therapeutic agents, ensuring that drugs are released precisely when and where they are needed, enhancing treatment effectiveness and minimizing side effects [42]. HA-based nanoparticles can be engineered with pH-sensitive polymers to enable controlled drug release in the acidic tumor microenvironment, which is common in many cancers. Another advancement includes the use of HA-functionalized nanoparticles for combination therapy [57]. For instance, HA can be linked to both chemotherapy drugs and imaging agents, allowing for real-time tracking of drug delivery and monitoring the therapeutic response. Additionally, the use of HA in combination with nucleic acid-based treatments like RNA interference, miRNA, and CRISPR technologies is emerging as an innovative strategy in cancer therapy [58]. Hydrogels made from HA are being investigated for targeted drug delivery, offering sustained release while reducing systemic side effects. These hydrogels can be injected directly into the tumor, enabling controlled drug release over an extended period, which is especially beneficial for treating localized cancers like glioblastoma or pancreatic cancer [33].

7.8 Challenges in Advancing HA-Based Delivery Systems from Preclinical to Clinical Stages

While HA-based DDS offer promising solutions for targeted cancer therapy, transitioning these systems from preclinical research to clinical application presents several challenges. Key obstacles include scalability, regulatory hurdles, and ensuring consistent quality and efficacy in large-scale production.

- **Scalability:** One of the primary challenges in transitioning HA-based DDS to clinical stages is scalability. The production of HA-based nanocarriers, such as nanoparticles, micelles, and hydrogels, often involves complex and sensitive processes that are well suited to small-scale laboratory settings but difficult to reproduce on a larger industrial scale. Ensuring uniformity in particle size, drug loading efficiency, and surface modification across large batches is crucial to maintaining the therapeutic efficacy and safety of the DDS [59]. Additionally, the sourcing of high-quality HA with consistent molecular weight and purity can be challenging when scaling up production, as variations in these parameters can affect the performance of the DDS [60].
- **Regulatory Hurdles:** Regulatory approval presents a major challenge in the clinical translation of HA-based DDS. Regulatory bodies like the U.S. Food and Drug Administration (FDA) and the European Medicines Agency (EMA) demand comprehensive preclinical and clinical evidence to establish the safety, efficacy, and quality of new drug delivery platforms. The innovative nature of HA-based DDS, often involving novel formulations and mechanisms of action, means that these systems may not fit neatly into existing regulatory frameworks [61, 62]. This can lead to additional requirements for demonstrating biocompatibility,

long-term stability, and the absence of immunogenic reactions. Furthermore, the use of HA, a naturally occurring polymer, raises questions about its metabolic pathways and potential off-target effects that must be thoroughly investigated [63].

- **Quality Control and Standardization:** Maintaining strict quality control and standardization across all production stages is essential for the clinical success of HA-based DDS. Variability in HA's molecular weight and the degree of chemical modification can lead to differences in the DDS's behavior in biological systems [64]. Developing robust methods for characterizing and controlling these parameters is necessary to ensure consistent product performance [65]. Additionally, integrating good manufacturing practices in the production process is critical to meet the regulatory standards required for clinical use [66].

Addressing these challenges is crucial for the successful clinical translation of HA-based DDS. Advances in manufacturing technologies, such as microfluidics and scalable nanoparticle synthesis techniques, can help overcome scalability issues [67]. Collaboration with regulatory agencies early in the development process can facilitate a clearer path to approval by addressing specific regulatory concerns. By tackling these obstacles, HA-based DDS can move closer to becoming a viable and widely used option in oncology, offering targeted, efficient, and less toxic therapeutic alternatives to traditional cancer treatments.

7.9 Conclusion

7.9.1 Summary of the Role of HA in Targeted Delivery of Anticancer Agents

HA has emerged as a powerful biomaterial in the targeted delivery of anticancer agents due to its unique properties and its ability to selectively interact with cancer cells. HA's versatility stems from its natural biocompatibility, biodegradability, and ability to be easily modified for various drug delivery applications. Its primary role in targeted delivery is based on its high affinity for the CD44 receptor, which is overexpressed on various types of cancer cells, including breast, ovarian, and colorectal cancers. HA-based DDS offer several advantages for cancer therapy, including enhanced drug accumulation at tumor sites, reduced systemic toxicity, and improved therapeutic efficacy. The ability of HA to interact with the tumor microenvironment allows for both passive and active targeting. Through receptor-mediated endocytosis, HA-coated nanoparticles can be internalized by cancer cells, leading to localized drug release. Moreover, HA can be conjugated with specific targeting ligands, chemotherapeutic agents, or RNA-based therapies, further improving the precision of treatment. Furthermore, HA's role in the ECM helps to enhance drug delivery by improving cellular uptake, modifying drug release kinetics, and facilitating penetration through the tumor stroma. HA-based systems are also being integrated with other nanomedicine technologies, such as liposomes, micelles, and nanoparticles, for better pharmacokinetic profiles and tumor specificity. These advances make HA a promising candidate for personalized and combination cancer therapies.

7.9.2 Promising Future of HA-Based DDS in Oncology

The future of HA-based DDS in oncology looks promising, fueled by ongoing progress in nanomedicine and biomaterial engineering. HA's inherent biocompatibility and its capacity to target tumor-specific receptors position it as an ideal candidate for the development of personalized cancer therapies. Modifying HA with various targeting moieties and therapeutic agents, such as chemotherapeutic drugs, gene therapies, or immunotherapies, presents significant potential for enhancing the precision and effectiveness of cancer treatments. A promising direction is the development of HA-based nanomedicines that combine drug delivery with imaging or diagnostic capabilities, enabling real-time monitoring of treatment progress. These "smart" DDS can be designed to respond to specific cues in the tumor microenvironment, like pH or enzyme activity, for controlled drug release and improved therapeutic outcomes. Furthermore, HA-based systems can be combined with other nanomedicines, such as liposomes, micelles, and nanoparticles, to address challenges like drug resistance, tumor heterogeneity, and limited bioavailability. HA's potential in personalized medicine is particularly noteworthy. For instance, integrating HA-based DDS with CRISPR-Cas9 technology could facilitate targeted gene editing directly within tumor cells, offering a novel approach to cancer treatment. Similarly, HA's role in delivering immune checkpoint inhibitors could revolutionize immunotherapy by enhancing the specificity and efficacy of immune responses against cancer cells. These combination strategies represent a multimodal approach to cancer therapy, addressing various aspects of tumor biology and treatment resistance.

Furthermore, clinical studies and preclinical trials have demonstrated the potential of HA-based delivery systems in specific cancers, such as breast cancer, ovarian cancer, and melanoma. As research progresses, HA-based DDS are expected to play a significant role in precision oncology, offering targeted, efficient, and less toxic therapeutic options. This continued evolution underscores the importance of HA as a versatile platform for next-generation cancer therapies.

AI disclosure statement: The author acknowledges the use of AI-based tools for minor language editing or grammatical correction. However, all intellectual contributions, analyses, and conclusions presented in this chapter are entirely the author's own.

References

1. Sung, H., *et al.*, Global Cancer Statistics 2020: GLOBOCAN Estimates of Incidence and Mortality Worldwide for 36 Cancers in 185 Countries. *CA Cancer J. Clin.*, 71, 3, 209–249, May 2021, doi: 10.3322/caac.21660.
2. Chabner, B.A. and Roberts, T.G., Chemotherapy and the war on cancer. *Nat. Rev. Cancer*, 5, 1, 65–72, Jan. 2005, doi: 10.1038/nrc1529.
3. Sawyers, C., Targeted cancer therapy. *Nature*, 432, 7015, 294–297, Nov. 2004, doi: 10.1038/nature03095.
4. Ferrara, N., Hillan, K.J., Novotny, W., Bevacizumab (Avastin), a humanized anti-VEGF monoclonal antibody for cancer therapy. *Biochem. Biophys. Res. Commun.*, 333, 2, 328–35, Jul. 2005, doi: 10.1016/j.bbrc.2005.05.132.
5. Peer, D., Karp, J.M., Hong, S., Farokhzad, O.C., Margalit, R., Langer, R., Nanocarriers as an emerging platform for cancer therapy. *Nat. Nanotechnol.*, 2, 12, 751–760, Dec. 2007, doi: 10.1038/nnano.2007.387.
6. Chabner, B.A. and Roberts, T.G., Timeline: Chemotherapy and the war on cancer. *Nat. Rev. Cancer*, 5, 1, 65–72, Jan. 2005, doi: 10.1038/nrc1529.
7. Maeda, H., Wu, J., Sawa, T., Matsumura, Y., Hori, K., Tumor vascular permeability and the EPR effect in macromolecular therapeutics: a review. *J. Control. Release*, 65, 1–2, 271–84, Mar. 2000, doi: 10.1016/s0168-3659(99)00248-5.
8. Barenholz, Y., Doxil®–the first FDA-approved nano-drug: lessons learned. *J. Control. Release*, 160, 2, 117–34, Jun. 2012, doi: 10.1016/j.jconrel.2012.03.020.
9. van der Meel, R., Sulheim, E., Shi, Y., Kiessling, F., Mulder, W.J.M., Lammers, T., Smart cancer nanomedicine. *Nat. Nanotechnol.*, 14, 11, 1007–1017, Nov. 2019, doi: 10.1038/s41565-019-0567-y.
10. Allen, T.M. and Cullis, P.R., Liposomal drug delivery systems: from concept to clinical applications. *Adv. Drug Deliv. Rev.*, 65, 1, 36–48, Jan. 2013, doi: 10.1016/j.addr.2012.09.037.

11. Stern, R., Asari, A.A., Sugahara, K.N., Hyaluronan fragments: an information-rich system. *Eur. J. Cell Biol.*, 85, 8, 699–715, Aug. 2006, doi: 10.1016/j.ejcb.2006.05.009.
12. Toole, B.P., Hyaluronan: from extracellular glue to pericellular cue. *Nat. Rev. Cancer*, 4, 7, 528–39, Jul. 2004, doi: 10.1038/nrc1391.
13. Burdick, J.A. and Prestwich, G.D., Hyaluronic acid hydrogels for biomedical applications. *Adv. Mater.*, 23, 12, H41–56, Mar. 2011, doi: 10.1002/adma.201003963.
14. Yu, M., Jambhrunkar, S., Thorn, P., Chen, J., Gu, W., Yu, C., Hyaluronic acid modified mesoporous silica nanoparticles for targeted drug delivery to CD44-overexpressing cancer cells. *Nanoscale*, 5, 1, 178–83, Jan. 2013, doi: 10.1039/c2nr32145a.
15. Misra, S., *et al.*, Hyaluronan-CD44 interactions as potential targets for cancer therapy. *FEBS J.*, 278, 9, 1429–43, May 2011, doi: 10.1111/j.1742-4658.2011.08071.x.
16. Turley, E.A., Noble, P.W., Bourguignon, L.Y.W., Signaling properties of hyaluronan receptors. *J. Biol. Chem.*, 277, 7, 4589–92, Feb. 2002, doi: 10.1074/jbc.R100038200.
17. Fraser, J.R., Laurent, T.C., Laurent, U.B., Hyaluronan: its nature, distribution, functions and turnover. *J. Intern. Med.*, 242, 1, 27–33, Jul. 1997, doi: 10.1046/j.1365-2796.1997.00170.x.
18. Stern, R., Hyaluronan catabolism: a new metabolic pathway. *Eur. J. Cell Biol.*, 83, 7, 317–25, Aug. 2004, doi: 10.1078/0171-9335-00392.
19. Day, A.J. and Prestwich, G.D., Hyaluronan-binding proteins: tying up the giant. *J. Biol. Chem.*, 277, 7, 4585–8, Feb. 2002, doi: 10.1074/jbc.R100036200.
20. Lee, J.Y. and Spicer, A.P., Hyaluronan: a multifunctional, megaDalton, stealth molecule. *Curr. Opin. Cell Biol.*, 12, 5, 581–6, Oct. 2000, doi: 10.1016/s0955-0674(00)00135-6.
21. Jiang, D., Liang, J., Noble, P.W., Hyaluronan in tissue injury and repair. *Annu. Rev. Cell Dev. Biol.*, 23, 435–61, 2007, doi: 10.1146/annurev.cellbio.23.090506.123337.
22. Misra, S., Hascall, V.C., Markwald, R.R., Ghatak, S., Interactions between Hyaluronan and Its Receptors (CD44, RHAMM) Regulate the Activities of Inflammation and Cancer. *Front. Immunol.*, 6, 201, 2015, doi: 10.3389/fimmu.2015.00201.
23. Zöller, M., CD44: can a cancer-initiating cell profit from an abundantly expressed molecule? *Nat. Rev. Cancer*, 11, 4, 254–67, Apr. 2011, doi: 10.1038/nrc3023.
24. Pandey, M.S., Baggenstoss, B.A., Washburn, J., Harris, E.N., Weigel, P.H., The Hyaluronan Receptor for Endocytosis (HARE) Activates NF-κB-mediated Gene Expression in Response to 40–400-kDa, but Not Smaller or Larger, Hyaluronans. *J. Biol. Chem.*, 288, 20, 14068–14079, May 2013, doi: 10.1074/jbc.M112.442889.

25. Tammi, R.H., Kultti, A., Kosma, V.-M., Pirinen, R., Auvinen, P., Tammi, M.I., Hyaluronan in human tumors: pathobiological and prognostic messages from cell-associated and stromal hyaluronan. *Semin. Cancer Biol.*, 18, 4, 288–95, Aug. 2008, doi: 10.1016/j.semcancer.2008.03.005.
26. Price, Z.K., Lokman, N.A., Ricciardelli, C., Differing Roles of Hyaluronan Molecular Weight on Cancer Cell Behavior and Chemotherapy Resistance. *Cancers (Basel)*, 10, 12, 482, Dec. 2018, doi: 10.3390/cancers10120482.
27. Lee, S.Y., Kang, M.S., Jeong, W.Y., Han, D.-W., Kim, K.S., Hyaluronic Acid-Based Theranostic Nanomedicines for Targeted Cancer Therapy. *Cancers (Basel)*, 12, 4, 940, Apr. 2020, doi: 10.3390/cancers12040940.
28. Seidu, T.A., Kutoka, P.T., Asante, D.O., Farooq, M.A., Alolga, R.N., Bo, W., Functionalization of Nanoparticulate Drug Delivery Systems and Its Influence in Cancer Therapy. *Pharmaceutics*, 14, 5, 1113, May 2022, doi: 10.3390/pharmaceutics14051113.
29. Jiao, Y., Pang, X., Zhai, G., Advances in Hyaluronic Acid-Based Drug Delivery Systems. *Curr. Drug Targets*, 17, 6, 720–30, 2016, doi: 10.2174/1389450116666150531155200.
30. Zhang, N., Wardwell, P., Bader, R., Polysaccharide-Based Micelles for Drug Delivery. *Pharmaceutics*, 5, 2, 329–352, May 2013, doi: 10.3390/pharmaceutics5020329.
31. Wang, H., *et al.*, PLGA/polymeric liposome for targeted drug and gene co-delivery. *Biomaterials*, 31, 33, 8741–8, Nov. 2010, doi: 10.1016/j.biomaterials.2010.07.082.
32. Chi, Y., *et al.*, Redox-sensitive and hyaluronic acid functionalized liposomes for cytoplasmic drug delivery to osteosarcoma in animal models. *J. Controlled Release*, 261, 113–125, Sep. 2017, doi: 10.1016/j.jconrel.2017.06.027.
33. Kim, J., Choi, Y., Kim, D.-H., Yoon, H.Y., Kim, K., Injectable Hydrogel-Based Combination Cancer Immunotherapy for Overcoming Localized Therapeutic Efficacy. *Pharmaceutics*, 14, 9, 1908, Sep. 2022, doi: 10.3390/pharmaceutics14091908.
34. Yang, Y., *et al.*, Drug conjugate-based anticancer therapy - Current status and perspectives. *Cancer Lett.*, 552, 215969, Jan. 2023, doi: 10.1016/j.canlet.2022.215969.
35. Mohammadinejad, R., *et al.*, *In vivo* gene delivery mediated by non-viral vectors for cancer therapy. *J. Control. Release*, 325, 249–275, Sep. 2020, doi: 10.1016/j.jconrel.2020.06.038.
36. Çağdaş Tunalı, B., Çelik, E., Budak Yıldıran, F.A., Türk, M., Delivery of siRNA using hyaluronic acid-guided nanoparticles for downregulation of CXCR4. *Biopolymers*, 114, 4, e23535, Apr. 2023, doi: 10.1002/bip.23535.
37. Paunovska, K., Loughrey, D., Dahlman, J.E., Drug delivery systems for RNA therapeutics. *Nat. Rev. Genet.*, 23, 5, 265–280, May 2022, doi: 10.1038/s41576-021-00439-4.
38. Nel, J., *et al.*, Functionalized liposomes for targeted breast cancer drug delivery. *Bioact. Mater.*, 24, 401–437, Jun. 2023, doi: 10.1016/j.bioactmat.2022.12.027.

39. Wang, L., Xu, H., Weng, L., Sun, J., Jin, Y., Xiao, C., Activation of cancer immunotherapy by nanomedicine. *Front. Pharmacol.*, 13, 1041073, Dec. 2022, doi: 10.3389/fphar.2022.1041073.
40. Yang, F., Shi, K., Jia, Y., Hao, Y., Peng, J., Qian, Z., Advanced biomaterials for cancer immunotherapy. *Acta Pharmacol. Sin.*, 41, 7, 911–927, Jul. 2020, doi: 10.1038/s41401-020-0372-z.
41. Mokhtari, R.B., *et al.*, Combination therapy in combating cancer. *Oncotarget*, 8, 23, 38022–38043, Jun. 2017, doi: 10.18632/oncotarget.16723.
42. Hossen, S., Hossain, M.K., Basher, M.K., Mia, M.N.H., Rahman, M.T., Uddin, M.J., Smart nanocarrier-based drug delivery systems for cancer therapy and toxicity studies: A review. *J. Adv. Res.*, 15, 1–18, Jan. 2019, doi: 10.1016/j.jare.2018.06.005.
43. Yao, Y., *et al.*, Nanoparticle-Based Drug Delivery in Cancer Therapy and Its Role in Overcoming Drug Resistance. *Front. Mol. Biosci.*, 7, 193, Aug. 2020, doi: 10.3389/fmolb.2020.00193.
44. Fu, C.-P., *et al.*, Hyaluronic Acid-Based Nanocarriers for Anticancer Drug Delivery. *Polymers (Basel)*, 15, 10, 2317, May 2023, doi: 10.3390/polym15102317.
45. Buckley, C., Murphy, E.J., Montgomery, T.R., Major, I., Hyaluronic Acid: A Review of the Drug Delivery Capabilities of This Naturally Occurring Polysaccharide. *Polymers (Basel)*, 14, 17, 3442, Aug. 2022, doi: 10.3390/polym14173442.
46. Zhong, L., *et al.*, Exploring the relationship of hyaluronic acid molecular weight and active targeting efficiency for designing hyaluronic acid-modified nanoparticles. *Asian J. Pharm. Sci.*, 14, 5, 521–530, Sep. 2019, doi: 10.1016/j.ajps.2018.11.002.
47. Luo, Z., Dai, Y., Gao, H., Development and application of hyaluronic acid in tumor targeting drug delivery. *Acta Pharm. Sin. B*, 9, 6, 1099–1112, Nov. 2019, doi: 10.1016/j.apsb.2019.06.004.
48. Hu, T., Gong, H., Xu, J., Huang, Y., Wu, F., He, Z., Nanomedicines for Overcoming Cancer Drug Resistance. *Pharmaceutics*, 14, 8, 1606, Aug. 2022, doi: 10.3390/pharmaceutics14081606.
49. Yerushalmi, N., Arad, A., Margalit, R., Molecular and cellular studies of hyaluronic acid-modified liposomes as bioadhesive carriers for topical drug delivery in wound healing. *Arch. Biochem. Biophys.*, 313, 2, 267–73, Sep. 1994, doi: 10.1006/abbi.1994.1387.
50. Bai, X., Smith, Z., Wang, Y., Butterworth, S., Tirella, A., Sustained Drug Release from Smart Nanoparticles in Cancer Therapy: A Comprehensive Review. *Micromachines (Basel)*, 13, 10, 1623, Sep. 2022, doi: 10.3390/mi13101623.
51. Sakurai, Y. and Harashima, H., Hyaluronan-modified nanoparticles for tumor-targeting. *Expert Opin. Drug Deliv.*, 16, 9, 915–936, Sep. 2019, doi: 10.1080/17425247.2019.1645115.

52. Maboudi, A.H., *et al.*, Micelle-based nanoparticles with stimuli-responsive properties for drug delivery. *Nanotechnol. Rev.*, 13, 1, 20230218, Mar. 2024, doi: 10.1515/ntrev-2023-0218.
53. Uthappa, U.T., Suneetha, M., Ajeya, K.V., Ji, S.M., Hyaluronic Acid Modified Metal Nanoparticles and Their Derived Substituents for Cancer Therapy: A Review. *Pharmaceutics*, 15, 6, 1713, Jun. 2023, doi: 10.3390/pharmaceutics15061713.
54. Ganesan, K., *et al.*, Targeting Engineered Nanoparticles for Breast Cancer Therapy. *Pharmaceutics*, 13, 11, 1829, Nov. 2021, doi: 10.3390/pharmaceutics13111829.
55. Kramer, M., Criswell, A., Marzette, K., Cutcliffe, E., Sewell-Loftin, M.K., Strain and hyaluronic acid interact to regulate ovarian cancer cell proliferation, migration, and drug resistance. *Mechanobiol. Med.*, 2, 4, 100094, Dec. 2024, doi: 10.1016/j.mbm.2024.100094.
56. Li, Y., Gao, Y., Zhang, X., Guo, H., Gao, H., Nanoparticles in precision medicine for ovarian cancer: From chemotherapy to immunotherapy. *Int. J. Pharm.*, 591, 119986, Dec. 2020, doi: 10.1016/j.ijpharm.2020.119986.
57. Gao, W., Chan, J.M., Farokhzad, O.C., pH-Responsive Nanoparticles for Drug Delivery. *Mol. Pharm.*, 7, 6, 1913–1920, Dec. 2010, doi: 10.1021/mp100253e.
58. Liu, T., *et al.*, CRISPR-Cas9-Mediated Silencing of CD44 in Human Highly Metastatic Osteosarcoma Cells. *Cell. Physiol. Biochem.*, 46, 3, 1218–1230, 2018, doi: 10.1159/000489072.
59. Sercombe, L., Veerati, T., Moheimani, F., Wu, S.Y., Sood, A.K., Hua, S., Advances and challenges of liposome assisted drug delivery. *Front. Pharmacol.*, 6, DEC, 163819, Dec. 2015, doi: 10.3389/FPHAR.2015.00286/BIBTEX.
60. Kesharwani, P., Jain, K., Jain, N.K., Dendrimer as nanocarrier for drug delivery. *Prog. Polym. Sci.*, 39, 2, 268–307, Feb. 2014, doi: 10.1016/J.PROGPOLYMSCI.2013.07.005.
61. Ventola, C.L., Progress in Nanomedicine: Approved and Investigational Nanodrugs. *Pharm. Ther.*, 42, 12, 742, Dec. 2017, Accessed: Jan. 24, 2025. [Online]. Available: https://pmc.ncbi.nlm.nih.gov/articles/PMC5720487/.
62. Ho, D., *et al.*, Enabling Technologies for Personalized and Precision Medicine. *Trends Biotechnol.*, 38, 5, 497–518, May 2020, doi: 10.1016/J.TIBTECH.2019.12.021.
63. Dhand, C., *et al.*, Bio-inspired *in situ* crosslinking and mineralization of electrospun collagen scaffolds for bone tissue engineering. *Biomaterials*, 104, 323–338, Oct. 2016, doi: 10.1016/J.BIOMATERIALS.2016.07.007.
64. Jiang, W., Gupta, R.K., Deshpande, M.C., Schwendeman, S.P., Biodegradable poly(lactic-co-glycolic acid) microparticles for injectable delivery of vaccine antigens. *Adv. Drug Deliv. Rev.*, 57, 3, 391–410, Jan. 2005, doi: 10.1016/J.ADDR.2004.09.003.
65. Kumari, A., Yadav, S.K., Yadav, S.C., Biodegradable polymeric nanoparticles based drug delivery systems. *Colloids Surf. B Biointerfaces*', 75, 1, 1–18, Jan. 2010, doi: 10.1016/J.COLSURFB.2009.09.001.

66. Bobo, D., Robinson, K.J., Islam, J., Thurecht, K.J., Corrie, S.R., Nanoparticle-Based Medicines: A Review of FDA-Approved Materials and Clinical Trials to Date. *Pharm. Res.*, 33, 10, 2373–2387, Oct. 2016, doi: 10.1007/S11095-016-1958-5/METRICS.
67. Shang, J., *et al.*, Recent developments in nanomaterials for upgrading treatment of orthopedics diseases. *Front. Bioeng. Biotechnol.*, 11, 1221365, Aug. 2023, doi: 10.3389/FBIOE.2023.1221365/BIBTEX.

8

Beta Glucagon: Immunomodulatory Effects and Anti-Cancer Applications

Mehwish Rafiq[1], Muhammad Asmat Ullah Saleem[2*], Ali Raza[3], Abdullah Ahmed Butt[4], Farhat Bano[5], Muhammad Ahsan Ullah Danish[6] and Ji-Xin Tang[7†]

[1]*National Institute of Food Science and Technology (NIFSAT), University of Agriculture, Faisalabad, Pakistan*
[2]*Institute of Nephrology, Affiliated Hospital of Guangdong Medical University, Zhanjiang, Guangdong, China*
[3]*Department of Food Sciences and Technology, Government College University, Faisalabad, Pakistan*
[4]*Department of Dairy Technology, University of Veterinary and Animal Sciences, Lahore, Pakistan*
[5]*Department of Allied Health Sciences, The University of Agriculture, Dera Ismail Khan, Khyber Pakhtun khwa, Pakistan*
[6]*Department of Clinical Sciences, Gomal University, Dera Ismail Khan, Khyber Pakhtun khwa, Pakistan*
[7]*Guangdong Provincial Key Laboratory of Autophagy and Major Chronic Noncommunicable Diseases, Key Laboratory of Prevention and Management of Chronic Kidney Diseases of Zhanjiang City, Institute of Nephrology, Affiliated Hospital of Guangdong Medical University, Zhanjiang, Guangdong, China*

Abstract

Beta-glucan is a type of polysaccharide found in the cell walls of various organisms, including fungi, yeast, bacteria, and cereals like oats and barley. Known for its immunomodulatory and anti-cancer properties, beta-glucan has garnered significant attention in recent years. This chapter explores the mechanisms by which beta-glucan exerts its effects on the immune system and its potential as an anti-cancer agent. Beta-glucan's immunomodulatory effects are primarily

**Corresponding author*: Dr.asmat_neau@yahoo.com
†*Corresponding author*: Tangjixin@gdmu.edu.cn

Luqman Jameel Rather, Showkat Ali Ganie and Mohammed A. Assiri (eds.) Polysaccharide Biomaterials in Cancer Research and Therapy: From Lab to Life, (223–266) © 2026 Scrivener Publishing LLC

mediated through its interaction with specific receptors on immune cells, such as dectin-1, complement receptor 3 (CR3), and toll-like receptors. These interactions trigger a cascade of immune responses, enhancing the activity of macrophages, neutrophils, and natural killer (NK) cells. Macrophages, upon activation by beta-glucan, exhibit increased phagocytic activity, improved antigen presentation, and the secretion of pro-inflammatory cytokines. Neutrophils show enhanced microbial killing abilities, while NK cells demonstrate increased cytotoxicity against tumor cells. These immune responses collectively contribute to a strengthened immune system capable of combating infections and malignancies. In addition to its immunomodulatory effects, beta-glucan has shown promising anti-cancer properties. Several preclinical and clinical studies have reported beta-glucan's ability to inhibit tumor growth and metastasis. Beta-glucan enhances the immune system's ability to recognize and destroy cancer cells by promoting the maturation and activation of dendritic cells, which are crucial for initiating adaptive immune responses. Furthermore, beta-glucan induces the production of specific cytokines, such as interferon-gamma and tumor necrosis factor-alpha, which play critical roles in antitumor immunity. One of the notable advantages of beta-glucan as an anti-cancer agent is its ability to modulate the tumor microenvironment. By altering the tumor microenvironment, beta-glucan can reduce immunosuppression and improve the efficacy of existing cancer therapies. For instance, beta-glucan can enhance the effectiveness of monoclonal antibody therapies by facilitating the recruitment and activation of immune cells at the tumor site. Additionally, beta-glucan's ability to enhance the gut microbiota's composition further contributes to its anti-cancer effects, as a healthy gut microbiome is associated with improved immune function and reduced cancer risk. Recent advancements in beta-glucan research have led to the development of novel delivery systems and formulations to improve its bioavailability and therapeutic potential. Encapsulation techniques, such as liposomes and nanoparticles, have been employed to enhance beta-glucan's stability and absorption in the body. These innovations hold promise for optimizing beta-glucan's clinical applications in immunotherapy and oncology. Beta-glucan is a potent immunomodulatory agent with significant anti-cancer potential. Continued research and clinical trials are essential to fully understand beta-glucan's mechanisms of action and to develop effective strategies for its integration into cancer treatment protocols.

***Keywords*:** Beta-glucan, immunomodulation, anti-cancer, immune response, tumor micro-environment

8.1 Introduction

Beta-glucans are a type of natural polysaccharide found in glucose molecules linked together by β-glycosidic bonds. They are found throughout nature, in the cell walls of bacteria, fungi, yeast, algae, and some plants (such as oats and barley) [58]. Because of the different sources and ways beta-glucans are structured, they have been subject to lots of attention for their potential health benefits as well as applications in food, pharmaceuticals, and all other kinds of industries. Mushroom-derived beta-glucans are widely consumed and tend to have primarily (1→3)-β-D-glucan backbones with variable levels of (1→6) branching, which display lower triple-helix content than cereal-based β(1–3)glucan [15]. Yeast beta-glucans, mainly (1→3)-β-D-glucan with a variable distribution of additional units such as 6-O-linked β- D-glucose oligomers, attached to every third residue in the backbone structure, whereas others linked through branching are isolated from yeast, particularly *Saccharomyces cerevisiae*. Beta-glucans present in oats and barley are mixed-linkage (1→3), (1→4)-β-D-glucans. This linear structure, with random (1→3) linkages interspersed in the main chain of consecutive (1→4)-linked glucopyranosyl residues, affects its water solubility and viscosity. Algal beta-glucans are an example of algal polysaccharides, found in algae such as *Laminaria* and show types where they possess a (1→3)-linked backbone with over 50% branching from β-(1→4)-linked glucose components, making them structurally distinct from terrestrial plant-derived beta-glucans. Linear and branched are so far known to be producers of bacterial beta-glucans; however, in the case of Agrobacterium, they exist also with some non-glycan components modifying their properties. With the exceptions of linkage changes and solvent differences in solubility, other cereals such as rye and sorghum also contain β-glucans that have similar structures.

The solubility, viscosity, and bioactivity of β-glucans depend on their structural properties including the type of glycosidic linkages formed between monomeric units, branching patterns within each molecular chain, and finally molecular size [26]. Beta-glucan solubility and molecular interactions with other food components are influenced by the presence of (1→3) linked glucose residues interspersed between longer stretches of mainly consecutive or regularly interspersed beta-(1-4)-linked regions, to which minor amounts, such as 6%–10%, in cereal fibers affect all model foods. β-glucans have potential health benefits such as they can modulate the immune system from an anti-inflammatory direction (not so much as fungi-derived peptides, e.g., yeast) by upregulating macrophages, neutrophils, or cell activities potentially useful for both immunological support and cancer therapy applications [36].

β-glucans from oats and barley including cereals have been shown to reduce blood cholesterol [47]. They are viscous in that they turn into a gel in the intestines and that is how they can bind with cholesterol, as well as bile acids lowering its absorption. Furthermore, taking beta-glucans can help slow down the breakdown and absorption of carbohydrates in individuals with diabetes, which leads to better blood sugar control [29]. They also serve as prebiotics, nourishing the good bacteria in your gut and supporting the general well-being of the intestines. Owing to the aforementioned health benefits, beta-glucans are used in a plethora of applications. In the food industry, they are mainly used to increase fiber content in functional foods and dietary supplements with cholesterol-lowering effects as well as immune-boosting activity. In the pharmaceutical field, β-glucans are being studied in many realms of sort; they can be used as preventive dealers inclusive of most cancer treatments or immune modulation. This is just another example of how important beta-glucans are and why they can be used in skincare products because they are extremely hydrating and soothing as well. It is a multifaceted bioactive compound with many health benefits, as well as other applications.

8.2 Importance of Immunomodulatory and Anti-Cancer Properties

8.2.1 Immunomodulatory Properties

This receptor-binding triggers downstream immunomodulatory effects of β-glucans. In this regard, multiple innate immune receptor types (e.g., Dectin-1, complement receptor 3 [CR3], and toll-like receptors [TLRs]) are expressed by various host immune cells such as macrophages, neutrophils dendritic cells, natural killer (NK) cells, etc. Beta-glucans begin a cascade of immune response when they bind to these with immune cell receptors. It activates innate immunity, one of the most important benefits. Macrophages and neutrophils are the primary responders in phagocytosis, which is used to engulf and destroy pathogens or dead/dying cells; this activity can be enhanced by immunomodulant compounds like beta-glucans (CC). β-glucans strengthen the action of these phagocytic cells to help diminish infections in the body [61]. In addition to activating innate immune components, beta-glucans can modulate adaptive immunity. Adjuvants induce the maturation and activation of dendritic cells, which are essential for antigen presentation to T and B lymphocytes. This improves the body, encouraging directed reactions toward specific pathogens or abnormal cells. β-glucans also influence cytokine expressions (signaling molecules that coordinate the immune response). They are capable of balancing pro-inflammatory and anti-inflammatory cytokines, thus promoting immune homeostasis to prevent more inflammation.

8.2.2 Anti-Cancer Properties

The cancer-fighting properties of β-glucans go hand in hand with their immune system-modulating effects. They are being characterized as adjuvant therapeutic agents in cancer because they may help the body defend itself better against tumors. One way this is achieved is by the promotion of antitumor immunity. β-glucans are responsible for the activation of NK cells and cytotoxic T cells, which play a central role in cancer immune defense [35]. This mechanism helps train the immune system to recognize and respond to abnormal cells, how to identify and kill cancer cells, leading to tumor reduction. β-glucans may also directly promote apoptosis, or programmed cell death, in cancer cells. This quality of the plant is very beneficial for cancer therapies as killing particular cells without damaging normal ones can prevent elevated-term characteristics from strengthening [65]. Also, β-glucans are traditionally studied along with common cancer treatments such as chemotherapy and radiation. In theory, they could help current treatments work better by stimulating the immune system to destroy cancer and also decrease many treatment-related side effects. β-glucans, on the other hand, can reduce cancer metastasis by changing not only immune responses but also tumor microenvironments [18]. Beta-glucans are immunomodulating effects that have been studied widely for clinical applications including anti-cancer strategies. This immune-enhancing ability of beta-glucans is a natural and promising treatment for infections as well as cancer. The aforementioned compounds are being actively investigated to realize their full therapeutic potential, potentially offering better outcomes for patients as well as a greater repertoire of immune-based therapies.

8.3 Understanding Beta-Glucan

Beta-glucans are various kinds of naturally occurring polysaccharides located in the cell walls of bacteria, fungi, fungus infection, and cereals such as oats plus barley. To comprehend beta-glucans, we have to consider the sources of these polysaccharides along with their structural features and action on the physiological level, rendering them a highly investigated subject within nutrition, medicine, as well as biotechnology. The popularity of natural and functional foods is causing beta-glucans to be increasingly studied for their potential ability to benefit human health.

8.3.1 Chemical Structure and Sources

Beta-glucans are a family of carbohydrates found in the cell walls or cereal fibers but also other plant sources such as mushrooms and bacteria, with well-known health-promoting attributes including cholesterol reduction (for which oat beta-glucan claims an EFSA-approved health claim) and blood sugar regulation. Oat beta-glucans have a mixed-linkage β-D-structure of (1→3) and (1→4)-linked D-glucose units. It consists of a linear backbone with β-D-glucose backbones connected by (1→4) linkages and containing single (1→3) connections distributed among the main chain. These (1→3) linkages cause the (1→4)-linkage to angle, and this irregular pattern is thought by many researchers to be responsible for certain unique biological functions of beta-glucans. Barley (*Hordeum vulgare*) is another important source of beta-glucans, analogous to oats but with minor differences in structure and solubility. Barley beta-glucans, like those of oats, are not water-soluble but can form high-viscosity solutions in cell-free extracts [29]. However, the proportion and distribution of these linkages might vary a little so it would slightly change their physicochemical properties. The increased molecular weight and the more 1→3 (units) linkages of barley beta-glucans could lead to gameplay due compared to oats. It is this arrangement of structures that gives them their ability to create viscous solutions in the GI tract, which slows down digestion and absorption (a good thing for controlling blood sugar levels as well as supporting heart health) [41].

Yeasts, especially for *Saccharomyces cerevisiae*, are also well known to provide a high concentration of immunomodulatory beta-glucans. The (1→3)-β-D-glucan is the major component of yeast β-glucans and contains many branched points in its skeletal chains, which are connected by β-(1→6) glycosidic linkage. This forked structure is unique and important for immune recognition. The branches form an intricate three-dimensional angle that enables the beta-glucans to better lock onto immune cell receptors like Dectin-1. This process then activates a broad range of immune responses, creating the potential for yeast beta-glucans to assist to increase our innate immunity and perhaps protect us from infections or diseases [49]. Well-known adjunctive remedies include mushrooms such as Reishi or Shiitake, which are brimming with bioactivity *via* beta-glucans. Fungal β-glucans are usually (1→3)-β-D-glucan backbones with sporadic branches of between 100 and 200 glucose units, essentially a higher-molecular-weight version of yeast beta-1,6 glucan (Figure 8.1). The most commonly known bioactive components of oats are the beta-glucans that frequently occur as triple-helix structures. Fungal β-glucans have

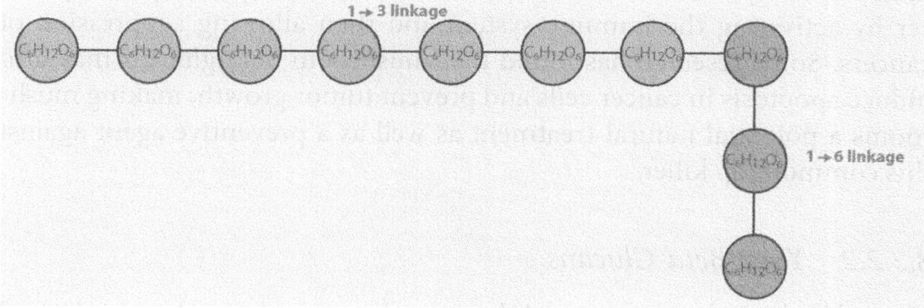

Figure 8.1 Chemical structure of beta-glucan from fungi showing the typical molecular structure.

additional solubility and immune-enhancing features from their structural complexity. Characterized by their ability to modulate immune responses, NK cells have been investigated for potential anti-cancer effects given that they can activate immune and induce tumor cell apoptosis [62]. Algae, particularly species of *Laminaria*, offers beta-glucans with structural characteristics that are not terrestrial. On the other hand, algal β-glucans consist mainly of (1→3)- linkages but also rare (1→2) branching, which illustrates that they have different features as well. This branching pattern makes the beta-glucan much less insoluble and a bio-actin form, which is being studied in health-supportive properties. As dietary fibers and possibly as modulators of the immune system, algal beta-glucans have a unique structure. The ability of some fibers to form gels and their high-water-binding capacity are advantageous in the food industry along with nutraceuticals because they modify nutritional profiles and cause changes in functional foods.

8.3.2 Types of Beta-Glucans

8.3.2.1 Fungal Beta-Glucans

Fungal beta-glucans are found in Reishi, Shiitake, and Maitake mushrooms, known for their immunomodulatory and anti-cancer properties. Research also suggests that beta-glucans combined with aloe vera enhance immune function by acting as polysaccharide powders that regulate the immune response of macrophages and dendritic cells [48]. This stimulation of activity promotes the secretion of cytokines, responsible for coordinating immune responses. Beta-glucans present in fungi boost immunity, which helps activate the body's natural defense mechanisms against infections.

Moreover, they have been demonstrated to be effective in preventing cancer by activating the immune system and then allowing suppression of cancers. Some research has found that mushroom beta-glucans may also induce apoptosis in cancer cells and prevent tumor growth, making mushrooms a potential natural treatment as well as a preventive agent against this common top killer.

8.3.2.2 *Yeast Beta-Glucans*

Natural biological response modulators such as yeast beta-glucans, derived from *Saccharomyces cerevisiae*, are some of the most potent immunomodulators we know. Immune cell receptors, like Dectin-1, kick off a response in the immune system by binding to commensal carbohydrates, and these interactions turn on macrophages (white round dots) as well as other cells involved in immunity [32]. This interaction triggers the molding of cytokines and promotes phagocyte activity further enhancing the body's ability to fight pathogens. Yeast beta-glucans have been shown to activate our body's NK cells, cytotoxic T lymphocytes that are particularly important in identifying and destroying cancerous cells. Consequently, yeast β-glucans prevent tumor growth by activating innate immune cells to participate in antitumor activity and creating conditions that promote apoptosis within the tumor.

8.3.2.3 *Oat Beta-Glucans*

Although oat beta-glucans are most well known for their cardiovascular and metabolic health benefits, they have also been shown to exert immunomodulatory effects. They can boost the immune system by activating macrophages and induce beneficial cytokines to be secreted. Oat beta-glucans (Figure 8.2), which lower cholesterol and improve blood

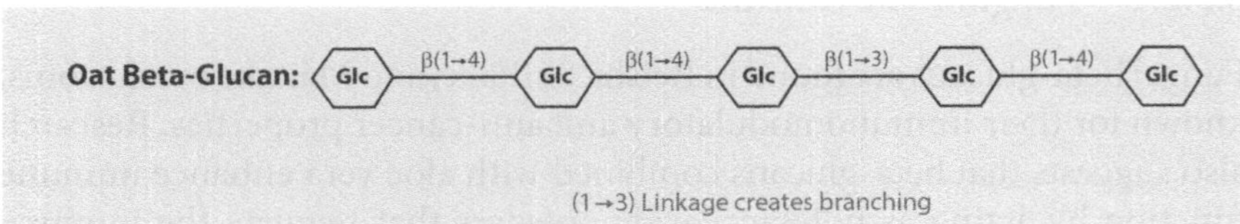

Figure 8.2 Chemical structure of oat beta-glucan.

glucose control, support the immune system through their contribution to good health [69]. While expanded research on these alternative forms of beta-glucans has focused mainly on their anti-cancer properties, oats have been shown to improve metabolic health, which, in turn, may lessen cancer risk. Oat beta-glucans have been shown to protect the cardiovascular system, and reductions in blood cholesterol may contribute to their anti-cancer properties.

8.3.2.4 Barley Beta-Glucans

The effects of barley beta-glucans have many similarities with oats, which have been the nutritional focus to date, indicating immunomodulatory properties. They are capable of stimulating macrophages and increasing host cytokine production, thus supporting the immune responses a body needs to combat infections [34]. The functionality of barley beta-glucans in reducing cholesterol and facilitating glycemic control also directly contributes to better health quality, which results in a reduced risk for certain diseases. About anti-cancer attributes, the barley beta-glucans bring enzymatic changes, therefore decreasing tumor threat. It is also suggested that their role in reducing inflammation and oxidative stress supports both aspects of development for cancer prevention.

8.3.2.5 Cereals Beta-Glucans

Immunomodulatory and health-beneficial effects have also been described for beta-glucans from other cereals, such as rye or sorghum. They also exert immunomodulatory activities by ingestion of the surrounding milieu including activation of macrophages and regulation of cytokine production. Consumption of these cereals leads to better gut health and metabolic regulation, aiding immune function and reducing disease susceptibility indirectly. While there is little research on the anti-cancer properties specifically in these beta-glucans, it would make sense that a compound that arguably helps prevent cancer (through weight loss and inflammation reduction) could both fight against and slow its progression. Dietary fiber and antioxidants in these cereals add to their health-protecting properties, which may impede the onset of cancer. The details of the different types of beta-glucans are provided in Table 8.1 along with the sources and structural characteristics.

Table 8.1 A table listing different types of beta-glucans (e.g., from fungi, yeast, oats, and barley) and their sources, along with structural characteristics.

Types of beta glucagon	Source	Structural characters
Fungal beta-glucan	Mushrooms	Predominantly (1→3)-β-D-glucans with some (1→6) branching; forms a triple-helix structure.
Yeast beta-glucan	*Saccharomyces cerevisiae*	Mostly (1→3)-β-D-glucans with (1→6) branching; known for a highly branched structure.
Oat beta-glucan	Oats (*Avena sativa*)	Mixed-linkage (1→3), (1→4)-β-D-glucans; linear structure with random (1→3) linkages breaking (1→4) sequence.
Barley beta-glucan	Barley (*Hordeum vulgare*)	Like oat beta-glucan with mixed-linkage (1→3), (1→4)-β-D-glucans; more linear than fungal or yeast glucans.
Algal beta-glucan	Algae (*Laminaria*)	Predominantly (1→3)-β-D-glucans with unique (1→2) branching; distinct from terrestrial sources.
Bacterial beta-glucan	Bacteria (*Agrobacterium*)	Linear or branched (1→3)-β-D-glucans; often with unique non-glucan components.
Cereal beta-glucan	Rye, sorghum	Similar to oat and barley with mixed-linkage (1→3), (1→4)-β-D-glucans; varies slightly in structure and solubility.

8.4 Methods of Extraction

8.4.1 Hot Water Extraction

Hot water extraction is one of the oldest and most common methods for beta-glucans isolation, especially from fungi and yeast. This process consists of heating the raw material with water at temperatures ranging from 80 to 100°C so that in this way cell wall will break down and beta-glucans will dissolve into the medium. After that extract, it was filtered for the removal of insoluble materials, which are proteins, lipids, and cell debris. The main advantage of hot extraction is the preservation of the functional properties of beta-glucans, which remain active and are suitable as bioactive substances [33]. On the other hand, it may be necessary to further purify this process in subsequent stages due to beta-glucans from such a raw material being water-soluble with other components, which inversely dissolved.

8.4.2 Alkaline Extraction

The most classic method, alkaline extraction with sodium hydroxide or potassium hydroxide solution, enabled selective solubilization of beta-glucans from cereal sources mainly oats and barley. Gut bacteria prefer an alkaline environment, probably in part because it makes cellulose and hemicellulose, which comprise the bulk of plant cell walls, water-soluble. Usually, the raw material is steeped in a heated (c. 60°C to c. 80°C) alkaline solution at concentrations of 1–2% for several hours (more problematical sources like cassava need more rigorous treatments). Following extraction, the solution is acidified to precipitate contaminants that can then be filtered or centrifuged. While high levels of beta-glucans can be achieved using this method, extreme care should be taken to carefully control the conditions so as not to degrade said polysaccharides.

8.4.3 Enzymatic Extraction

Enzymatic extraction incorporates special enzymes that specifically degrade cell wall components without damaging beta-glucans. Cellulases, hemicellulases, and proteases are the widely known enzymes for this extraction [56]. This method of using enzymes is done by incubating the raw material with an enzyme at optimal pH and temperature for several hours. This method is useful since it sustains the basic structure and bioactivity of beta-glucans. One of its main applications is the handling of sensitive materials, or whenever high purity is a concern. Enzymatic extraction is an environment-friendly process that utilizes enzymes to selectively remove or modify cell wall components, offering a sustainable approach to extraction.

8.4.4 Acid Extraction

Acids such as acetic acid or citric acid are used to solubilize beta-glucans. Beta-glucans are released following the breakdown of the cell wall matrix due to acidic conditions. This usually involves treatment of the material at low to moderate temperature (50–70°C), with a dilute acid solution. Although acid extraction is not as common and less suitable than others, it may be advantageous when keeping the beta-glucan structure under certain conditions. The solution is then filtered or precipitated to remove impurities and is usually neutralized after extraction.

8.5 Methods of Purification

8.5.1 Alcohol Precipitation

For the isolation of beta-glucans, the simplest and best method is alcohol precipitation. Ethanol (or methanol) is mixed with water extract in such quantity that helps precipitation of beta-glucans. The problem is alcohol is a nonpolar solvent, and beta-glucans are hydrophilic. The mixture is left for some time, and beta-glucans are settled separately, thus isolated by centrifugation or filtration. The precipitate can then be resuspended and washed with alcohol to remove the remaining impurities. This is a very scalable and easy-to-control process for industrial uses. Nevertheless, stringent controlling the content of alcohol and temperature is essential to acquire a maximal output with high purity.

8.5.2 Ultrafiltration

The membranes used in ultrafiltration have pores of specific sizes that the beta-glucans are separated by weight as well [17]. Cellulose mixed with water is pumped onto the membrane before it sets, and through osmosis (water moving from lower concentration to higher), beta-glucan solution surrounds that cellulose catching smaller molecules as a result. It is a very high potential method for concentrating and purifying beta-glucans. It is typically combined with other purification methods to obtain the kind of purities being talked about. The bioactivity of beta-glucans is noteworthy, especially for food and pharmaceutical applications; hence, chemical-free ultrafiltration processing is able to preserve their characteristic structural property.

8.5.3 Chromatography

Beta-glucans can be separated easily from by-product components with high resolution in chromatography techniques, for example, gel filtration and ion exchange chromatography [67]. Gel filtration chromatography filters molecules according to their size and allows the isolation of larger beta-glucans from smaller impurities. On the other hand, ion exchange chromatography separates molecules based on charge differences removing charged impurities [63]. These are high-precision methods that yield higher purity levels and are perfect for research or the needs of applications requiring beta-glucans in a purer form. However, they are often more involved and expensive when compared with other purification techniques.

8.5.4 Dialysis

However, dialysis uses semi-permeable membranes to separate beta-glucans from low-molar-mass compounds and impurities. The beta-glucan solution was put into a dialysis bag that is immersed in a large volume of water or buffer. Small molecules exit the bag, leaving behind purified beta-glucans. This is an example of dialysis, which, in general, does not interfere with the chemical nature of beta-glucans, and due to its non-invasive character preserves both their structure and functionality. They are excellent for lab-scale purification as they provide a mild and delicate process of purification to guarantee that the bioactivity of beta-glucans is not lost during the process. But dialysis is slow and not useful for industrial-scale operations.

8.6 Beta-Glucan Immunomodulatory Effects

8.6.1 Mechanism of Action

8.6.1.1 Dectin-1 Receptor

Dectin-1 is a pattern recognition receptor, and the role it plays is very important in the ability of the immune system to recognize the presence of most pathogen antigens. It is especially affiliated with fungal ones [2]. It belongs to the C-type lectin receptor family and is expressed at the cellular surface mainly in dendritic cells, macrophages, and neutrophils, but to a lesser degree in T cells. Thus, Dectin-1 recognizes not only the major components of fungal cell walls, including beta-glucan, but also beta-glucan coming from yeast, bacteria, or, in some forms, even higher plants [2]. It has also been associated with other very key cytokines (pro-inflammatory), including TNF-α, IL-6, and

IL-23, relevant to the effective response of immunity to infections [59]. Further studies have also shown that this Dectin-1/Syk pathway not only induces a response against the pathogen but also is competent to activate dendritic cells by way of a maturation process [9]. It is expected that enhancing dendritic cell maturation will have the potential for beta-glucans to potentiate the immune system with a capacity to mount long-lasting antigen-specific responses. It has been demonstrated that Dectin-1 is capable of enhancing immunity recognition and killing of tumor cells by the activation of macrophages and dendritic cells, which can bring tumor antigens to T cells and can further induce immune response against the tumor [10, 30].

8.6.1.2 Complement Receptor 3

It plays a very essential role in the immune system, particularly during the operation of phagocytosis and immune surveillance. Expressions of CR3 have been found on different immune cells: neutrophils, macrophages, and NK cells [8]. It is paramount in the recognition and phagocytosis of foreign-invading organisms and in the control of immune responses [52]. CR3 is one of the integrin proteins implicated in cell adhesion and signaling. The basic role of CR3 is to perform the phagocytosis of the opsonized pathogen. Opsonization is the marking of a pathogen for destruction by the immune system, usually coating their surface with complement proteins or antibodies [53]. These opsonized pathogens will then bind to the CR3, allowing the phagocytes to engulf and destroy it [1]. The ligation of beta-glucan with CR3 will induce a variety of intracellular signaling events, which activate the immune cell [31]. These include initiation of the Syk kinase pathway and the creation of reactive oxygen species (ROS)—events necessary for killing ingested pathogens [31]. Besides, in connection with their role in clearing pathogens, the members of the integrin receptor family, which include CR3, are being considered to play a role in how the immune system handles cancer as well [54]. In these circumstances, there are reports that CR3 can, in fact, facilitate the recognition and phagocytosis of tumor cells [66].

8.6.1.3 Toll-Like Receptors

TLRs belong to the protein family whose major function pertains to the innate immune system. Basically, the functions of these proteins deal with the recognition of molecules associated with pathogens. Their expression in terms of receptors is mainly on immune cells like macrophages, dendritic cells, and neutrophils. This identification of the presence of microbial components by them takes place through an activated immune response after going through a signaling pathway [24]. As such, TLRs present the first line of defense against host infection and trigger cytokine induction upon stimulation to direct immune responses [60]. This TLR recognizes it and triggers the intracellular pathways of activated NF-κB (nuclear factor kappa-light-chain-enhancer of activated B cells) [2]. NF-κB is generally considered a transcription factor involved in controlling genes encoding immune responses, cytokines, chemokines, and other inflammatory mediators [53]. In this way, such TLR-mediated activation allows for the expression of TNF-α, IL-1, and IL-6 (proinflammatory cytokines) able to generate the possibility required by an initializing and chronic inflammatory response to keep infections under control [54, 64]. Other cytokines like IL-1 and IL-6 activate the T cells and B cells, which make up the immune cells of the adaptive immunity [23, 64]. It binds to TLRs, hence increasing the system's ability to identify and destroy tumor cells. This is due to the fact that cytokines activate NK cells and cytotoxic T lymphocytes [51].

8.6.2 Activation of Immune Cells

8.6.2.1 Macrophages

One of the crucial members of the immune system, macrophages participate equally in both innate and adaptive immunity. Cells identify, engulf, and destroy microorganisms through phagocytosis and further activate other immune cells [7, 14]. The binding to the surface receptors of macrophages triggers intracellular events that heighten its ability to engulf and destroy pathogens [10]. Phagocytosis thus becomes an integral part in controlling the course of the infection or, at the least, controlling pathogen dissemination. The primary effect of β-glucan is to increase cytokine production by macrophages [19]. The latter are signaling molecules mediating and regulating immunity, inflammation, and hematopoiesis [20]. These cytokines initiate and amplify the host inflammatory response by bringing more immune cells to the infection site or damage, making them more potent in their immune response state [30]. A very important role of macrophages, apart from fighting infection, is in cancer immunity. Beta-glucan enhances the killing ability of macrophages against encountering tumor cells [54, 59]. On the other hand, beta-glucan-treated macrophages exhibited an enhanced antigen presentation. That is to say, they would most likely have procedures for presenting antigens to T cells and cause an adaptive immune response [52].

8.6.2.2 Neutrophils

There are five types of WBCs. Neutrophils form the maximum number of leukocytes in circulation, around 70%, and hence make up the majority of WBCs of the innate immune system. They form the first line of defense in host immunity, which works to counter infection due to the very fast process of response and phagocytosis of the invading pathogen [55]. Thirdly, they are highly mobile and, as predominantly first-line defenders, reach the seat of infection/damage very quickly. Once neutrophils arrive at the site, they adopt other mechanisms. Phagocytosis, degranulation, and neutrophil extracellular trap release are some of the activities that neutrophils do [2, 66]. Hence, it results in increased chemotaxis and accumulation of these neutrophils in the site of infection [51]. One of the basic functions that neutrophils perform is phagocytosis, the engulfing and digestion of pathogens [4]. This effect is done through the binding of beta-glucan by CR3 in interaction with this effect upon the efficiency of pathogen uptake and destruction [30]. Besides stimulation of phagocytosis, beta-glucan also triggers the production of ROS by neutrophils [52, 59]. The other is that neutrophils release NETs, which is a network of extracellular fibers composed by DNA and histones complexed with antimicrobial proteins [19]. B-glucan increased the output of NETs and increased the potential of neutrophils to prevent the spreading of an infection [42].

8.6.2.3 NK Cells

It is one of the necessary arms of the innate immunity and represents an effective arm of host defense, responding rapidly to tissue cells infected by a virus or to tumor cells in the shortage of prior sensitization [16]. NK cells must swift a variety of initiating and inhibitory receptors, with their expression adjusted to the right level of cytotoxicity. In other words, NK cells must respond immediately to the threat without causing harm due to errors through fratricide or an exaggerated response to the infection [5]. Beta-glucan, a polysaccharide containing a β-1, 3 link with branches, has been isolated from the cell walls of fungi and yeast, and from plants;

it has been shown to activate NK cells [23, 51]. Such upregulation in cytotoxicity is mediated *via* the initiation of NK cells and expression at the cell surface of different activating NK cell receptors, including NKG2D, which are involved in the recognition of stress-induced ligands on the surface of infected or malignant cells [5]. Another important mechanism through which β-glucan enhances the activity of NK cells is the production of the cytokine interferon-gamma, which represents nearly the most potent factor of immune response against cancer and infections [2, 55].

8.6.3 Effect on Adaptive Immune Response

8.6.3.1 Dendritic Cell Activation

Dendritic cells are classified as major players of the immune system. They act as principal APCs and form a connection between innate and adaptive immunity. These cells internalize the antigens from pathogens or tumor cells and process them for presentation on T cells to elicit an adaptive immune reaction [1]. Maturation and initiation of DCs finally establish the preconditions for adequate immune functioning and arouse an antigen-specific, lasting immune response [1, 42]. It involves upregulation of major histocompatibility complex molecules like CD80 and CD86, and effective activation of T cells by cytokines [19, 28]. Antigen presentation by DCs is a very important process for activation of both helper and cytotoxic T lymphocytes [1, 52]. Though T helper cells regulate the immune response by activation of other immune cells, cytotoxic T lymphocytes themselves destroy tumor cells [1, 51]. It even induces the key cytokines, including IL-12 and TNF-α, in mediating T-cell differentiation and activation of the DC having treatments with beta-glucans [52]. Of these, IL-12 are major Th1-type immune response-inducing molecules that interlink with improved antitumor and antiviral immunity [30].

8.6.3.2 T-Cell Responses

T cells are the effector cells of the adaptive immune system and pertain to recognition and the T-cell response to antigens containing epitopes presented by antigen-presenting cells like dendritic cells. Two major subtypes are helper T cells, which help different immune cells, and cytotoxic T lymphocytes, which damage infected or malignant cells [65]. Major steps for the activation and proliferation of T cells are involved in the specific, long-lasting immune response to infection and tumors

(Figure 8.3) [50]. Beta-glucan has a direct effect on the activation and functions of T cells [10]. It activates the function of the dendritic cell; hence, T-cell responses are boosted indirectly, especially in the context of infection and cancer [7]. A major effect of beta-glucan on T cells is the basis towards a Th1 kind of immune response. Of the helper T cells, the Th1 cells make up a group of T cells that can produce cytokines, and among the latter, the regulation of macrophages and enhancing the cytotoxic activity especially of CD8+ T cells by IFN-γ are of paramount significance [54]. Such a response has been observed against intracellular pathogens, primarily viruses, as well as tumor cells. It stimulates the Th1 response, enhancing the body's ability to activate the immune system and defend against foreign invaders [42].

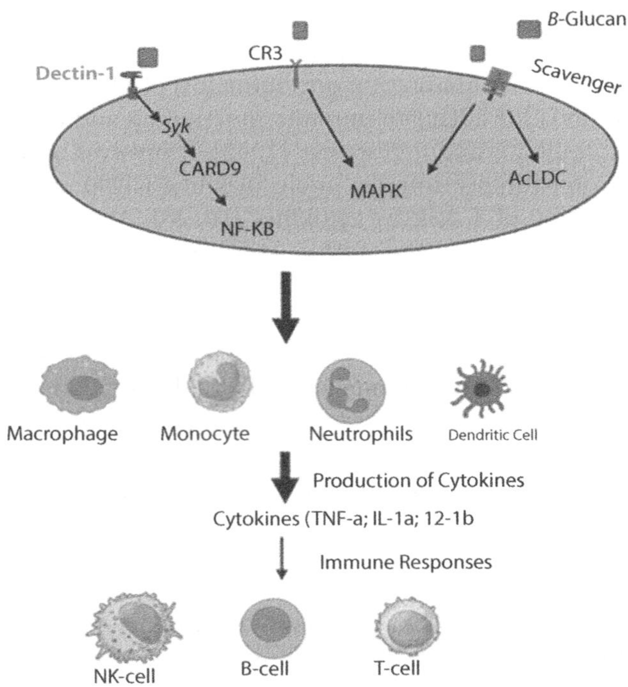

Figure 8.3 Immune activation through the induction of (1→3)-β-glucans: the (1→3)-β-glucans may exert their effect through the activation of numerous receptors, including Dectin-1, CR3, and scavenger, which are found within.

8.7 Anti-Cancer Properties

8.7.1 Preclinical and Clinical Studies

Indeed, only recently, at a preclinical and clinical level, extensive studies of beta-glucan as an anti-cancer agent have been performed, while very promising results on the efficacy of this compound against tumor growth and metastasis were obtained in recent years [4]. Studies at the preclinical levels using animal models have so far shown quite a great deal of evidence that beta-glucan had a significant effect in reducing the tumor burden, hence improving the overall survival rate of animals with different types of cancer [24]. Preclinical data testify that beta-glucan can also induce antitumor effects against several experimental models for breast, lung, colorectal, and melanoma cancers [7]. Indeed, in murine models of breast cancer, administration with β-glucan has affected the volume of the tumor and the number of sites of metastasis [50]. This effect is achieved primarily by enhancing the immune response through the activation of macrophages, neutrophils, and natural killer (NK) cells [30]. Research evidence based on studies of colorectal cancer models has similarly shown that beta-glucan is able to suppress tumor growth and metastasis, mediated possibly through the activation of immune cells and control of the tumor microenvironment [2, 23] . This higher immune activity correlated with disease stabilization, and some patients even displayed partial tumor regression.

8.7.2 Immune Surveillance

This can be annotated through most of the anti-cancer mechanisms of beta-glucan that are mediated through the enhancement of immune surveillance [51]. Immune surveillance is a process in which elements of the immunity recognize and eliminate malignant cells before their replicative or invasive events happen, before they develop into recognizable tumors, or metastasize in different parts of the body [14]. Immune surveillance is significantly augmented by beta-glucan through activities embodied in various immune cells, particularly macrophages and NK cells [1]. Macrophages become central in the body's defense against cancer since they can sense, ingest, and dispose of malignant cells [19, 54]. This will result in the activation of macrophages, which turn highly phagocytic as well as cytokine producers. Most of these cytokines,

Table 8.2 Specific immune cells affected by beta-glucan.

Immune cell type	Mechanism of action	Relevant outcomes
Macrophages	Enhanced phagocytosis, increased cytokine secretion (IL-1, IL-6, TNF-α)	Increased pathogen clearance, enhanced immune response [4].
Neutrophils	Improved chemotaxis, increased ROS production	Improved pathogen elimination, faster immune response.
NK cells	Increased cytotoxicity, upregulation of activating receptors (NKG2D), IFN-γ production	More effective targeting of tumor and virally infected cells [65].
Dendritic cells	Enhanced maturation and antigen presentation, increased cytokine production (IL-12, TNF-α)	Improved T-cell activation and adaptive immunity [19].
T cells	Promoted Th1-type response, activation of cytotoxic T lymphocytes	Enhanced immune surveillance and antitumor response [4].

including TNF-α, IL-6, and IL-12, will play their part in managing this immune response against cancer through activation of immune cells to this area of the tumor and eventually creating a rather adverse inflammatory milieu for the survival of the tumor cancer cells (Table 8.2) [53]. The reason NK cells offer a first line of defense against tumors is that it is integral to their function to identify and kill cancer cells without any necessary sensitization [7].

8.7.3 Antigen Presentation

In a tumor setting, DCs are the main inducer and regulator of adaptive immune responses. DCs, as the most potent APC, can take internal and processing of antigens, or "antigens from tumor cells," to be presented to T cells. Such activation will include the CTLs, which would have the ability of precognition and elimination of cancer cells [59]. It has been considered to increase the activity of dendritic cells, which then offer the antigen for an amplified antitumor response in the host's immune system [28]. In this regard, beta-glucan activates the respective signaling pathways downstream and therefore induces DC maturation and activation through its binding to surface receptors, such as Dectin-1 and CR3 [52]. Mature dendritic cells upregulate the major histocompatibility complex molecules and co-stimulatory molecules that will help trigger T cells [42].

In this way, another important effect of beta-glucan on dendritic cells is to favor a Th1-type immune response [30]. This type of response is effective against intracellular pathogens and tumors and is characterized by the cytokines that have to be produced, such as IL-12 and IFN-γ, involved in the activation and differentiation of CTLs. It could ensure that the effect of the immunity on cancer cells, to cause their destruction through an avid attack assay, basically gives an advantage to the Th1 response [7]. Apart from enhancing antigen presentation, beta-glucan also induces dendritic cell migration into the lymphoid tissues in which the cell interacts with T cells [59].

8.7.4 Tumor Microenvironment

It is also correct that the TME contains several cellular and molecular constituents, including immune cells, stromal cells, blood vessels, and extracellular matrix elements in a complex and dynamic milieu. Indeed, the TME has an extremely main role in development, progression, and resistance of a tumor to therapies [64]. These quite frequently result in immunosuppressive conditions under which cancer cells are allowed to evade the immune system and hence go on growing and metastasizing. The above effects of beta-glucan on TME set up a more permissive environment for effective antitumor immunity [52, 66]. The different tumors have evidenced differences in IT inhibiting through recruitment into the TME of Tregs and MDSCs [7]. While Tregs dampen effector T cells, MDSCs impair the function of many immune cells (including T cells and NK cells), thus dampening anti-cancer immune responses [2]. The line β-glucan reduces the count of Tregs and MDSCs in the TME to reduce immunosuppression and guarantee effectiveness in the antitumor response [54]. Other than decreasing the immunosuppressive cells in the TME, β-glucan skews the cytokine profiling in the tumor environment and finally induces the generation of pro-inflammatory cytokines

IL-12 and TNF-α [19]. Both these cytokines take part in the activation of immune cells and enhancement of their cytotoxicity [1]. Especially, IL-12 is believed to have the capacity for the production of the Th1-type immune response that is regarded as a precondition for effective anti-tumor immunity [51]. Moreover, this β-glucan markedly inhibited the release of other immunosuppressive cytokines, such as IL-10 and TGF-β, produced by the tumor [2].

8.7.5 Current Chemotherapy

Beta-glucan will help to enhance the effect of chemotherapy by strengthening protective immune responses (Table 8.3) [30]. However, it is often burdened by serious side effects that drastically diminish the effectiveness of application and increase the risk of development of chemoresistance [7]. It acts by boosting an immune response; therefore, it acts as an immunomodulatory agent, hence overcoming some of the limitations of conventional cancer treatments (Cardenas). One of the primary mechanisms through which beta-glucan potentiates chemotherapy is mitigation of its immunosuppressive effect [51]. Chemotherapy often depletes the immune cells [24]. Beta-glucan reduces the effectiveness of chemotherapy by stimulating more and activating the very similar immune cells [54]. It stimulates the general immune response during chemotherapy. This is very important since a working immune system is needed to clear the remaining cancerous cells that were left over after chemotherapy that initially was insufficient [42]. Beta-glucan also potentiates the effect of chemotherapy by altering TME. This has already been elucidated: it can be so highly immunosuppressive as to set up a barrier through which chemotherapy cannot effectively penetrate to hit the cancer cells [52]. Decrease in Treg and MDSC count sets up a situation whereby the immune response can happen robustly and turn out sensitizing in appearance at the TME for its combined effect with chemotherapy to bring both modes of attack to bear upon the cancer population [28].

8.8 Beta-Glucan and the Gut Microbiota

Beta-glucans are complex carbohydrates (polysaccharides) commonly present in oats, fungi, algae, and bacteria. Beta-glucans are acknowledged

Table 8.3 Table summarizing key preclinical and clinical studies demonstrating beta-glucan's efficacy in inhibiting tumor growth, enhancing immune responses, and improving cancer treatment outcomes.

Authors	**Objective**	**Results**
Adachi *et al.* [1]	To explore the synergistic effects of mushroom-derived β-glucans and antibody drugs on NK cell activity against lymphoma.	Mushroom-derived β-glucans enhanced NK cell-mediated cytotoxicity against lymphoma cells when combined with antibody drugs.
Benlier *et al.* [4]	To assess the combination of β-glucan with PD-1/PD-L1 checkpoint inhibitors in advanced cancer patients.	β-glucan significantly reduced oxidative DNA damage, suggesting a protective role in colorectal cancer therapy.
Bhosale [5]	To assess the antimicrobial, antioxidant, and anti-cancer effects of β-glucan derived from *Agaricus bisporus* on cervical cancer cells.	*Agaricus bisporus*–derived β-glucan showed significant anti-cancer activity by inducing apoptosis in cervical cancer cells.
Cheung *et al.* [8]	To investigate the impact of oral beta-glucan on antibody titers after ganglioside vaccination in neuroblastoma patients.	Oral beta-glucan significantly increased antibody titers, with no additional toxicities observed.
Cheung *et al.* [9]	To evaluate the adjuvant effect of oral β-glucan on antibody response to GD2/GD3 vaccine in high-risk neuroblastoma patients.	Oral β-glucan enhanced anti-GD2 IgG1 titers, indicating improved immune response without added toxicities.

(*Continued*)

Table 8.3 Table summarizing key preclinical and clinical studies demonstrating beta-glucan's efficacy in inhibiting tumor growth, enhancing immune responses, and improving cancer treatment outcomes. (*Continued*)

Authors	Objective	Results
Corso *et al.* [14]	To investigate the radio protective and anti-cancer effects of β-glucan derived from *Enterococcus faecalis* in mice.	β-glucans showed antitumor effects through apoptosis and inhibition of cellular proliferation.
de Graaff *et al.* [16]	To investigate the effects of different β-glucans on the polarization of tumor-associated macrophages.	Certain β-glucans reprogrammed macrophages to produce inflammatory chemokines, enhancing anti-cancer immunity.
Gu [20]	To evaluate the antioxidant effects of β-glucan on DNA damage in colorectal cancer patients.	β-glucan reduced tumor growth and improved survival in irradiated mice, showing radio protective and anti-cancer effects.
Lo *et al.* [31]	To explore β-glucan's effect on myeloid-derived suppressor cells (MDSCs) in oral cancer patients.	Preoperative β-glucan administration reduced MDSC levels, enhancing antitumor immunity and recurrence-free survival.
Peymaeei *et al.* [43]	To evaluate the anti-cancer effects of *Candida albicans*–derived beta-glucan on mesenchymal stem cells *in vitro*.	Beta-glucan enhanced apoptosis of lung cancer cells *in vitro*, indicating potential as an anti-cancer agent.
Špaček *et al.* [50]	To evaluate the immunomodulatory effects of *Pleurotus ostreatus*–derived β-glucan in breast cancer patients in remission.	β-glucan enhanced immune cell counts, suggesting a role in immune rehabilitation and better prognosis for breast cancer patients.

(*Continued*)

Table 8.3 Table summarizing key preclinical and clinical studies demonstrating beta-glucan's efficacy in inhibiting tumor growth, enhancing immune responses, and improving cancer treatment outcomes. (*Continued*)

Authors	Objective	Results
Upadhyay *et al.* [60]	To review the effects and mechanisms of polysaccharides, including β-glucans, in breast cancer models.	Yeast-derived β-glucan induced apoptosis in cervical cancer cells, demonstrating potential as a cancer therapy.
Wang *et al.* [64]	To assess the antioxidant and anti-cancer properties of yeast-derived β-glucan against cervical cancer cells *in vitro*.	The combination therapy improved immune cell recruitment, delayed tumor progression, and enhanced progression-free survival.
Wani *et al.* [65]	To review the dual role of β-glucan in regulating apoptosis and cell proliferation in cancer therapy.	β-glucan was found to induce apoptosis and inhibit cell proliferation, suggesting its potential as a therapeutic agent.

as functional food components due to their biological characteristics such as antioxidant, anti-inflammatory, antidiabetic, cholesterol lowering, immune-modulating response, and tumor suppressor (anti-cancer). Several studies have shown a remarkable impact of beta-glucan on gut microbiota fluctuations and human immune system (Figure 8.4). A bioactive form of beta-glucan, known as Ganoderma lucidum (GL) polysaccharide, has played an essential role in defeating cancer cells due to its immunostimulatory potentiality [11].

8.8.1 Relationship Between Gut Health and Immune Function

Gut and immune system develops a unified structure to protect from ingested toxins and disease-causing bacteria. This structure is helpful in providing a strong defensive mechanism in inflammatory environment. A well-performing immune system is essential for existence; it always remains alert in order to response to any danger. Widely, cells of immune system have been divided into innate as well as adaptive immune responses; these two work simultaneously and perform different functions. Phagocytes,

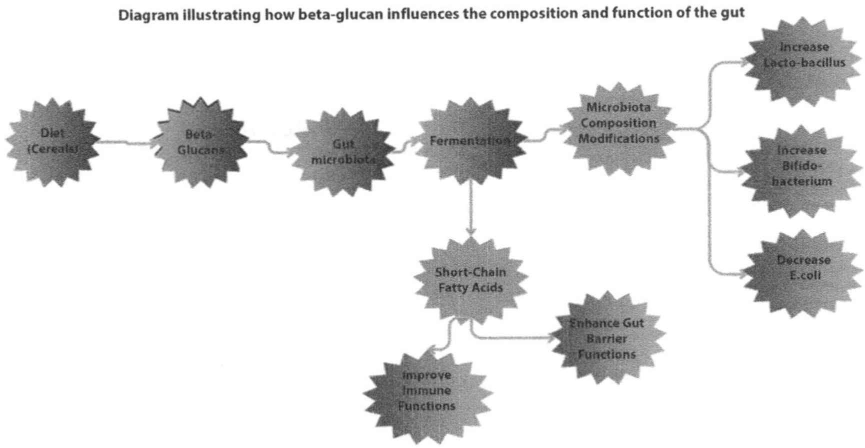

Figure 8.4 Diagram illustrating how beta-glucan influences the composition and function of the gut.

neutrophils, eosinophils, and dendrites are cells of innate immune response that responds rapidly on the spot to infectious attacks. Meanwhile, T cells and lymphocytes are adaptive immune response that are more powerful in recognizing specific pathogens; they recall and attack them whenever they are exposed in the body. T cells consist of cytotoxic T cells (CD8 receptors) and T-helper (Th) cells, are hypercritical in identifying the antigens, and are involved in the direct execution of inflammatory and tumor cells. T-helper (CD4 receptors) cells are pivotal in synchronizing the reactions of other immune cells. Th cells are further divided into two subsets as Th1 cells and Th2 cells. These Th1 cells play their important role in antiviral and other cellular immune responses by producing interferon gamma (IFN-γ) and interleukin (IL-2). Th2 cells are known for allergic, anti-parasites, and antibody (humoral) responses due to yielding of IL-4, IL-5, and IL-13. On the other hand, lymphocytes, also called as B-cells, are accountable for immunoglobulin (Ig) or antibody formation, which reacts to a specific antigen and assists the immune system to identify and kill pathogens. Ig is divided into five classes, IgM, IgD, IgG, IgA, and IgE; each of these performs specific function. IgA is involved in preventing bacterial and viral infections and food allergy [3].

To sustain intestinal homeostasis and slow down infectious pathogens, this dynamic relationship between gut microbiota and immune system is very crucial as well as an active area of research this time. Gut microbiota convert proteins and complex carbohydrates into vitamins and other metabolic products to make a communication pathway between immune cells and the gut epithelium. These metabolites help in inflammation detection by interacting with immune cells. While defective interconnection between gut bacteria and immune cells results in inflation of pathogens, these relevant metabolic alterations disrupt epithelial barrier, which causes to increase vulnerability to infection. This condition, known as gut dysbiosis (dysbacteriosis), causes immune dysregulation and boosts chances of insulin resistance, chronic inflammation, and oxidative stress in the body. In the long run, gut dysbiosis conditions get worse, and this can lead to high incidence of diabetes, obesity, autoimmune disorders, cardiac failure, Crohn's disease, and cancer [70]. Overall, this shows interaction between gut health and immunity responses and functions; microbiome assists in further expansion of innate and adaptive immune system; at the same time, immune system harmonizes to preserve the main features of the symbiotic host–microbe relationship. In a heritable vulnerable host, unbalanced microbiota–immunity collaboration under specific environment is considered as the main cause of multiple pathogenic immune-related illness. Therefore, maintenance of gut health plays a fundamental role in the proper functioning of the immune system [72].

8.8.2 Role of Beta-Glucan in Modulating Gut Microbiota

Beta-glucan (β-glucan) is a soluble fiber that has been famous for its healthier benefits and capability of modulating the composition of gut microbiota and controlling metabolic diseases. β-glucan and gut microbiota show strong associations that result in alterations in the formation of gut microbiota, enrichment of useful bacteria, along with the formulation of functional metabolite products through which gut microbial fermentation occurs. This modulating gut microbiota and its related products proved beneficial in promoting the beta-gut supplementations for healthy gut benefits and help in preventing and treating therapy for different metabolic disorders [11, 12, 38]. β-glucan acts as prebiotics (good for digestive-support mechanism). Bifidobacterium and lactobacillus are healthy beneficial bacteria that are promoted by β-glucan; these bacteria undergo fermentation process of β-glucans to produce short-chain fatty acids (acetate, butyrate, and propionate); are then involved in the nourishment of internal gut lining; control inflammation; and assist the immune system to restore the gut health. In the immune system, gut-associated lymphoid tissue is present, and β-glucans interact with this tissue and play a role in the modulation of gut immune responses.

Another feature of β-glucans is that they promote strong gut barrier function to restrain the discharge of deleterious products into bloodstream. During this modulating gut microbiota, β-glucans have shown anti-inflammatory characteristics in the gut to protect against pathogens and advance gut defense mechanism through antimicrobial peptides. They serve in the management of metabolic disorders as type 2 diabetes and obesity. This can be concluded that a well-balanced gut microbiota is necessary to maintain overall good health as it enhances digestion-nutrient consumption, improves immune responses, and minimizes the probability of inflammatory issues [27, 37].

8.8.3 Implications for Cancer Prevention and Therapy

β-glucan has been recognized as a powerful immune stimulant and serves as an antagonist against benign and malignant tumors. One of the key developments of β-glucan is its immunomodulatory effect that shows a strong link with cancer context by activating and stimulating the body's natural defense system including macrophages, T cells, and NK cells. This feature also favors the potency of immunotherapy and other cancer therapies. Recent studies have indicated that β-glucans possess antitumor and antioxidant properties to slow down tumor growth by controlling angiogenesis and inducing apoptosis among cancer cells. Due to its anti-inflammatory and chemo-preventive traits, β-glucan protects internal organs from chronic inflammation as well as carcinogens by suppressing the tumor incidence or destroying tumor cells with the help of white blood cells. Dietary fibers in β-glucan provide healthy gut microbiota to reduce the exposure of certain cancers. All this shows interaction among β-glucan, gut microbiota, and cancer, which can lead to advancement of preventive therapies and other strategies.

8.9 Advances in Beta-Glucan Research and Applications

Research studies have progressively highlighted that the advances in β-glucan improved the extraction techniques, structure–function relationship (providing deep knowledge about interaction between β-glucan structure and its biological functions), and novel delivery systems. Due to its exclusive features and biological activities, β-glucan has appeared as a favorable biomolecule having advanced variety of future health advantages and applications in various fields including pharmaceuticals (vaccines, metabolic diseases, cancer), food and beverages (dairy, bakery products), dietary supplements, and cosmetics (skin care products). Clinical trials are ongoing on the developments of beta-glucan supplements to identify their association in the management of diabetes mellitus, cardiovascular disorders, high cholesterol, and certain cancers. Through genetic engineering, genetic modifications in plants are made to generate large concentration of highly effective β-glucans as well as raise their bioactivities [40, 45].

8.9.1 Novel Delivery Systems and Formulations

The latest developments in β-glucan research have contributed to the advancement of novel delivery systems and formulations such as nanoparticles, liposomes, and hydrogel to improve stability, target delivery, and bioavailability. The consumption, tissue distribution, and preservation of β-glucan can be achieved through these innovatory formulations to optimize therapeutic potency. Hence, researchers have analyzed these novel delivery systems to cope with the challenges of β-glucan as enzymatic degradation in the gastrointestinal tract (GIT), unable to target specific cells, resistance to dissolution, and limited oral bioavailability [68]. In nanoparticle-based delivery system, nanoparticles serve as a "carrier" for β-glucan to make a pathway for resolvability and absorption and find its specified location of tumor cells by altering their outermost area with ligands that bind to receptor cells to deliver the therapeutic agents in moderate and sustained method. This is especially useful in cancer therapy during which long time revelation to immunomodulatory factors boosts the tumor inhibitory responses. Lipids, chitosan, and alginate are components of nanoparticles that have been explored as operative vehicles for β-glucan delivery.

Stability and productiveness of β-glucans have been enhanced by encapsulating them in nanoparticles to protect them from biological environmental deterioration. Due to basic characteristics of having high encapsulating power, controlled drugs discharge, and integration of distinctive agents, these nanoparticles are widely applied in drug delivery operations. Among metallic nanoparticles, gold and silver nanoparticles showed unique visual attributes and capability to assist the cellular absorption; therefore, these are used to speed up the delivery of β-glucans. Meanwhile, silica-based nanoparticles allow sufficient storing and release profiles due to their ability of possessing large surface area and adaptable pore sizes [21, 22]. In liposomal encapsulation, liposomes are vesicles made up of phospholipids and play a crucial role as a delivery system for β-glucans to advance effective treatments with less or no side effects. To prevent them from declination, enhance their pharmacokinetics features, and promote targeted delivery to specified sites, a strategy is used in which β-glucans are encapsulated in liposomes. This encapsulation efficiency depends upon various aspects such as lipid composition, preparatory method type, lipid–cholesterol proportion, and physiochemical conditions of β-glucans. Furthermore, these formulations strengthen cellular absorption, refine biodistribution phenomena, and accelerate tumor-suppressing activities. Liposomes are used to supply therapeutic agents as antitumor drugs and other biomolecules. To lessen the toxicity and foster the efficacy, liposomal formulations are applied for enhancement of therapeutic response of drugs against cancer cells [39].

8.9.2 Improved Bioavailability and Therapeutic Potential

Bioavailability refers to a substance/nutrient/drug that can be absorbed in bloodstream and stored or used by body to perform its function. Molecular masses, source, structure, composition, extraction techniques, and its collaboration with other nutrients are factors that can show significant effect on the bioavailability of β-glucans. Small-size β-glucans are easily soluble and absorbed as compared to β-glucans with large size and weight, which undergo hydrolysis to convert themselves to smaller fragments. To protect β-glucans from deterioration during digestion, they are encapsulated or fermented to also improve their solubility and stability. Studies have indicated that efficiency and cellular uptake of β-glucans increased when they work in a synergistic way. Under supportive microbiomics conditions, β-glucans combine with probiotics to enhance gut health outcomes and improve bioavailability. Nanoparticles and liposomal encapsulation are best examples to yield from internal environmental degradation and boost the bioavailability [45].

Recent advances in β-glucans have shown remarkable potential in magnifying their effectiveness and comprehending the modes of action in therapeutic applications. β-glucans possess immunomodulatory effects through Dectin-1 & TLRs and boost the responses of neutrophils, NK cells, and macrophages; foster the body's power to fight against the infections; and play their crucial role in cancer treatment in a synergistic way to enhance the effectiveness of therapy with other immunomodulatory agents including vaccines and cytokines. In high cholesterol patients, these β-glucans are involved in adhering the bile acids in the intestine, which results in increasing the discharge of cholesterol and visibly lower LDL cholesterol levels.

These β-glucans provide favorable conditions to prevent atherosclerosis and cardiac problems. In diabetic patients, β-glucans serve as an antihyperglycemic agent to manage the blood sugar levels by reducing the absorption of carbohydrates in the body, increasing insulin sensitivity, and regulating appetite hormones in the obese. As a prebiotic, they improve the gut health by promoting the growth of useful bacteria and act as an anti-inflammatory agent. This all indicates that these novel delivery systems have improved the bioavailability of β-glucans as well as enhanced therapeutic potency to work effectively within human physiology [6, 44].

8.9.3 Current and Future Clinical Applications in Immunotherapy and Oncology

β-glucans have the capability to modulate the immune responses and upgrade the humans' natural defense system against carcinogenic pathogens; therefore, β-glucans are investigated in immunotherapy and oncology. In current clinical applications, β-glucans are used as adjuvants in cancer therapy to increase the quality and ability of cancer vaccines during treatments such as chemotherapy and radiotherapy by regulating the immune responses against cancer tumors. To control hematological malignancies including lymphoma and leukemia, β-glucans are specially formulated to increase the chances of patient survival along with these therapies. β-glucans act as anti-metastatic to inhibit the tumor growth in certain cancers such as colorectal and breast cancers. β-glucans are assimilated into vaccines to formulate the nano-vaccines to improve antigen presentation and to enhance immune action against specific tumors. As research on β-glucans advances, future applications are emerging, including the development of personalized β-glucan-based immunotherapies. The exploration of synergistic strategies involves combining β-glucan therapies with other cancer treatments, such as immunotherapy or targeted therapy, for enhanced efficacy in cancer patients. Ongoing research also examines the role of β-glucans in managing chronic diseases associated with immune system disruptions, including autoimmune disorders [13].

8.10 Challenges and Future Directions

Meanwhile, therapeutic functions of beta-glucans are encouraging, but still there are various ongoing challenges such as complexity in standardization due to variations in the source and structure of β-glucans, inverse relation of their molecular weight and bioavailability, insecurity of safely using beta-glucan dietary supplements, complication of their mode of action, and feeling of discomfort after their intake due to side effects. For future directions, there is a requirement for proper research to overcome these described challenges to improve the effectiveness of beta-glucans in cancer treatments. There is demand for proper standardization, understanding its mechanism, formulation techniques, development of combined therapies consisting of β-glucans, gut microbiota modulation, and standard cancer medications. Apart from these challenges, the future of β-glucans is bright due to progressive improvements in considering the composition, bioavailability, and immunotherapeutic system that will open the way for the evolution of innovative and powerful β-glucan-based therapies for a vast number of disorders [71].

8.10.1 Manufacturing Limitations and Variability in Bioactivity

Large-scale production of β-glucans involves a challenging process. β-glucans' function and structural integrity through extraction processes, e.g., enzymatic hydrolysis or alkaline extraction, depend on precise conditions to prevent damage. High costs, complex procedures, and using environmentally impacting chemicals are the rules for industrial-scale production. Furthermore, consistency of quality and purity from batch to batch are difficult because of variations in raw materials and processing conditions [46]. Because of these factors, there are limits on how affordable and accessible β-glucan products can be manufactured and made available; both would be key for low-cost consumer goods and medium to widespread therapeutic use. The bioactivity of such β-glucans is dramatically dependent on the source, molecular weight, solubility, and structural linkage of the glycosidic carbohydrates [45]. For example, β-glucans from oats have different immunomodulatory or cholesterol-lowering effects than those from other fungi or yeast. β-glucans' variation makes standardizing products and their use in health and disease-related management challenging. Additionally, variations in the extraction and purification processes can introduce variability into a final product, making it impossible to ensure efficacy among various formulations. **Health effects of excessive use:** β-glucans are generally safe to consume; however, their consumption can have potential side effects, including at high doses and for people with certain health conditions. Because β-glucans contain a fair bit of fiber, some studies suggest that the fiber in beta-glucans, when consumed in excess, can cause discomfort to the gastrointestinal system, such as bloating, gas, and diarrhea. Furthermore, they have immunomodulatory properties, so individuals with compromised immune systems or having autoimmune conditions may experience unpredicted immune responses to beta-glucans. These risks must be evaluated regarding dosage, safety profile, and personalized beta-glucan consumption recommendations. **Regulatory and consumer acceptance problems:** Another complication is that β-glucans have yet to gain regulatory or consumer acceptance. Global variables in health claims, regulatory frameworks, and labelling recommendations can delay the global commercialization of beta-glucan-based products. Furthermore, consumers must be more educated about the health effects and safety of β-glucans obtained from nonconventional sources (such as fungi or yeast) [57]. These are, other than the traditional domains, bioactive compounds with potential intracellular applications. Meanwhile, TCR integration in cutting-edge technologies (e.g., CAR-T cell therapies) and its use in health and medicine for emerging fields (e.g., precision medicine, personalized immunotherapy) make new fields possible.

8.10.2 Limitations of Current Research

The quality of product can be affected due to the deficiency of standardization methods used for the extraction and analysis of β-glucans. No large-scale clinical trial studies are available for the safety and efficiency of different therapies in case of certain disorders. Due to variations in β-glucans' source and structure, their biological activity is affected, and it creates a complicated situation to produce a standardized dose for clinical practice. Another limitation is the use of inconsistent experimental designs and procedures during research, such as using animal models instead of human clinical trials to investigate the influence of β-glucans, due to diversity in metabolic system, immune actions, and infection development in these two species (animals and humans). In addition to these conditions, alterations in medication, intake orally or intravenously, therapy time period, and other controlling measures, all these cause contradictions in the results of therapeutic agents. The limitations in understanding the mode of actions of β-glucans make it difficult to enhance their therapy's effects.

Unavailability of large-scale clinical trials cause adverse situation for medical professionals to prescribe β-glucans for standard therapy choice for cancer treatments. There is limited research about the potential side effects after using β-glucans for long duration. There is a need to overcome these limitations of beta-glucans before their extensive clinical applications are concluded [40].

8.10.3 Areas Requiring Further Investigation

There are several areas demanding for additional research to fully understand the phenomena of mechanism of action and efficacy of beta-glucans: to explore the structural variability of β-glucans and interaction between a particular structure's characteristics and their correlative biological effects to enhance the selection plan of β-glucan therapies; to investigate and understand the molecular mode of action of β-glucans and their signal transduction pathways by which immune systems get activated to suppress the tumor cells and other metastasis; to analyze the combined therapies of β-glucans, treatment duration, dosage, and administration pathways of these synergistic therapies to exaggerate the therapeutic efficiency in cancer treatment; to examine the adverse effects of long-term use of large quantity of β-glucans and their association with other medications taken by patients for cure of different medical conditions; and to observe the influence of genetic variations, dietary habits, and environmental elements on the strength, bioavailability, and stability of β-glucans. Hence, it can be concluded that exploring these areas can result in the evolution of productive and safe beta-glucans in immunomodulatory and anti-cancer applications [13].

8.10.4 Potential for Integration Into Standard Cancer Treatment Protocols

Due to their exclusive tumor-inhibiting and immune-modulatory characteristics, there are several reasons that show the potential integration of β-glucans into conventional cancer therapies to improve immunotherapeutic outcomes. Immune advancements (activate defense mechanism), enhanced efficiency of standard treatments (chemotherapy, radiation therapy), minimized adverse effects (vomiting, weakness, nausea), and better quality of life are major potential advantages. There are three main potential integration approaches that can be applied along with these standard anti-cancer protocols. Firstly, adjunctive therapy is the administration of β-glucans (orally or IV) into patients when they are already getting normally antitumor medications to boost their effectiveness and probably preventing the side effects. Secondly, preservative therapy is to support the prime cancer therapeutics and application of β-glucans supplement to intercept the reappearance of tumors and refine the survivance rate of patients. Thirdly, supportive measures are implemented to deal and control hospitalization-related complexities and enhance the quality of life to make it remarkable.

Beyond these benefits, there are some challenges and consideration for the use of β-glucans in cancer treatments such as shortage of standardized dosage and quality of extracted β-glucans, no full command on their mechanistic reactions, personalized variations (relevant to genetics, cancer type, level of illness), variations in their source and consistency, and short-term effects on survival chances. Further research and clinical trials are required to overcome the above-mentioned challenges to develop the effective β-glucans-based therapies for the better recovery of cancer patients [40].

8.10.5 Precision Medicine and Beta Glucan-Based Personalized Immunotherapy

It is also known as precision medicine, which tailors treatment strategies to individual patients using genetic, environmental, and lifestyle factors. In this scenario, the immunomodulatory properties of β-glucans are of paramount importance. The researchers then use advanced molecular profiling techniques to pinpoint patients most likely to profit from beta-glucan-based therapies. For example, an individual who may more effectively respond to β-glucans is shown as an individual with specific immune receptor polymorphisms, such as dectin polymorphism or TLR polymorphism. This can increase β-glucans' ability to reduce the risk of disease and species threats from generic treatments. β-glucans appear promising in personalized immunotherapy, mainly as they can regulate and modulate immune responses. Therefore, they are ideal therapeutic candidates to enhance the antitumor potential of the cancer-targeted immune system. The possibility of a biological immunotherapeutic pathway incorporating the treatment of β-glucans in combination with another agent can be tailored to the patient profile, especially when they possess an immune status. Polymeric β-glucans, for example, can be used as an adjuvant to vaccines or monoclonal antibody therapies to augment the specificity and potency of tumor or pathogen responses [25].

8.10.6 Emerging CAR-T Cell Therapy and Its Role in Integrative Treatments

Chimeric antigen receptor T-cell (CAR-T) therapy is a revolutionary cancer treatment approach that involves engineering one's T cells to recognize and destroy certain antigens in cancer cells. It is based on the elementary idea of engineering the patient's T cells to recognize and kill cancer. Adding β-glucans to CAR-T therapy can boost the tumor microenvironment to be immunogenic [35]. In solid tumors, traditionally hard to treat, β-glucans help innate immune cells that create cytokines that activate the needs of our CAR-T cells for infiltration and efficacy. In addition, they may enhance the effective CAR-T cell killing of a tumor by overcoming immunosuppression of the tumor microenvironment. However, future research could explore beta glucan interaction with CAR-T cells to help in better cancer treatments. As described earlier, β-glucans are another innovative application of a specific nanotechnology-based delivery system; if β-glucans are encapsulated into nanoparticles or liposomes, they will show improved bioavailability, stability, or regulated intracellular or intravascular delivery [73]. Such approaches are particularly relevant for developing β-glucan-based cancer treatment and immunotherapy. In addition, β-glucans released from these nanocarriers can be controlled to optimize their effects on immune cells and sustain the therapeutic impact. Beta-glucans' versatility allows them to be included in combination therapies and other emerging technologies. For example, maybe scientists can conjugate beta-glucans with checkpoint inhibitors to circumvent cancer, or researchers can conjugate them with probiotics and prebiotics to promote gut health and immunity. There should be scope for β-glucans in modern medicine to explore these synergies.

8.11 Conclusion

Beta-glucans are heterogeneous groups of natural polysaccharides, which are powerful bioactive compounds. They belong to those natural components that feature a large number of health benefits. Being the least soluble, these ingredients are compelled from different sources, which include fungi, yeast, oats, barley, and other cereals. At the same time, however, the significant feature that determines the properties $\beta 1 \rightarrow 3$ and $\beta 1 \rightarrow 4$ linkages is unspecific. They have to combine the structure β-glucan because of its guaranteed biological activity. In addition, these features determined the way materials will interact with the human immune system to be able to decrease cholesterol levels and demonstrate anti-cancer behavior. To get the desired bioactivity, as well as a high magnitude, it was critical to create highly effective extraction and purification techniques that supply the desired characteristics to the resulting substances. Thus, the commonly used extract takes beta-glucans by hot water, enzymes, or alkali, and afterward, the polysaccharide is fermented by alcohol and separated with ultrafiltration. In this context, the right way is critical to achieve the most general and most reliable compound extraction and protection against damaged substances and subsequent need events. β-glucans affect the immune system's functioning, causing a cascade of measures for human protection against pathogens, viruses, or cancer cells. At the same time, however, these materials have many health advantages, and those include a decreased danger of cardiovascular diseases, diabetes, and severe illnesses such as cancer. For the reason that they are natural and non-toxic to humans, they are worth receiving detailed studies as natural anti-cancer cell agents. With the winning level of evidence and an overall increasing number of health advantages related to these polysaccharides, it is expected that they will have a prominent position in the clinical and dietary areas of human source application in terms of preventing the onset of many human diseases and developing their drugs.

AI disclosure statement: The author acknowledges the use of AI-based tools for minor language editing or grammatical correction. However, all intellectual contributions, analyses, and conclusions presented in this chapter are entirely the author's own.

References

1. Adachi, Y., Momose, F., Momose, H., Tada, R., Ohno, N., Potentiation of antitumor activity by antibody drugs and mushroom-derived β-glucans in natural killer cell mediated tumoricidal activities against non-Hodgkin's B-cell lymphoma. International. *J. Med. Mushrooms, 25*, 3, 1–19, 2023.
2. Ahmad, F., Ahmad, F., Khan, M.I., Alsayegh, A., Wahab, S., Alam, M.I., Ahmed, F., Ganoderma lucidum: A potential source to surmount viral infections through β-glucans immunomodulatory and triterpenoids antiviral properties. *Int. J. Biol. Macromol.*, 186, 37–47, 2021.
3. Barrea, L., Muscogiuri, G., Frias-Toral, E., Laudisio, D., Pugliese, G., Castellucci, B., Colao, A., Nutrition and immune system: from the Mediterranean diet to dietary supplementary through the microbiota. *Crit. Rev. Food Sci. Nutr.*, *61*, 18, 3066–3090, 2021.

4. Benlier, N., Uçar, N., Öğüt, E., Çınkır, H., Yıldırım, M., Karadeniz, P., Akkol, E., Khan, H., Saygili, E., Assessment of antioxidant effect of beta-glucan on the whole blood oxidative DNA damage with the comet assay in colorectal cancer. *Curr. Mol. Pharmacol.*, 15, 2, 446–553, 2022.
5. Bhosale, A., Trivedi, R., Upadhyay, T.K., Gurjar, D., Aghaz, F., Khan, F., Pandey, P., Zeyaullah, M., Alam, M.S., Al-Najjar, M.A.A., Siddiqui, S., Investigation on antimicrobial, antioxidant, and anti-cancerous activity of Agaricus bisporus derived β glucan particles against cervical cancer cell line. *Cell. Mol. Biol.*, *68*, 9, 150–159, 2022.
6. Bobade, H., Gupta, A., Sharma, S., Beta-glucan, in: *Nutraceuticals and Healthcare*, Academic Press, pp. 343–358, 2022.
7. Cheng, H., Sun, L., Shen, D., Ren, A., Ma, F., Tai, G., Zhou, Y., Beta-1,6 glucan converts tumor-associated macrophages into an M1-like phenotype. *Carbohydr. Polym.*, *247*, 116715, 2020.
8. Cheung, I., Mauguen, A., Feng, Y., Ragupathi, G., Basu, E., Roberts, S., Modak, S., Kushner, B., Cheung, N., Oral beta-glucan enhanced anti-ganglioside antibody titer after vaccination against high-risk neuroblastoma. *Cancer Res.*, 82, 12, 5218, 2022.
9. Cheung, I., Mauguen, A., Modak, S., Ragupathi, G., Basu, E., Roberts, S., Kushner, B., Cheung, N., Effect of oral β-glucan on antibody response to ganglioside vaccine in patients with high-risk neuroblastoma: A phase 2 randomized clinical trial. *JAMA Oncol.*, 9, 2, 242–250, 2023.
10. Comer, J., Bassette, M., Burghart, R., Loyd, M., Ishiguro, S., Singam, E.R.A., Tamura, M., Beta-1,3 oligoglucans specifically bind to immune receptor CD28 and may enhance T cell activation. *Int. J. Mol. Sci.*, *22*, 6, 3124, 2021.
11. Chen, C., Huang, X., Wang, H., Geng, F., Nie, S., Effect of β-glucan on metabolic diseases: A review from the gut microbiota perspective. *Curr. Opin. Food Sci.*, *47*, 100907, 2022.
12. Chen, G., Chen, D., Zhou, W., Peng, Y., Chen, C., Shen, W., Zeng, X., Yuan, Q., Improvement of metabolic syndrome in high-fat diet-induced mice by yeast β-Glucan is linked to inhibited proliferation of Lactobacillus and Lactococcus in gut microbiota. *J. Agric. Food. Chem.*, *69*, 27, 7581–7592, 2021.
13. Cognigni, V., Ranallo, N., Tronconi, F., Morgese, F., Berardi, R., Potential benefit of β-glucans as adjuvant therapy in immuno-oncology: A review. *Explor. Target. Anti-tumor Ther.*, *2*, 2, 122, 2021.
14. Corso, C.R., Mulinari Turin de Oliveira, N., Moura Cordeiro, L., Sauruk da Silva, K., da Silva Soczek, S.H., Frota Rossato, V., Maria-Ferreira, D., Polysaccharides with antitumor effect in breast cancer: a systematic review of non-clinical studies. *Nutrients*, *13*, 6, 2008, 2021.
15. Cerletti, C., Esposito, S., Iacoviello, L., Edible mushrooms and beta-glucans: Impact on human health. *Nutrients*, *13*, 7, 2195, 2021.
16. de Graaff, P., Berrevoets, C., Rösch, C., Schols, H., Verhoef, K., Wichers, H., Debets, R., Govers, C., Curdlan, zymosan and a yeast-derived β-glucan

reshape tumor-associated macrophages into producers of inflammatory chemo-attractants. *Cancer Immunol., Immunother., 70*, 547–561, 2021.

17. del Carmen Razola-Díaz, M., Ochando-Pulido, J.M., Guerra-Hernández, E.J., García-Villanova, B., Verardo, V., Influence of Membrane Separation Processes on Food Bioactives, in: *Retention of Bioactives in Food Processing*, Springer, pp. 511–546, 2022.
18. Del Cornò, M., Gessani, S., Conti, L., Shaping the innate immune response by dietary glucans: any role in the control of cancer? *Cancers, 12*, 1, 155, 2020.
19. Duan, X., Ding, J., Qi, C., Research progress of dendritic cell-associated C-type lectin 1 (Dectin-1) in anti-tumor immunology. *Xi bao yu fen zi mian yi xue za zhi = Chin. J. Cell. Mol. Immunol., 39*, 11, 1039–1043, 2023.
20. Gu, Y.-H., New screening for the development of radioprotectors: Radioprotection and anti-cancer effect of β-glucan (Enterococcus faecalis), IntechOpen, 2020. doi: 10.5772/intechopen.95016.
21. Guo, W., Zhang, X., Wan, L., Wang, Z., Han, M., Yan, Z., Li, J., Deng, R., Li, S., Mao, Y., β-glucan-modified nanoparticles with different particle sizes exhibit different lymphatic targeting efficiencies and adjuvant effects. *J. Pharm. Anal.*, 14, 12, 100953, 2024.
22. Huang, J., Wu, C., Tang, S., Zhou, P., Deng, J., Zhang, Z., Wang, Y., Wang, Z., Chiral active β-Glucan nanoparticles for synergistic delivery of doxorubicin and immune potentiation. *Int. J. Nanomed.*, 15, 5083–5095, 2020.
23. Hadiuzzaman, M., Moniruzzaman, M., Shahjahan, M., Bai, S., Min, T., Hossain, Z., B glucan: Mode of action and its uses in fish immunomodulation. *Front. Mar. Sci.*, 9, 905986, 2022.
24. Iliev, D., Strandskog, G., Sobhkhez, M., Bruun, J., Jørgensen, J., Secretome profiling of Atlantic salmon head kidney leukocytes highlights the role of phagocytes in the immune response to soluble β-glucan. *Front. Immunol., 12*, 736964, 2021.
25. Ikewaki, N., Dedeepiya, V.D., Raghavan, K., Rao, K.-S., Vaddi, S., Osawa, H., Kumar, S.R.B., βglucan vaccine adjuvant approach for cancer treatment through immune enhancement (BVACCIEN) in specific immunocompromised populations. *Oncol. Rep., 47*, 1, 1–9, 2022.
26. Jan, N., Wani, T.A., Masoodi, F., Gani, A., Naik, H., Beta-Glucans, in: *Food biopolymers: Structural, functional and nutraceutical properties*, pp. 93–125, 2021.
27. Karimi, R., Homayoonfal, M., Malekjani, N., Kharazmi, M.S., Jafari, S.M., Interaction between β-glucans and gut microbiota: a comprehensive review. *Crit. Rev. Food Sci. Nutr.*, 64, 22, 7804–7835, 2023.
28. Kalia, N., Singh, J., Kaur, M., The role of dectin-1 in health and disease. *Immunobiology, 226*, 2, 152071, 2021.
29. Lante, A., Canazza, E., Tessari, P., Beta-glucans of cereals: Functional and technological properties. *Nutrients, 15*, 9, 2124, 2023.

30. Liu, X., Xu, Y., Li, Y., Pan, Y., Zhao, S., Hou, Y., Ferumoxytol-β-glucan inhibits melanoma growth *via* interacting with Dectin-1 to polarize macrophages into M1 phenotype. *Int. J. Med. Sci.*, *18*, 13, 3125–3139, 2021.
31. Lo, Y.-W., Lee, A., Liu, Y.-C., Ko, H., Peng, H.-H., Lee, H.-C., Pan, P.-Y., Chiang, C., Cheng, S.-J., β-glucan therapy converts the inhibition of myeloid-derived suppressor cells in oral cancer patients. *Oral Dis.*, 28, 6, 1484–1495, 2022.
32. Mata-Martínez, P., Bergón-Gutiérrez, M., Del Fresno, C., Dectin-1 signaling update: new perspectives for trained immunity. *Front. Immunol.*, *13*, 812148, 2022.
33. Mejía, S.M.V., de Francisco, A., Bohrer, B., A comprehensive review on cereal β-glucan: Extraction, characterization, causes of degradation, and food application. *Crit. Rev. Food Sci. Nutr.*, *60*, 21, 3693–3704, 2020.
34. Mio, K., Otake, N., Nakashima, S., Matsuoka, T., Aoe, S., Ingestion of high β-glucan barley flour enhances the intestinal immune system of diet-induced obese mice by prebiotic effects. *Nutrients*, *13*, 3, 907, 2021.
35. Mishra, V., Tripathi, V., Yadav, P., Singh, M., Beta glucan as an immune stimulant in tumor microenvironment—Insight into lessons and promises from past decade. *Int. J. Biol. Macromol.*, *234*, 123617, 2023.
36. Murphy, E.J., Rezoagli, E., Pogue, R., Simonassi-Paiva, B., Abidin, I.I.Z., Fehrenbach, G.W., O'Neil, E., Major, I., Laffey, J.G., Rowan, N., Immunomodulatory activity of β-glucan polysaccharides isolated from different species of mushroom–A potential treatment for inflammatory lung conditions. *Sci. Total Environ.*, *809*, 152177, 2022.
37. Ma, L., Luo, Z., Huang, Y., Li, Y., Guan, J., Zhou, T., Du, Z., Yong, K., Yao, X., Shen, L., Modulating gut microbiota and metabolites with dietary fiber oat β-glucan interventions to improve growth performance and intestinal function in weaned rabbits. *Front. Microbiol.*, *13*, 1074036, 2022.
38. Murphy, E.J., Rezoagli, E., Major, I., Rowan, N.J., Laffey, J.G., β-glucan metabolic and immunomodulatory properties and potential for clinical application. *J. Fungi*, *6*, 4, 356, 2020.
39. Niaz, T. and Mackie, A., Effect of beta glucan coating on controlled release, bioaccessibility, and absorption of β-carotene from loaded liposomes. *Food Funct.*, *15*, 3, 1627–1642, 2024.
40. Noorbakhsh Varnosfaderani, S.M., Ebrahimzadeh, F., Akbari Oryani, M., Khalili, S., Almasi, F., Mosaddeghi Heris, R., Payandeh, Z., Li, C., Nabi Afjadi, M., Alagheband Bahrami, A., Potential promising anticancer applications of β-glucans: a review. *Biosci. Rep.*, *44*, 1, BSR20231686, 2024.
41. Northrop, G., D'costa, A.S., Tosh, S.M., Bordenave, N., Viscosity development from oat bran β-glucans through *in vitro* digestion is lowered in the presence of phenolic compounds. *Food Funct.*, *13*, 7, 3894–3904, 2022.
42. Patidar, A., Mahanty, T., Raybarman, C., Sarode, A., Basak, S., Saha, B., Bhattacharjee, S., Barley beta-Glucan and zymosan induce Dectin-1 and Toll-like receptor 2 colocalization and anti-leishmanial immune response

in Leishmania donovani-infected BALB/c mice. *Scand. J. Immunol., 92*, 1, e12952, 2020.

43. Peymaeei, F., Sadeghi, F., Safari, E., Khorrami, S., Falahati, M., Roudbar Mohammadi, S., Roudbary, M., Candida albicans Beta-Glucan Induce Anti-Cancer Activity of Mesenchymal Stem Cells against Lung Cancer Cell Line: An *In-Vitro* Experimental Study. *Asian Pac. J. Cancer Prev. APJCP, 21*, 3, 837–843, 2020.
44. Şengül, M. and Ufuk, S., Therapeutic and functional properties of beta-glucan, and its effects on health. *Eurasian J. Food Sci. Technol., 6*, 1, 29–41, 2022.
45. Singla, A., Gupta, O.P., Sagwal, V., Kumar, A., Patwa, N., Mohan, N., Ankush, Kumar, D., Vir, O., Singh, J., Beta-Glucan as a Soluble Dietary Fiber Source: Origins, Biosynthesis, Extraction, Purification, Structural Characteristics, Bioavailability, Biofunctional Attributes, Industrial Utilization, and Global Trade. *Nutrients, 16*, 6, 900, 2024.
46. Shimada, Y., Ishida, T., Kato, Y., Uwagami, H., Kato, Y., Kanematsu, Y., ... Ohara, S., Material balance and energy consumption in the factory-scale coproduction of glucan and mannan from yeast extract residue. *Food Sci. Technol. Res., 27*, 6, 871–880, 2021.
47. Schmidt, M., Cereal beta-glucans: An underutilized health endorsing food ingredient. *Crit. Rev. Food Sci. Nutr., 62*, 12, 3281–3300, 2022.
48. Sindhu, R.K., Goyal, A., Das, J., Choden, S., Kumar, P., Immunomodulatory potential of polysaccharides derived from plants and microbes: A narrative review. *Carbohydr. Polym. Technol. Appl., 2*, 100044, 2021.
49. Singh, R.P. and Bhardwaj, A., β-glucans: A potential source for maintaining gut microbiota and the immune system. *Front. Nutr., 10*, 1143682, 2023.
50. Špaček, J., Vočka, M., Zavadova, E., Konopasek, B., Petruželka, L., Immunomodulation with β-glucan from Pleurotus ostreatus in patients with endocrine dependent breast cancer. *Immunotherapy*, 14, 1, 31–40, 2021.
51. Stothers, C., Burelbach, K.R., Owen, A.M., Patil, N., McBride, M.A., Bohannon, J., Sherwood, E.R., β-Glucan induces distinct and protective innate immune memory in differentiated macrophages. *J. Immunol., 206*, 8, 1768–1779, 2021.
52. Su, C.-H., Lu, M.-K., Lu, T., Lai, M., Ng, L., A (1→6)-branched (1→4)-β-D-glucan from Grifola frondosa inhibits lipopolysaccharide-induced cytokine production in RAW264.7 macrophages by binding to TLR2 rather than Dectin-1 or CR3 receptors. *J. Nat. Prod., 83*, 9, 2730–2738, 2020.
53. Su, C.-H., Tseng, Y.-T., Lo, K., Lai, M., Ng, L., Differences in anti-inflammatory properties of water soluble and insoluble bioactive polysaccharides in lipopolysaccharide-stimulated RAW264.7 macrophages. *Glycoconjugate J., 37*, 4, 565–576, 2020.
54. Su, Y., Chen, L., Yang, F., Cheung, P., Beta-D-glucan-based drug delivery system and its potential application in targeting tumor-associated macrophages. *Carbohydr. Polym., 253*, 117258, 2021.

55. Su, Y., Yang, F., Chen, L., Cheung, P., Mushroom carboxymethylated β-D-glucan functions as a macrophage-targeting carrier for iron oxide nanoparticles and an inducer of proinflammatory macrophage polarization for immunotherapy. *J. Agric. Food. Chem.*, *70*, 11, 3234–3247, 2022.
56. Streimikyte, P., Viskelis, P., Viskelis, J., Enzymes-assisted extraction of plants for sustainable and functional applications. *Int. J. Mol. Sci.*, *23*, 4, 2359, 2022.
57. Sushytskyi, L., Synytsya, A., Čopíková, J., Lukáč, P., Rajsiglová, L., Tenti, P., Vannucci, L.E., Perspectives in the Application of High, Medium, and Low Molecular Weight Oat β-d-Glucans in Dietary Nutrition and Food Technology—A Short Overview. *Foods*, *12*, 6, 1121, 2023.
58. Thomas, S., Rezoagli, E., Abidin, I.Z., Major, I., Murray, P., Murphy, E.J., β-Glucans from yeast—Immunomodulators from novel waste resources. *Appl. Sci.*, *12*, 10, 5208, 2022.
59. Thongsiri, C., Nagai-Yoshioka, Y., Yamasaki, R., Adachi, Y., Usui, M., Nakashima, K., Nishihara, T., Schizophyllum commune β-glucan: Effect on interleukin-10 expression induced by lipopolysaccharide from periodontopathic bacteria. *Carbohydr. Polym.*, *253*, 117285, 2021.
60. Upadhyay, T., Trivedi, R., Khan, F., Al-Keridis, L.A., Pandey, P., Sharangi, A., Alshammari, N., Abdullah, N.M., Yadav, D., Saeed, M., *In vitro* elucidation of antioxidant, antiproliferative, and apoptotic potential of yeast-derived β-1,3-glucan particles against cervical cancer cells. *Front. Oncol.*, 18, 12, 94207512, 2022.
61. Van Steenwijk, H.P., Bast, A., De Boer, A., Immunomodulating effects of fungal beta-glucans: From traditional use to medicine. *Nutrients*, *13*, 4, 1333, 2021.
62. Vogler, M., Shanmugalingam, S., Särchen, V., Reindl, L.M., Grèze, V., Buchinger, L., Kühn, M., Ullrich, E., Unleashing the power of NK cells in anticancer immunotherapy. *J. Mol. Med.*, *100*, 3, 337–349, 2022.
63. Wallace, R.G. and Rochfort, K.D., Ion-Exchange Chromatography: Basic Principles and Application. *Methods Mol. Biol.*, 2699, 161–177, 2023.
64. Wang, M., Bai, Y., Pei, J., Li, D., Pu, X., Zhu, W., Xia, L., Qi, C., Jiang, H., Ning, Y., β-glucan combined with PD-1/PD-L1 checkpoint blockade for immunotherapy in patients with advanced cancer. *Front. Pharmacol.*, 25, 13, 887457, 2022.
65. Wani, S.M., Gani, A., Masoodi, F., Mir, S., Khanday, F., β-glucan: A dual regulator of apoptosis and cell proliferation. *Int. J. Biol. Macromol.*, 1, 182, 1229–1237, 2021.
66. Wu, Z., Yang, Y., Li, J., Bossier, P., Wei, X., Guo, Z., Han, B., Ye, J., β-Glucans in particulate and solubilized forms elicit varied immunomodulatory and apoptosis effects in teleost macrophages in a dose-dependent manner. *Front. Immunol.*, *14*, 1243358, 2023.
67. Yang, W. and Huang, G., Extraction methods and activities of natural glucans. *Trends Food Sci. Technol.*, *112*, 50–57, 2021.

68. Yang, F. and Cheung, P.C.K., Fungal β-Glucan-based nanotherapeutics: from fabrication to application. *J. Fungi*, *9*, 4, 475, 2023.
69. Yu, J., Xia, J., Yang, C., Pan, D., Xu, D., Sun, G., Xia, H., Effects of oat beta-glucan intake on lipid profiles in hypercholesterolemic adults: A systematic review and meta-analysis of randomized controlled trials. *Nutrients*, *14*, 10, 2043, 2022.
70. Yoo, J.Y., Groer, M., Dutra, S.V.O., Sarkar, A., McSkimming, D.I., Gut microbiota and immune system interactions. *Microorganisms*, *8*, 10, 1587, 2020.
71. Zhao, L.-Y., Mei, J.-X., Yu, G., Lei, L., Zhang, W.-H., Liu, K., Chen, X.-L., Kołat, D., Yang, K., Hu, J.-K., Role of the gut microbiota in anticancer therapy: from molecular mechanisms to clinical applications. *Signal Transduct. Target. Ther.*, *8*, 1, 201, 2023.
72. Zheng, D., Liwinski, T., Elinav, E., Interaction between microbiota and immunity in health and disease. *Cell Res.*, *30*, 6, 492–506, 2020.
73. He, L., Zhu, Z., Qi, C., β-glucan—A promising immunocyte-targeting drug delivery vehicle: Superiority, applications and future prospects. *Carbohydr. Polym.*, 339, 122252, 2024.

9

Guar Gum: Structural Modification Strategies for Therapeutic Anticancer Effect

Bushra Munir[1], Iqra Noor[2], Maimoona Nazir[2], Abdul Ghaffar[2*], Shazba Aziz[2], Sadia Falak[3] and Hunaira Nasreen[2]

[1]Institute of Chemistry, University of Sargodha, Sargodha, Pakistan
[2]Department of Biochemistry, Government College University, Faisalabad, Pakistan
[3]Department of Biochemistry, University of Jhang, Jhang, Pakistan

Abstract

Guar gum is a potent agrochemical polysaccharide consisting of galactomannan and proteins, which is processed from cluster bean. The use of guar gum has been increased as additive in food, pharmaceuticals, cosmetics, textile, paper, explosive, and oil drilling industries. The beneficial effects of guar gum have been found in diseases like diabetes, cardiovascular, howel movements, and cancer. It is used as natural biodegradable biopolymer in drug delivery (DD) of many medicines including anticancer drugs. Easy availability, non-toxicity, eco-friendly, and biodegradable nature of GG have made it an ideal candidate for DD applications. GG-based hydrogels, films, scaffolds, and nanoparticles have been explored widely for their targeted DD applications. Guar gum has been modified through thermal, sonochemical, and crosslinking agents to enhance the material's properties and commercial application. The modified guar gum contains the grafted chain through a C–N a side chain or carboxymethylation, oxidized crosslinking, and enzymatic modification on the guar gum and can be determined through FTIR (Fourier Transform Infrared Spectroscopy), XRD, FESEM, and UV-vis spectra analysis. Anticancer activities of guar gum have been linked to antioxidant, anti-initiation, carcinogen activator enzymes, carcinogen metabolism through cytochrome P450 1A (CYPTA), and detoxification through glutathione-S-transferases (GSTs). Remarkable improvements have been found in treatment

**Corresponding author*: aghaffaruaf@yahoo.com; abdulghaffar@gcuf.edu.pk

Luqman Jameel Rather, Showkat Ali Ganie and Mohammed A. Assiri (eds.) Polysaccharide Biomaterials in Cancer Research and Therapy: From Lab to Life, (267–300) © 2026 Scrivener Publishing LLC

of hepatocellular carcinoma using modified guar gum in combinatorial therapy. This chapter describes composition, processing, properties, and DD properties of modified GG as a natural therapeutic agent to augment the applications of phytochemicals in medical.

Keywords: Guar gum, agrochemical polysaccharide, galactomannan, proteins

9.1 Introduction

Natural polysaccharides have gained great attention, as the increasing focus on biodegradable, renewable, biocompatible, and nontoxic material synthesis, among others [86, 93]. Glycosidic bonds are complex chemical compounds that function as complex chemical structures and are widely used in different forms of applications. The most important factors to classify these compounds are structural complexity, origin, molecular weight, and hydrophilicity. It has wide biological applications and galactomannans, and its derivatives are extracted from guar, cassia, and locust beans. It is a linear carbohydrate polymer consisting of a backbone of mannose, with galactose side chains. This structure provides unique properties and functionality and is therefore very suitable for many uses. The endosperm of the leguminous plants *Cyamopsis tetragonolobus* and *Cyamopsis psoraloides* is used to get guar gum as an inexpensive galactomannan source. This natural substance is an all-around valued substance and a broadly used thing in various businesses. Alternate names for it are Glucotard, Calcutta lucern, Cyamopsis, Guaran, Cluster bean, and Cuarina. It is light-colored to pale yellow, scentless, macromolecular weight glycans. The guar bean plant grows to about 0.6 m in height and produces pods of 5 to 12.5 cm long [85]. Application of this technology spans in various industries in the field of pharmaceuticals, cosmetics, food, textiles, paper, explosives, and toiletry [66].

Mortality related to cancer is one of the most important global causes. Each year, 19.3 million new cases of cancer are diagnosed and about 10 million people die of cancer worldwide. Worldwide cancer incidence is predicted to elevate to 28.4 million cases by 2040 [81]. There are various treatment options available for cancer, including surgical procedures, hormonal treatments, chemotherapy, radiation therapy, and immunotherapy [11, 35]. While chemotherapy is commonly employed, it is associated with considerable adverse effects, including neuropathy, anemia, fluctuations in weight, sexual issues, and hair loss. Additionally, chemotherapy requires heavy doses since it lacks specificity for the target site. It primarily works by disrupting DNA formation and the mitosis to eliminate cancer cells [78]. However, this approach also harms healthy cells, leading to undesirable complications. In turn, there is a critical desire to develop new agents that can specifically target cancer cells without damaging normal tissues. Since the 1980s, researchers have explored drug delivery systems utilizing polymers to boost the therapeutic index and bioactivity of traditional treatments [39]. Polymeric drug delivery systems have gained significant prominence in cancer treatment over the last two decades [77].

Phytochemicals in plants have a wide range of therapeutic applications. The alkaloids, flavonoids, polyols, and polysaccharides have been used to treat different cancers. Guar gum is a natural biopolymer that has shown promising potential in cancer treatment, particularly as a component in drug delivery systems. Guar gum has demonstrated cancer chemopreventive activity by inhibiting enzymes like glutathione-S-transferases (GSTs) and cytochrome P450 1A (CYPIA), both involved in carcinogen metabolism [24]. C-glycosylated guar gum and sulfated derivatives of guar gum (SGG) effectively inhibited the carcinogen-activating enzyme CYP1A, while SGG showed stronger radical scavenging and anti-proliferative effects against cancer cells. Both derivatives also modulated macrophage functions toward an anti-inflammatory response [19]. A hydrogel responsive to pH and salt, created from guar gum, was developed for the delivery of curcumin, a natural anticancer drug. The hydrogel, characterized by physiochemical techniques, demonstrated favorable swelling behavior and drug release kinetics, highlighting its potential as an organic drug delivery system sourced from agriculture goods [25]. Moreover, it also shows its ability to reduce toxicity in cancer cells and pH-responsive drug delivery making it possible as a natural treatment option in cancer treatment.

Hydrogels, films, scaffolds, nanoparticles, and their use to deliver anticancer medications are possible with modified guar gum. Thermal treatment, crosslinking, sonochemical processes, etc. give chemical modifications to guar gum making it effective in medical applications. These modifications are analyzed through techniques like physiochemical techniques to assess structural and drug-binding changes. The present chapter describes guar gum, its sources, chemical composition, and structural modifications. The use of these modified products has been discussed for treatment of cancer [30].

9.2 Structure and Composition of Guar Gum

Gum plants store nutrients that embryo uses as a food source during germination. These plants originate from the Indian subcontinent, the southern region, including the semiarid regions of Brazil, South Africa, Australia, and southern United States, particularly Texas and Arizona. Pakistan and India dominate global guar production, together supplying nearly all of it, with India as the largest contributor. This region plays a crucial role in meeting the worldwide demand for guar. India is the largest global producer of guar. India produced about 650,000 tonnes of guar extract in the 2013–2014 period, with 6,010,000 tons traded, and more than 50% exported to the United States. Guar gum is not soluble in substances like hydrocarbons, fats, alcohols, esters, or ketones, aside from certain organic solvents such as formamide. Its primary solvent is water [53]. The natural carbohydrate gum in guar gum consists of 34.5% D-galactose anhydride and 63.4% D-mannose anhydride (Figure 9.1).

A linear backbone of β-D-mannopyranosyl linkages units and α-D-galactopyranosyl side chains with galactose-to-mannose averages of 1:1.6

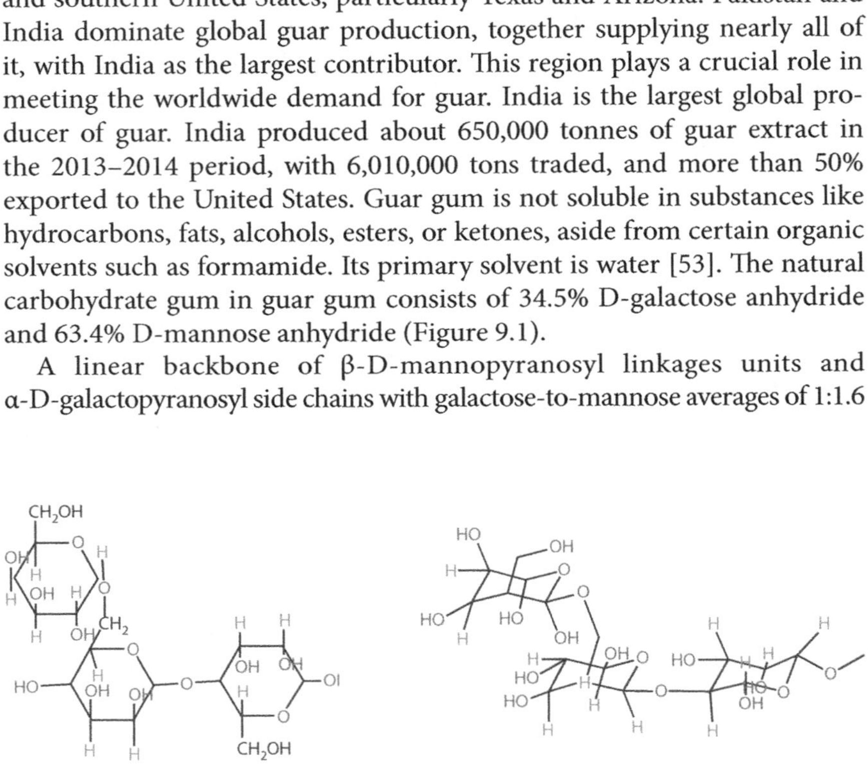

Figure 9.1 Structure of guar gum.

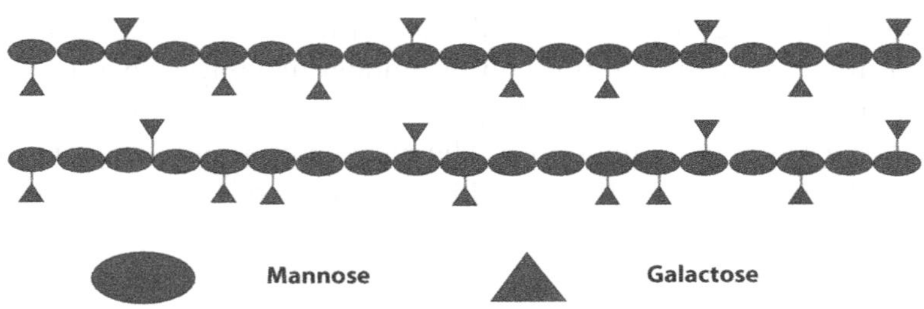

Figure 9.2 Guar gum showing mannose backbone and galactose as branch.

Table 9.1 General composition of guar gum.

Constituents	Percentage
Protein (N × 6.25)	5.0–6.0
Fiber	2.0–3.0
Moisture	8.0–14
Ash	0.5–1.0
Galactomannan	75–85

to 1:2 makes up the structure of guar gum, which is a type of galactomannan (Figure 9.2) [75, 91].

Additionally, ketoses or uronic acids were not found in the polysaccharide material (guaran). The guar grain comprises multiple layers of the outer husk (16–18%), the endosperm (34–40%), and the germ (43–46%). The seed is primarily composed of proteins, while the endosperm is rich in galactomannan (Table 9.1).

9.3 Physical and Chemical Properties of Guar Gum

The characteristics of guar galactomannan and similar polymers are influenced by their interactions in moist environments (Table 9.2). Guar gum expands and dissolves in water and other polar solvents, creating stable hydrogen bonds, whereas in hydrophobic solvents, it creates weak intermolecular hydrogen attractions. Its dissolving rate and viscosity tend to increase as particle size decreases, pH lowers, and temperature rises. The soluble salts and other agents that bind water, like sucrose, slow the hydration process.

9.3.1 Guar Gum Processing

The commercial extraction of guar gum involves several mechanical processes, including sieving, polishing, attrition, and roasting. The separation of the endosperm from its other components is facilitated by the varying hardness of these components. Once the hull and germ are eliminated, guar splits are procured. The hull can be easily separated after thermal treatment using attrition milling or other types of impact mills, allowing for efficient processing.

Table 9.2 Characteristics of guar gum.

Property	Description
Chemical composition	Linear chains of β-D-mannopyranosyl and α-D-galactopyranosyl units
Appearance	Whitish to golden powder
Solubility	Viscose gel is formed when dissolved in cold water
Viscosity	High viscosity in solution; temperature- and concentration-dependent
Texture	Hydrated, smooth, and creamy
Average molecular weight	Typically ranges from 200,000 to 800,000 Da
Decomposition temperature	Decomposes at temperatures above 200 degrees Celsius
Moisture content	Usually approximately 8–12%
pH	pH ranges from 6 to 8
Stability	Stable in acidic and neutral media, less stable in highly alkaline medium
Reactivity	Enzymatic hydrolysis oxidation sensitive
Thickening agent	Used in food and medicine
Emulsifying agent	Aids with the stabilization of emulsions in different formulations
Water retention	Superior ability to retain water

The finer fractions of the seed and hull are retrieved from the endosperm through separating, and the endosperm is then ground to produce powdered guar gum. Guar gum can be further purified by first dissolving it in water, then precipitating and recovering it using ethanol or isopropanol. This refining process enhances its quality for various applications. The final product, referred to as clarified (or purified) guar gum, is often formulated with sugar content (Figure 9.3) [87, 94].

Guar can absorb significant quantities of water producing a highly viscous dispersion. Temperature significantly influences fundamental characteristics of guar gum. As temperature increases, the hydration water

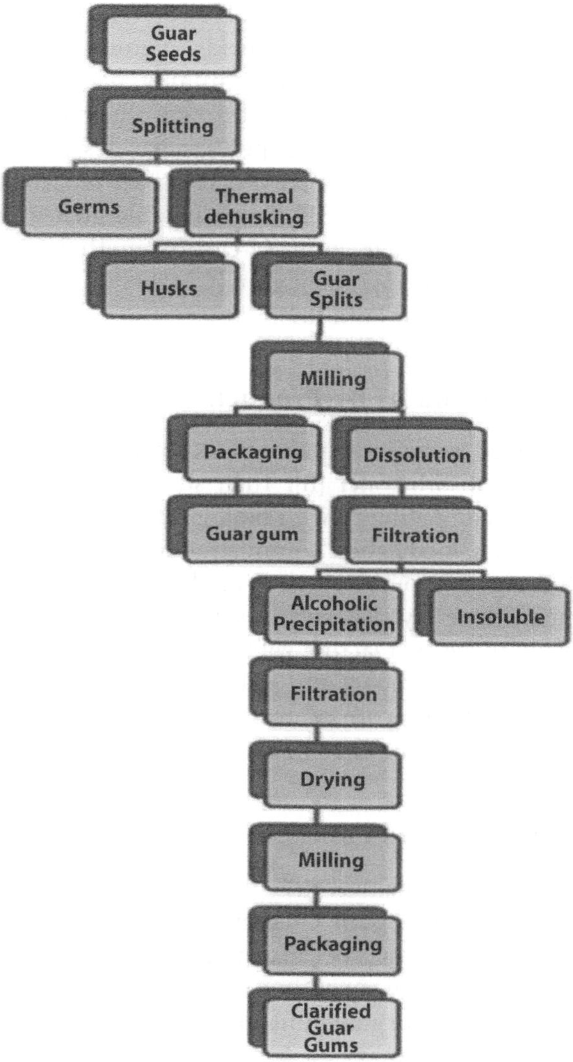

Figure 9.3 Processing of guar gum.

surrounding the polymer molecules is lost [15, 44, 47]. Being biocompatible, it exhibits varying solubility rates and viscosity under different solution conditions [8, 44]. The fluidity of guar gum is primarily changed by impurities, temperature, and pH, which are used to classify it into edible and commercial-grade materials [80]. Guar gum has few applications due to its thick fluidity and moisture content. However, its industrial uses, particularly in the food sector, paints, oilfields, pigments, pharmaceuticals, personal care products, water treatment, mining, paper, and superabsorbent materials, are greatly expanded through chemical modifications, which enhance its properties. Natural polysaccharides, like guar gum, can easily be converted into carboxymethyl derivatives, offering a wide range of applications for researchers [31]. Some notable guar gum derivatives include hydroxymethyl guar gum O-carboxymethyl-O-2-hydroxy-3-(trimethylammonium propyl) guar gum (CMHTPG) [96], meth-acryloyl guar gum and sulfated guar gum [89].

9.3.2 Guar Gum and Its By-Products

Highly cross-linked polymeric networks known as hydrogels have an amazing ability to absorb water [8]. Their strong swelling ability, hydrophilic nature, and compatibility with biological systems make them ideal for use in biosensors, medication administration, and agricultural applications. Crosslinking compounds, such as methylene bis-acrylamide, glutaraldehyde, and ethylene-glycol derivatives, interconnect the polysaccharide chains inside hydrogels by reacting with the hydroxyl groups on the polymer chains to create a compact and stable structure. Their water absorption and structural strength are controlled by these interrelated networks, and as such, hydrogel can be used in many different industries [68].

9.3.3 Guar Gum-Based Films

Excellent barrier and mechanical strength and germ resistance are possible with films made using guar gum. Guar gum and legume starch biological-composite edible packaging is because of their antibacterial qualities that can be applied as ingredients in culinary packaging [63]. The solvent casting method is used to make guar gum and silver–copper nanocomposites, which are suitable for culinary packaging due to their high mechanical, thermal, antibacterial, and oxygen barrier qualities [2]. In this research, films of different ratios of guar gum were prepared and the films' properties were investigated. The mechanical, antibacterial, and transparency/opacity features of the films were affected due to the inclusion of guar gum. By varying the proportion contained in a guar gum film, good tensile and puncture strength, low oxygen permeability, and noticeable antibacterial action against common microorganisms were achieved [5].

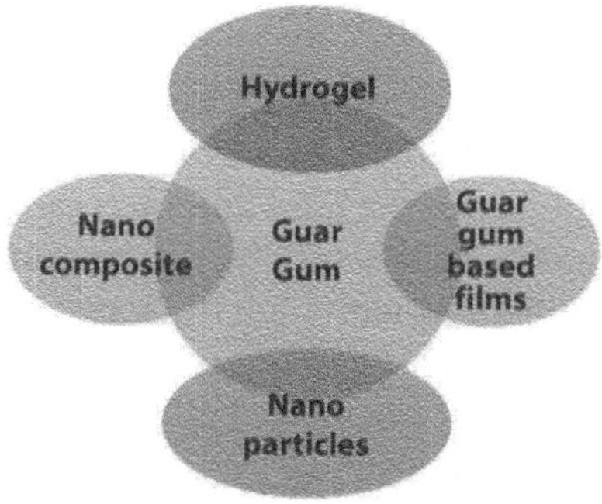

Figure 9.4 Derivatives of guar gum.

Because they are biodegradable, the composite films formed of guar gum and chitosan may help lessen environmental issues related to synthetic packaging [60].

9.3.4 Silica-Based Nanocomposites of Guar Gum

Silica is a colorless mineral in the earth's crust and can be used to create various useful materials, including guar gum–based nanocomposites (Figure 9.4). Modified guar gum/silica composites have been developed that can remove anionic dyes with great efficacy and high reusability for water treatment [47]. A colonic enzyme-responsive system was demonstrated in a study on the application of mesoporous silica nanocomposites for medication administration. Other formulations, such as guar gum–capped mesoporous silica, demonstrate the ability to load medicinal medicines, while hydrolyzed guar gum silica made with sol-gel techniques has good adsorption qualities for metal ions and dyes in water [52].

9.4 Chemical Modification of Guar Gum

Although guar gum is readily accessible and inexpensive, its uncontrolled hydration rate reduces its viscosity over time, and microbial contamination restricts its extended use. To overcome these limitations, guar gum has been chemically altered to enhance its properties. Guar gum is aimed at improving guar gum solubility, stability, and versatility for different industrial applications by means of derivatives [34].

9.4.1 Carboxy Methyl Guar Gum

Carboxy methyl groups are introduced into the hydroxyl groups of guar gum with the reaction of the hydroxyl groups with chloroacetic acid to increase the water solubility of the gum and increase its viscosity. The gelling properties and stability of this modified guar gum make it very useful in aqueous-based formulations with high thickness requirements like food and pharmaceutical products [17].

9.4.2 O-Carboxymethyl-o-Hydroxypropyl Guar Gum

The inclusion of both carboxymethyl and hydroxypropyl groups formed by reaction with chloroacetic acid and propylene oxide results in enhanced solubility and viscosity of CMHPG. These properties make it also a good thickening agent in formulation with high stability such as adhesives, textiles, and enhanced oil recovery [70].

9.4.3 O-Carboxymethyl-o-2-Hydroxy-3- (Trimethylammonium Propyl) Guar Gum

The derivative is a carboxymethyl and trimethylammonium combination that increases the water solubility and cationic properties. CMHTPG possesses these characteristics, which make it a good choice for use in the enhanced oil recovery and water treatment processes in which it can more readily interact with anionic substances and enhance viscosity in aqueous environments [37].

9.4.4 Ammonium Hydroxylpropyl Trimethyl Chloride of Guar Gum

Ammonium functional groups are added to the guar gum by rendering it to interact with trimethylchlorosilane or similar reagents to improve water retention and gel-forming properties. It is useful in applications that need to sustain moisture retention in agriculture, cosmetics, and personal care products [84].

9.4.5 Acryloyloxy Guar Gum

Acryloyloxy groups ($COOCH{=}CH_2$) are introduced into guar gum through reaction with acryloyloxy chloride and guar gum is thus rendered reactive for polymerization. It is often modified to achieve high absorbency and stability and is used in controlled release and superabsorbent applications, e.g., water-absorbing materials, diapers, and soil conditioners [69].

9.4.6 Methacryloyl Guar Gum

As acryloylation goes, so does guar gum when reacted with methacryloyl chloride to add methacrylate groups ($COOCH_2C\ (CH_3)\ {=}CH_2$) to create hydrogels and to improve binding properties. In medical and personal care products such as wound dressings and hydrogel patches, which require high water retention and adhesion, methacryloyl guar gum is particularly useful [92].

9.4.7 Sulfated Guar Gum

The guar gum reacts with sulfur trioxide or chlorosulfonic acid to introduce sulfate groups ($-OSO_3H$) forming this derivative. The sulfate groups increase water solubility and properties of the gum as a dispersing agent, which are of use in detergents, paints, and dispersants [42].

9.4.8 Crosslinking of Guar Gums

Crosslinking guar gum with different precursors produces hydrogels for encapsulation of different drugs to analyze their release profiles. Controlled drug delivery systems are most advantageous with these aquatic gels. The potential of a colon targeted delivery mechanism using low expansion crosslinks guar gum (GG) hydrogel was studied after treating GG with trisodium tri-meta-phosphate (STMP). The findings showed that enzymatically biodegradable crosslinked guar gum is a proficient medium for colon therapeutic distribution systems [22]. The medicine diffusion capabilities of chemically bonded guar gum polyacrylamide network were examined. These hydrogel particles from guar gum were loaded with two blood pressure-lowering drugs (verapamil and nifedipine) to assess their regulated drug release ability [79].

9.4.8.1 Crosslinking Guar Gums in Treatment of Colorectal Cancer

Spherical, free-flowing microspheres cross-linked with glutaraldehyde were successfully created using the emulsification method. The release profile from these guar gum microspheres was influenced due to concentrations of guar gum and glutaraldehyde. Release studies indicated that the microspheres could delay the release of methotrexate (MTX) until it reaches the colon, where bacterial enzymes are abundant and can degrade guar gum, facilitating the administration of the target therapy. Therefore, guar gum microspheres present a promising system for the colon-specific release of MTX for colorectal cancer therapy [12].

9.4.8.2 *Crosslinking Guar Gums in Treatment of T-Cell Leukemia*

Nanoparticles, due to their dimensions and characteristics, represent promising agents for combating cancer. Guar gum nanoparticles incorporating tamoxifen citrate in the current study demonstrated the advantages of nanoencapsulation for the highly protein-binding medication tamoxifen citrate in passive targeting of malignancies [21]. The drug-entrapped nanoparticles were as effective as the unencapsulated drug when administered to cancerous cells. Nevertheless, the crosslinked guar gum nanoparticles loaded with tamoxifen citrate displayed a sustained release of the medication and postponed programmed cell death over an extended duration, rendering it suitable for oncological therapy [65].

9.4.8.3 *Grafting of Carboxymethyl Guar Gum*

Carboxymethylated guar gum is a negatively charged semi-synthetic derivative of guar-based polymer, a galactomannan complex carbohydrate. It is produced through the reaction of guar gum with NaCl with the help of NaOH [61]. CMGG is an inexpensive and highly water-soluble commercial polysaccharide. In the present research, CMGG is the main framework and polysaccharide onto which polyacrylamide (PAM) branches are grafted. Alteration of polymers is an important way of alteration of polymers, and grafting is an important method to combine synthetic and natural polymers [43, 83]. Such a process provides several factors of merit such as excellent coagulation, regulated biodecomposition, and elevated shear stability of resulting branch copolymer. Many polysaccharides such as dextran, guar gum, cashew gum, hydroxyl propylated guar polysaccharide, amylopectin, and glycogen have been grafted with different polymers such as acrylamide copolymer [1, 6, 28, 46]. The coagulation properties of these graft copolymers are optimized in different solution than linear PAM-derived polymers. The increased performance of these grafted PAM copolymers is related to the greater access of the branched polyacrylamide links to suspended microparticles [71–73]. The branch copolymerization of many of the monomers has been applied to various substrates using ceric ions [23, 46, 95]. Grafting typically occurs when radical sites formed on polymer surfaces propagate, which helps reduce the production of homopolymer. These data explore certain features of the formation and analysis of polyacrylamide branched CMGG (CMGG-g-PAM) and investigate the coagulation efficiency of the manufactured products [20].

9.5 Enzymatic Modifications of Guar Gum

Enzymatic modifications of guar gum, including depolymerization, deacetylation, crosslinking, transglycosylation, and partial hydrolysis, improve its drug delivery potential, particularly for cancer treatments. Solubility and absorption are enhanced by depolymerization, and deacetylation stabilizes drug carriers for controlled release. Transglycosylation allows for enzyme-specific drug release at cancer sites, and crosslinking produces a gel matrix for release of targeted drug. Breakdown of the extracellular barriers, through partial hydrolysis, facilitates tumor penetration. This versatility to be modified and the targeted nature of drug delivery makes guar gum a useful material (Table 9.3). Research has been done on enzymes such as proteases, lipases, and specific carbohydrate hydrolyzing enzymes for use in these areas.

Guar gum is changeable with enzymatic hydrolysis to improve its solubility and its molecular weight to facilitate better drug absorption and delivery. A central composite design (CCD) was used to test different combinations of factors such as enzyme concentration, pH, temperature, and reaction time, and to optimize the hydrolysis process. Cellulose from *Aspergillus niger* was used for the experiments, and the hydrolyzed guar gum was then assayed for fluidity to determine the effectiveness of different conditions. A strong correlation was found between predicted and experimental values for a second-order model, and so we showed that the process was modelled quite well. The effect of some factors, such as enzyme concentration and pH, on lowering viscosity was much greater than that of others. The optimized conditions obtained from this study can be utilized to produce guar gum of higher quality for drug delivery use [45]. Guar gum is a distinct complex carbohydrate frequently used in the nutraceuticals. C-glycosylated derivative of guar gum and its sulfated by-product

Table 9.3 Enzymatic modification of guar gum.

Modification	Enzymes	Effect on guar gum	Drug application	Potential side effects
Depolymerization	Mannanases, galactosidases	Decrease viscosity improves solubility	Enhances drug absorption as a solubilizing agent	Possible irritation in sensitive tissues
Deacetylation	Deacetylases	Improved solubility	Stabilizes drug carriers, enabling controlled drug release	Potential toxicity if over deacetylated
Crosslinking	Laccases, peroxidases	Increased gel strength	Acts as drug delivery matrix, providing controlled released	May reduce drug bioavailability if overcrosslinked
Transglycosylation	Transgly-cosidases	Improved emulsifying and stabilizing properties	Enables enzyme-specific drug release at cancer sites	Enzyme specificity could cause incomplete activation
Partial hydrolysis	Hydrolases	Reduced molecular weight improves digestibility	Aids in tumor penetration by breaking down extracellular barriers	Degraded forms may cause gastrointestinal disturbance

(SGG) were evaluated for potential cancer chemopreventive and soothing properties. The evaluation of cancer chemoprevention, particularly in the anti-initiation phase, showed that it was an efficient antagonist. It inhibited the mutagen-activating hepatic P450 enzyme but also increased the activity of mutagenic-detoxifying catalyst such as GST. In contrast, sodium stibogluconate inhibited both GSTs and CYP1A. Additionally, SGG exhibited superior reactive species scavenging ability compared to guar gum, effectively neutralizing peroxyl, superoxide, and hydroxyl radicals, which are harmful reactive species. Both guar gum and sulfated by-product were discovered to influence how macrophages work, leading to a response that reduces inflammation. They improved the growth of macrophages and their ability to engulf fluorescein isothiocyanate (FITC)-zymosan, while significantly inhibiting nitric oxide synthesis and the excretion of immune response regulator such as tumor necrosis factor alpha (TNF-α) in lipopolysaccharide (LPS)-activated RAW 264.7 immune cells. Interestingly, both guar gum and SGG markedly reduced the FITC-LPS interaction with RAW 264.7 cells, as demonstrated by cellular profiling [19].

9.6 Characterization Techniques

9.6.1 Fourier Transform Infrared Spectroscopy

Fourier transform infrared spectroscopy (FTIR) is a harm-free technique for analyzing the molecular structure of both organic and inorganic materials in earth material natural resources [36, 62, 90]. In medical applications, FTIR is essential in characterizing guar gum, a natural polymer explored for cancer treatment and drug delivery [16]. When chemically modified, such as through grafting with acrylic acid, guar gum becomes more stable and biocompatible. FTIR aids in confirming these modifications, particularly by identifying functional groups, which helps in developing advanced therapeutic delivery systems for targeted oncological therapies.

9.6.2 NMR Analysis of Guar Gum

Proton nuclear magnetic resonance (H NMR) is a very important analytical procedure to determine chemical composition, and hence to understand the nature of a substance, especially for complex biomolecules such as guar gum. H NMR is used to identify chemical groups such as methylene groups and hydroxyl groups within its cyclic structure in guar gum analysis. It is particularly useful for confirming modifications, such as the bonding of acrylic acid to form copolymers (e.g., GG-g-PAA) to improve drug-carrying properties. This technique verifies structural changes that enhance solubility, stability, and bioavailability of guar gum–based hydrogels and grafted polymers for drug delivery, especially for cancer treatment [63].

9.6.3 X-Ray Diffraction Analysis of Guar Gum

XRD was used to study the crystalline arrangement of guar gum and other substances. Free betulinic acid and hesperidin were crystalline, whereas materials such as guar gum, alginate, and linseed oil were amorphous [45]. Encapsulation of these compounds (e.g., MNED microcapsules) caused the active compounds to become molecularly dispersed and non-crystalline, as evidenced by the lack of crystalline crests present in the microcapsules.

It showed that the spray-drying encapsulation technique was effective also recorded a related outcome for lycopene microencapsulated with gelatine.

9.7 Application of Guar Gum in Health Management

Guar gum is frequently utilized in different industries; pharmacies, cosmetics, food, textiles, paper explosives, and toiletries are just a few of the industries (Figure 9.5). Its antibacterial, antiproliferative, bulk-forming, hypoglycemic, and hypolipidemic qualities are acknowledged from a therapeutic standpoint [66].

9.7.1 The Role of Guar Gum in Cancer Therapy

Guar gum and its by-products have also shown promise in cancer therapy, particularly in addressing colorectal cancer, one of the commonly prevalent forms linked to gastrointestinal disorders. The properties of guar gum may aid in supporting patients undergoing treatment and potentially improve outcomes. Cancer is still the world's major cause of death and is a serious public health issue [9]. The fundamental components of the cell's cytoskeleton are biopolymeric proteins. Cancer alters the cytoskeleton's and the extracellular matrix's architecture. Because altered protein structures affect the mechanics of deformation, cancer cells' capacity to stretch or contract is also affected. There are various types of cancer, including breast, lung, prostate, skin, and colon cancer, each affecting different organs and tissues

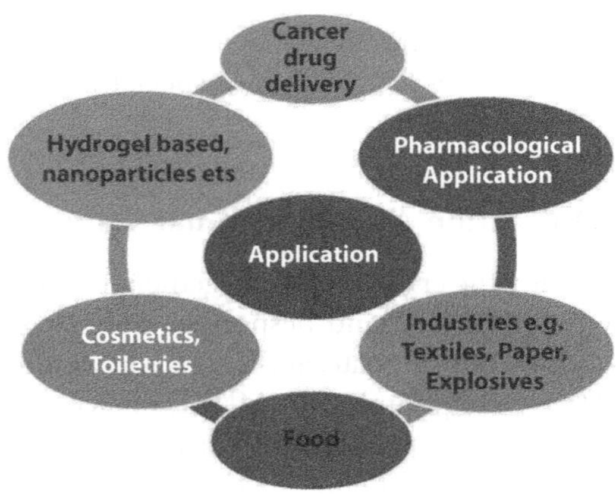

Figure 9.5 Applications of guar gum.

in the body. The groundbreaking discovery of the proto-oncogene by Varmus and Bishop, which offered insights into the function of molecules and genes in causing cancer in humans, is responsible for the cellular and molecular pathways dictating the origins of cancer [13].

The size of the microparticles is measured using a Zeta sizer, where the particles are mixed in a solution and analyzed by the machine's software. The shape and surface of the microparticles are studied with a scanning electron microscope (SEM). This involves scattering the particles onto sticky tape that is applied to a metal object, covering it with a thin layer of gold, and then magnifying the picture 1000 times to produce fine-grained details [45].

Drug encapsulation was assessed using the back-calculation approach following a previously published protocol [74]. The aqueous phase was collected in a separate sample tube after centrifuging the microparticle dispersion for 30 minutes at 12,000 rpm. The aqueous phase was collected after centrifuging and any remaining pellet subjected to three rounds of washing with water. In all, the total concentration area for the pharmaceuticals in each of the collected aqueous phase was analyzed by HPLC to determine drug incorporation and encapsulation efficiency.

In the development of drug delivery systems, such as nanoparticles or hydrogels, guar gum has been used in breast cancer treatment to provide modulated and controlled release of chemotherapeutic medicine. Incorporation of guar gum into pharmaceutical carriers increases the solubility, stabilization, and physiological availability of anticancer therapeutics [34]. These delivery systems guarantee that the drug is released slowly and its time to come; this effect is more preferable for the tumor site and at the same time will decrease the side effect of the drug so the treatment itself will be more efficient. Guar gum–based hydrogels are being studied for their use to deliver drugs, such as doxorubicin, a common chemotherapy drug used to treat breast cancer. The use of this approach minimizes the systemic toxicity of the drug while maintaining its efficacy against cancer cells.

The gel-forming properties of guar gum help drugs absorb better and prevent the rapid breakdown of drugs in the body for a controlled release over time. By doing so, it can improve overall therapeutic outcomes in breast cancer by delivering more consistent drug levels in the bloodstream and at the tumor site. Often times, chemotherapy drugs come with serious side effects like gastrointestinal problems that limit their use. The fiber content of guar gum helps to do this by promoting digestive health and, in turn, helping prevent side effects such as constipation.

However, guar gum may also improve body defense system response to metastatic cells. The exact mechanisms behind how this works are still in research, but that polysaccharides like guar gum have been shown to stimulate immune cells, such as macrophages and lymphocytes that may help track and fight cancer cells [14].

When used as part of combination therapy, guar gum has been found to make breast cancer cells more responsive to chemotherapy drugs. This means that lower doses of these drugs can be used, reducing toxicity while maintaining efficacy. Guar gum has been used in combination with other natural or synthetic agents to boost the cancer-killing potential of chemotherapy drugs by improving drug delivery to the tumor site.

9.7.1.1 Colorectal Cancer

Guar gum and its by-products are effective in metastatic treatment, particularly for colon cancer, the most prevalent type of cancer related to gut disorders. The effectiveness of methotrexate-containing glutaraldehyde crosslinked guar gum in the therapy of colon cancer. The manufacture of guar gum microspheres for local medication release inside the large intestine was prepared through crosslinking glutaraldehyde emulsification. The study suggests that conjugated guar has a high encapsulation in conjunction with methotrexate (MTX). The US Pharmacopeia paddle type (type 2) dissolution system was applied to deliver drug in monitored environment, and the findings change with concentration of guar gum and glutaraldehyde [12]. Synthetic guar gum can help inhibit cancer and should be taken as a dietary addition. Guar gum variants can both stimulate and inhibit the tumor inducer detox enzymes glutathione-S-transferases (GSTs) and cytochrome P450 IA (CYPIA) [19].

9.7.1.1.1 Colon-Specific Drug Delivery

Guar gum has gained attention for its use in site-specific therapy method, specifically for colorectal cancer treatment. Guar gum's biocompatibility and biodegradability make it an optimal carrier for therapeutics formulations aimed at the colon. Guar gum–based microspheres were prepared to co-deliver doxorubicin and metformin to the colon, enhancing the specificity and efficacy of the chemotherapy drugs. This approach minimizes systemic side effects, which is critical in colorectal cancer treatments where localized drug release can limit damage to healthy tissues [67]. Guar gum formulations have been studied for their ability to deliver drugs under regulated conditions within the large intestine. Polysaccharides like guar gum have demonstrated potential for delaying drug release until the drugs arrive in the colon, which is beneficial for treating gastrointestinal disorders. Exploration into guar gum–coated tablets and capsules for colon-targeted therapies demonstrated improved drug retention in the target area, thus enhancing treatment efficacy [7].

9.7.1.1.2 Dietary Fiber and Colon Health

Dietary fibers, including guar gum, are known to support colon health, which is important for lowering the chance of colorectal cancer. Guar gum is a soluble fiber that ferments in the colon, generating fatty acids with short chains such as butyrate. Butyrate has occurred to exhibit inflammation-reducing and cancer-fighting actions, especially in the colon where it can induce apoptosis (cell death) in cancerous cells. A study on the impact of hydrolyzed guar gum revealed that it acts as a prebiotic, fostering the proliferation of beneficial bacteria like Akkermansia and Faecali bacterium. These microbes help maintain a healthy gut microbiome, which is linked to reducing the chance of inflammation and cancerous changes in the colon [76]. The study found that PHGG supplementation increased levels of these bacteria, suggesting that guar gum may support the prevention of colorectal cancer through its prebiotic effects [21].

9.7.1.2 Breast Cancer

Anticancer drugs in breast cancer treatment and their interaction between guar gum (GG) revolve around the polymer's ability to modify the pharmacokinetics and pharmacodynamics of the drugs, enhancing their therapeutic efficacy and reducing side effects. Regardless of significant advancements in operative methods, effectively preventing breast cancer recurrence remains a challenge. This is mainly due to the possibility of remaining neoplastic cells being left behind in the surgical margins, specifically in those who have received conservative breast surgery [3, 4]. Surgeries like lumpectomies are successful in removing most of the tumor; there is a risk that some cancerous cells may remain at the edges of the removed tissue. These leftover cells can cause the cancer to come back, which is why preventing recurrence is difficult even with improved surgical methods [57].

Anticancer drugs have harmful toxic effects on healthy tissues, which is the main problem. These side effects often lead to reduced dosages, treatment delays, or even stopping the therapy altogether. Most anticancer drugs target specific receptors but face challenges in delivery because of their high molecular size, low water dissolvability, and short lifespan in the body [58]. Clinically, radiotherapy and chemotherapy are commonly given after neoplasm removal. However, both modalities come with significant harmfulness and adverse effects throughout the body [10, 82]. It is possible to avoid off-target toxic effects with local chemotherapy in relation to systemic therapies. Additionally, regional chemotherapy may reduce the waiting period before starting adjuvant chemotherapy [3, 88, 97]. Tamoxifen citrate, a non-steroidal anti estrogen, serves as the primary hormone treatment for breast carcinoma [41]. It mainly targets tissues that have a high concentration of estragon receptors (ER). For over 30 years, tamoxifen has been utilized for the therapy of estrogen receptor–positive breast cancer [32]. Tamoxifen is classified as an estrogen receptor modulator [40]. In mammary carcinoma cells, tamoxifen functions by inhibiting the action of estrogen, which is known for its antagonistic effect. However, in other tissues, such as the endometrium and bones, it can mimic estrogen's effects, referred to as its agonistic effect (Figure 9.6). Guar gum can help improve the effectiveness and safety of tamoxifen by controlling its release, enhancing solubility, and reducing systemic toxicity, benefiting breast cancer patients in the post-chemotherapy phase.

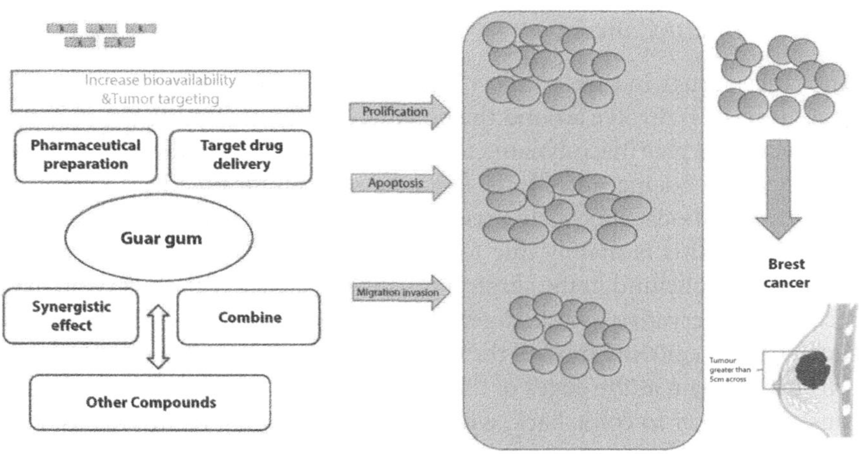

Figure 9.6 Guar gum shows potential to aid breast cancer care through better drug absorption.

It has been shown to be a potent drug medium for target drug release in tumor therapy. Controlled drug release is made possible by its polysaccharide structure, with drug delivery limited to cancer cells and minimized toxic effects on healthy tissue. Apoptosis of breast cancer cells can be induced by the modified guar gum, which activates, for example, enzymes like caspases that are important to prevent cancer proliferation. In addition, the anti inflammatory and antioxidant properties of the agent dampen inflammation and oxidative stress in the tumor environment, slowing cancer progression. Guar gum also strengthens the immune system to stimulate immune responses to kill tumor cells and may inhibit tumor vascularization, cutting off the tumor's blood supply to keep it from growing.

9.7.1.3 Hepatocellular Carcinoma

Natural, biodegradable delivery system for natural compounds in hepatocellular carcinoma is used with guar gum. The potential therapeutic thymoquinone and piperine are often hampered by their hydrophobic nature in clinical efficacy. To overcome this, a microvehicle was designed based on guar gum to encapsulate these compounds to increase their stability and bioavailability. It performs well with a lower median lethal dose (LD50) against hepatocellular carcinoma cells and with good antibacterial effects as well as improved anticancer response with a significant decrease in the minimum inhibitory concentration (MIC). Structural validation of the guar gum delivery system was done by advanced techniques such as FTIR, XRD, FESEM, and UV-visible spectroscopy. The guar gum delivery system was also released at a pH-dependent manner optimizing therapeutic delivery in combination therapeutics. It presents the use of guar gum microvehicles for improving the medical use of phytochemicals in cancer treatment [15].

Guar gum and sodium guar gum showed remarkable effects in minimizing the growth of human liver cancer cells (Hep G2), with SGG showing specific cytotoxicity toward mammary glands carcinoma cells (MCF-7). Not a single compound, however, displayed significant cytotoxicity against human lymphoblastic leukemia cells (1301). In Hep G2 cells, SGG caused significant disruptions in cell cycle progression, leading to hold in the S phase (synthesis phase) and G2/M (gap 2 and mitosis phase), which was involved with necrotic rather than programmed cell death, in both guar gum and SGG cells treated [19].

9.7.2 Guar Gum in Treatment of Other Diseases

Beyond diabetes and heart disease, guar gum has applications in treating a variety of other conditions. It has been utilized for managing cholera, functional constipation, and diarrhea. Additionally, its solutions are sometimes incorporated into eye-drop formulations, showcasing its versatility in medicinal applications.

9.7.2.1 Guar Gum in Diabetes Management

Guar gum is recognized for its efficacy in managing blood sugar concentrations. Research indicates that it can reduce postprandial (after-meal) spikes in blood sugar and insulin concentration. For example, a study with diabetic patients demonstrated that incorporating guar gum to their diet resulted in notable decreases in certain health markers, emphasizing its potential as a dietary approach for managing diabetes [50].

9.7.2.2 Guar Gum in Heart Disease Treatment

The soluble polysaccharides present in guar gum have attracted attention as potential components in the formulation of functional foods aimed at cardiovascular health. Water-soluble gums are widely utilized as solvents, thickening material, and aroma additive in pharmaceutical and culinary trades [29]. Guar gum, with its composition of soluble fiber (75%), has been found to reduce cholesterol levels, which may subsequently decrease the risk of cardiovascular diseases. It has crude protein (2.16%), insoluble fibers (7.6%), moisture content (9.55%), ash (0.54%), and fat (0.78%), making it a good source of nutrition in heart-healthy diets [38].

9.8 Drug–Polymer Interaction

9.8.1 Functional Group Modification in Doxorubicin and Metformin HCl

Guar gum interacts with drugs like doxorubicin and metformin HCl. Functional group modifications in these drugs can alter their binding with guar gum, influencing drug release profiles. FTIR analysis can identify shifts in the positions of the functional group peaks as a function of the pH indicating hydrogen bonding, electrostatic interactions, or clusters of these interactions. By this interaction, controlled and sustained release of the drugs is afforded, leading to improved therapeutic efficacy and reduced systemic toxicity [10]. Desiccated powdered samples of metformin HCl, doxorubicin, and the microparticles were made into potassium bromide (KBr) disks with which they were analyzed by Fourier transform infrared spectroscopy (FTIR) [51]. The disks were prepared using crushed 2 mg of the specimen with 98 mg of potassium bromide and then vacuum-compressed. Observed samples were recorded over a wavelength range of 500–4000 cm^{-1} using Nicolet Omnic software, and the IR spectrum was captured. The source spectra of metformin HCl and doxorubicin [59] were matched against the resulting infrared spectra and signals, and the results were analyzed [55].

9.8.2 pH-Responsive Drug Delivery in Cancer Therapy

A guar gum–based, pH, and salt responsive hydrogel is created for delivery of curcumin, a natural anticancer drug. An acrylic acid guar gum hydrogel was synthesized by attaching acrylic acid to guar gum with (NH4)2S2O8 as a catalyst and C7H10N2O2 as a binder to increase structural stability [64]. TGA, FTIR, SEM, and NMR were used to classify the hydrogels and evaluate the properties. In this work, we study swelling behavior and water diffusion in various pH and salt conditions, followed by curcumin release kinetics studies. The results show that this renewable hydrogel could act as a dependable and eco-friendly drug delivery system using both curcumin and guar gum from agricultural products [25].

9.9 Comparative Evaluation of Guar Gum with Other Biopolymers

Guar gum is more effective than other polymers to improve gut heath and activity. It also has antimicrobial activity and efficient drug delivery for cancer therapy. It ensures stability and excellent biocompatibility with minimum side effects. Unlike chitosan and alginate, it is cost-effective, highly versatile, abundant, and suitable for different formulations (Table 9.4).

Table 9.4 Comparison of guar gum versus another biopolymer.

Biopolymers	Targeted drug delivery	Biocompatibility and toxicity	Stability and resistant to degradation	Cost and availability
Guar gum	Ideal for colorectal cancer therapy	Biodegradable plants derived and exhibited minimal toxicity and immunogenicity	Protect drug payloads from premature degradation. Stable in acidic environment	Freely available cost-effective ideal for large-scale use
Chitosan	Primarily used for mucosal delivery but struggle with pH	Biocompatible but causes allergic reaction in some patients	Unstable in neutral and basic in pH, limited application in drug delivery system	Moderately priced, depends on crustacean sources
Alginate	Sensitive to ionic environment reduced target efficiency	Biocompatible but may have batch-to-batch variability in purity	Degradation in ionic environment, reduced its compatibility for drug delivery	Relatively affordable but subjected to geographical availability
Dextran	Chemically modified for active targeting but lacks inherent specificity	Biocompatible but required purification to remove impurity	Lacks inherent protection against premature degradation	Moderately priced

9.10 Synergistic Potential of Guar Gum Derivatives in Combinatorial Cancer Treatments

Natural compounds were modified to produce optimized versions, so called modified natural compounds that are enhanced in their therapeutic effects. They may enhance the delivery of drugs in combinatorial cancer treatments, lower side effects, and boost the efficacy of traditional treatment.

9.10.1 Guar Gum with 5-Fluorouracil

Colon carcinoma is treated with 5-fluorouracil (5FU) [48]. The bioavailability of drug was improved through a microsphere formulation using

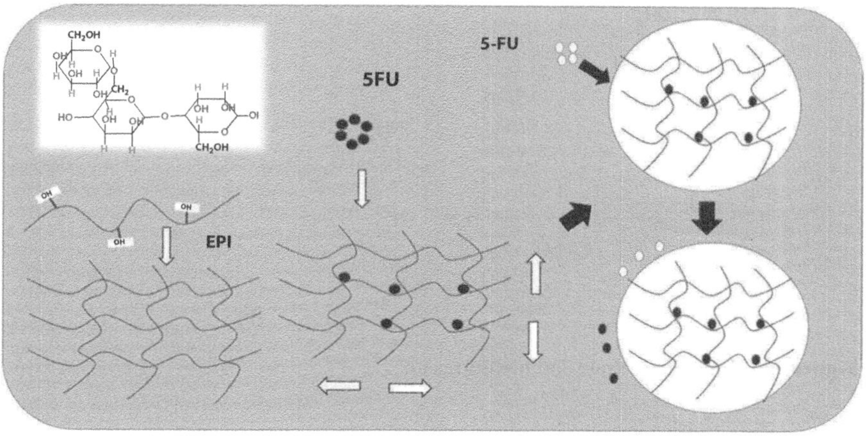

Figure 9.7 5-fluorouracil (5FU) bound to guar gum improves its bioavailability and facilitates controlled drug release over 24 hours. The process improves its efficacy against colorectal cancer.

guar gum and $Na_2 [B_4O_5 (OH)_4].8H_2O$ through the suspension linking process. This formulation enables controlled drug release over 24 hours, particularly targeting the colon, which improves its efficacy against colorectal cancer (Figure 9.7). The 5FU-filled microspheres demonstrated enhance reliability, with drug release occurring *via* zero-order kinetics through both breakdown and dissolution processes [56]. This approach allows for maximum and controlled drug delivery specifically for colon cancer. Administering 5FU directly to the colon is beneficial due to its ideal pH range of approximately 5.5 to 7 and low digestive enzyme activity, which together promote better drug absorption. This colon-specific drug delivery system had tested for effectiveness in the living system [26].

9.10.2 Guar Gum with Tamoxifen Citrate

Tamoxifen (TMX) reveals an opposing action in mammary carcinoma cells and is often applied in the treatment of estrogen receptor-positive (ER+) cancer [32]. TMX nanoparticles encapsulated in guar gum were created using the dispersion process. Guar gum has been utilized as a pharmaceutical carrier for various anticancer medications; there is little information available about this specific nanoformulation. When guar gum is chemically bound with tamoxifen citrate (Figure 9.8a), then this combination provides effective results against cancer. The analysis of TMX encapsulated guar gum nanocarriers was conducted in albino mice over a

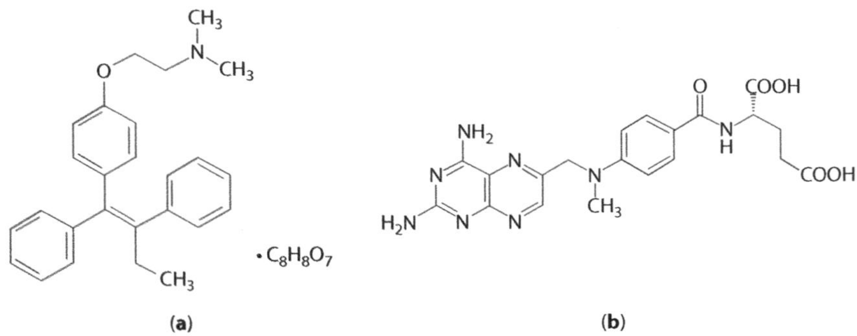

Figure 9.8 Tamoxifen citrate and methotrexate.

two-day period. Results indicated that the nanoparticles accumulated in both the mammary and ovarian tissues, with a significantly higher uptake and retention observed in the mammary glands [27, 33].

9.10.3 Guar Gum with Methotrexate

Guar gum microcapsule was designed to treat colon cancer [49]. The loading productivity of the MTX-filled microparticles was discovered to be 75.7%. These microcapsules were able to deliver the optimal quantity of the drug to the target position in colorectal cancer [54]. Albino rats were administered the formulation orally, and drug delivery was measured at various time intervals in the gastrointestinal track. When guar gum is chemically bound with methotrexate, then this combination provides effective results against cancer (Figure 9.8b). The research showed that guar gum microcapsule delivers MTX directly at the colon, proving to be an efficient delivery method for MTX in colorectal cancer treatment [12].

9.10.4 Guar Gum with Curcumin

Curcumin, known for its antioxidant properties, has been explored as an anticancer property, though its limited absorption in the gastrointestinal tract remains a significant challenge [18]. To address this, composition combining curcumin with varying concentrations of guar gum was developed and assessed for its impact on colon cancer (Figure 9.9). A solution with 40% guar gum released 91.1% of the drug, while the 50% guar gum solution had a lower deliver rate of 82.1% compared to the 40% solution [18]. The effectiveness of guar gum and its drug delivery capabilities opposing gut flora have been investigated using rat cereal contents, suggesting

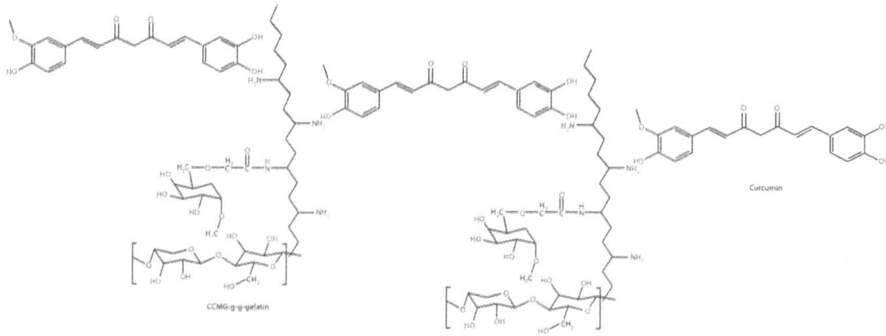

Figure 9.9 Guar gum with curcumin.

that guar gum might serve as a possible transporter for curcumin distribution in the treatment of colon cancer [55].

9.11 Future Prospective

Guar gum when combined with advanced technologies looks very promising in cancer treatment. Combined with nanotechnology, it improves drug delivery directly to tumors, reducing side effect on healthy tissues. It plays vital role in gut health could also lead to new diets that help in preventing cancers, specifically in digestive system. By modifying its structure researchers can enhance its ability to stick to the target cancer cells, making treatment more effective. More research on guar gum could become an important part of cancer treatment in safer and better ways.

9.12 Conclusion

Guar gum, a galactose-mannose polysaccharide extracted from *Cyamopsis psoraloides* and *Cyamopsis tetragonolobus*, has demonstrated substantial versatility across various fields such as pharmaceuticals, cosmetics, food, and textiles. Its natural abundance, especially in India and Pakistan, and water solubility make it a key biopolymer. In cancer therapy, guar gum's potential as a therapeutic distribution agent is notable due to its capability to be chemically modified, allowing targeted and controlled delivery of chemotherapeutic agents. Furthermore, guar gum derivatives have shown cancer chemopreventive properties, such as inhibiting carcinogenic enzymes and enhancing the efficacy of anticancer treatments.

With ongoing advancements in polymer-based drug delivery systems, guar gum is positioned as a promising compostable and safe biopolymer that may minimize the side effects of traditional chemotherapy while improving treatment effectiveness.

AI disclosure statement: The author acknowledges the use of AI-based tools for minor language editing or grammatical correction. However, all intellectual contributions, analyses, and conclusions presented in this chapter are entirely the author's own.

References

1. Adhikary, P., Tiwari, K.N., Singh, R.P., Synthesis, characterization, and flocculation characteristics of polyacrylamide-grafted glycogen. *J. Appl. Polym. Sci.*, 103, 2, 773–778, 2006.
2. Arfat, Y.A., Ejaz, M., Jacob, H., Ahmed, J., Deciphering the potential of guar gum/Ag-Cu nanocomposite films as an active food packaging material. *Carbohydr. Polym.*, 157, 65–71, 2017.
3. Askari, E., Seyfoori, A., Amereh, M., Gharaie, S.S., Ghazali, H.S., Ghazali, Z.S., Akbari, M., Stimuli-responsive hydrogels for local post-surgical drug delivery. *Gels*, 6, 2, 14, 2020.
4. Bastiancich, C., Bianco, J., Vanvarenberg, K., Ucakar, B., Joudiou, N., Gallez, B., Danhier, F., Injectable nanomedicine hydrogel for local chemotherapy of glioblastoma after surgical resection. *J. Control. Release*, 264, 45–54, 2017.
5. BeMiller, J.N. and Whistler, R.L. (Eds.), *Industrial gums: Polysaccharides and their derivatives*, Academic Press, 2012.
6. Biswal, D.R. and Singh, R.P., Characterisation of carboxymethyl cellulose and polyacrylamide graft copolymer. *Carbohydr. Polym.*, 57, 4, 379–387, 2004.
7. Black, J., Hickson, L., Black, B., Perry, C., Prognostic indicators in paediatric cochlear implant surgery: a systematic literature review. *Cochlear Implants Int.*, 12, 2, 67–93, 2011.
8. Brassesco, M.E., Valetti, N.W., Picó, G., Molecular mechanism of lysozyme adsorption onto chemically modified alginate guar gum matrix. *Int. J. Biol. Macromol.*, 96, 111–117, 2017.
9. Bray, F., Ferlay, J., Soerjomataram, I., Siegel, R.L., Torre, L.A., Jemal, A., Global cancer statistics 2018: GLOBOCAN estimates of incidence and mortality worldwide for 36 cancers in 185 countries. *CA Cancer J. Clin.*, 68, 6, 394–424, 2018.
10. Bu, L.L., Yan, J., Wang, Z., Ruan, H., Chen, Q., Gunadhi, V., Gu, Z., Advances in drug delivery for post-surgical cancer treatment. *Biomaterials*, 219, 119182, 2019.

11. Chakraborty, S. and Rahman, T., The difficulties in cancer treatment. *Ecancermedicalscience*, 6, ed 16, 2012.
12. Chaurasia, M., Chourasia, M.K., Jain, N.K., Jain, A., Soni, V., Gupta, Y., Jain, S.K., Cross-linked guar gum microspheres: A viable approach for improved delivery of anticancer drugs for the treatment of colorectal cancer. *AAPS PharmSciTech*, 7, E143–E151, 2006.
13. Chowdhary, M. and White, W., U.S. Patent Application No. 09/991,356, 2002.
14. Chudzikowski, R.J., Guar gum and its applications. *J. Soc. Cosmet. Chem.*, 22, 1, 43, 1971.
15. Das, S., Bera, D., Pal, K., Mandal, D., Karmakar, P., Dey, A., Hepatocellular carcinoma cells. *J. Dermatol. Res.*, Article 101994, 2020.
16. D'Angelo, J.A. and Zodrow, E.L., Chemometric study of functional groups in different layers of Trigonocarpus grandis ovules (Pennsylvanian seed fern, Canada). *Org. Geochem.*, 42, 9, 1039–1054, 2011.
17. Dodi, G., Hritcu, D., Popa, M.I., Carboxymethylation of guar gum: Synthesis and characterization. Cellulose Chemistry and Technology, characterization. *Cellul. Chem. Technol.*, 45, 3, 171, 2011.
18. Elias, E.J., Anil, S., Ahmad, S., Daud, A., Colon targeted curcumin delivery using guar gum. *Nat. Prod. Commun.*, 5, 6, 1934578X1000500621, 2010.
19. Gamal-Eldeen, A.M., Amer, H., Helmy, W.A., Cancer chemopreventive and anti-inflammatory activities of chemically modified guar gum. *Chem. Biol. Interact.*, 161, 3, 229–240, 2006.
20. Gerhäuser, C., Klimo, K., Heiss, E., Neumann, I., Gamal-Eldeen, A., Knauft, J., Frank, N., Mechanism-based *in vitro* screening of potential cancer chemopreventive agents. *Mutat. Res. Fundam. Mol. Mech. Mutagen.*, 523, 163–172, 2003.
21. Giannini, E.G., Mansi, C., Dulbecco, P., Savarino, V., Role of partially hydrolyzed guar gum in the treatment of irritable bowel syndrome. *Nutrition*, 22, 3, 334–342, 2006.
22. Gliko-Kabir, I., Yagen, B., Baluom, M., Rubinstein, A., Phosphated cross-linked guar for colon-specific drug delivery: II. *In vitro* and *in vivo* evaluation in the rat. *J. Control. Release*, 63, 1–2, 129–134, 2000.
23. Gupta, K.C. and Sahoo, S., Grafting of acrylonitrile and methyl methacrylate from their binary mixtures on cellulose using ceric ions. *J. Appl. Polym. Sci.*, 79, 5, 767–778, 2001.
24. Habig, W.H., Pabst, M.J., Jakoby, W.B., Glutathione S-transferases: the first enzymatic step in mercapturic acid formation. *J. Biol. Chem.*, 249, 22, 7130–7139, 1974.
25. Haq Asif, A., Karnakar, R.R., Sreeharsha, N., Gite, V.V., Borane, N., Al-Dhubiab, B.E., Meravanige, G., pH and salt responsive hydrogel based on guar gum as a renewable material for delivery of curcumin: A natural anti-cancer drug. *J. Polym. Environ.*, 29, 1978–1989, 2021.

26. Kamal, T., Sarfraz, M., Arafat, M., Mikov, M., Cross-linked guar gum and sodium borate-based microspheres as colon-targeted anticancer drug delivery systems for 5-fluorouracil. *Pak. J. Pharm. Sci.*, 30, 2017.
27. Krishnaiah, Y.S.R., Karthikeyan, R.S., Satyanarayana, V., A three-layer guar gum matrix tablet for oral controlled delivery of highly soluble metoprolol tartrate. *Int. J. Pharm.*, 241, 2, 353–366, 2002.
28. Krishnamoorthi, S., Mal, D., Singh, R.P., Characterization of graft copolymer based on polyacrylamide and dextran. *Carbohydr. Polym.*, 69, 2, 371–377, 2007.
29. Karim, A.A. and Bhat, R., Gelatin alternatives for the food industry: recent developments, challenges and prospects. *Trends Food Sci. Technol.*, *19*, 12, 644–656, 2008.
30. Kumar, P., Kumari, K., Chopra, H.K., Kaur, N., Sonochemical and thermal modification of guar gum: a comparative analysis. *Mater. Today Proc.*, 68, 1093–1100, 2022.
31. Kame, N. and Uchida, K., Seismic radiation from dynamic coalescence, and the reconstruction of dynamic source parameters on a planar fault. *Geophys. J. Int.*, 174, 2, 696–706, 2008.
32. Lashley, M.R., Niedzinski, E.J., Rogers, J.M., Denison, M.S., Nantz, M.H., Synthesis and estrogen receptor affinity of a 4-hydroxytamoxifen-labeled ligand for diagnostic imaging. *Bioorg. Med. Chem.*, 10, 12, 4075–4082, 2002.
33. Lee, J.W., Park, J.H., Robinson, J.R., Bioadhesive-based dosage forms: The next generation. *J. Pharm. Sci.*, 89, 7, 850–866, 2000.
34. Lemarchand, C., Gref, R., Couvreur, P., Polysaccharide-decorated nanoparticles. *Eur. J. Pharm. Biopharm.*, 58, 2, 327–341, 2004.
35. Liang, C., Zhang, X., Yang, M., Dong, X., Recent progress in ferroptosis inducers for cancer therapy. *Adv. Mater.*, 31, e1904197, 2019.
36. Lis, G.P., Mastalerz, M., Schimmelmann, A., Lewan, M.D., Stankiewicz, B.A., FTIR absorption indices for thermal maturity in comparison with vitrinite reflectance R0 in type-II kerogens from Devonian black shales. *Org. Geochem.*, 36, 11, 1533–1552, 2005.
37. Li-Ming, Z., Jian-Fang, Z., Peter, S.H., A comparative study on viscosity behavior of water-soluble chemically modified guar gum derivatives with different functional lateral groups. *J. Sci. Food Agric.*, 85, 2638–2644, 2005.
38. Lowry, O.H., Rosebrough, N.J., Farr, A.L., Randall, R.J., Protein measurement with the Folin phenol reagent. *J. Biol. Chem.*, 193, 1, 265–275, 1951.
39. Liechty, W.B., Kryscio, D.R., Slaughter, B.V., Peppas, N.A., Polymers for drug delivery systems. *Ann. Rev. Chem. Biomol. Eng.*, 1, 1, 149–173, 2010.
40. Marcsek, Z., Kocsis, Z., Jakab, M., Szende, B., Tompa, A., The Efficacy of Tamoxifen in Strogen Receptor–Positive Breast Cancer Cells Is Enhanced by a Medical Nutriment. *Cancer Biother. Radiopharm.*, 19, 6, 746–753, 2004.
41. Martin, E.A., Brown, K., Gaskell, M., Al-Azzawi, F., Garner, R.C., Boocock, D.J., White, I.N., Tamoxifen DNA damage detected in human endometrium using accelerator mass spectrometry. *Cancer Res.*, 63, 23, 8461–8465, 2003.

42. Mestechkina, N.M., Egorov, A.V., Shcherbukhin, V.D., Synthesis of galactomannan sulfates. *Appl. Biochem. Microbiol.*, 42, 4, 326–330, 2006.
43. Mishra, N., Yadav, K.S., Rai, V.K., Yadav, N.P., Polysaccharide encrusted multilayered nano-colloidal system of andrographolide for improved hepatoprotection. *AAPS PharmSciTech*, 18, 381–392, 2017.
44. Modasiya, M.K., Gadhawala, Z.M., Patel, V.M., Studies on design and development of colon specific drug delivery using sesbania gum. *Int. J. Pharm. Life Sci.*, 1, 389–395, 2010.
45. Mudgil, D., Barak, S., Khatkar, B.S., X-ray diffraction, IR spectroscopy and thermal characterization of partially hydrolyzed guar gum. *Int. J. Biol. Macromol.*, 50, 4, 1035–1039, 2012.
46. Nayak, B.R. and Singh, R.P., Synthesis and characterization of grafted hydroxypropyl guar gum by ceric ion induced initiation. *Eur. Polym. J.*, 37, 8, 1655–1666, 2001.
47. Pal, S., Patra, A.S., Ghorai, S., Sarkar, A.K., Mahato, V., Sarkar, S., Singh, R.P., Efficient and rapid adsorption characteristics of templating modified guar gum and silica nanocomposite toward removal of toxic reactive blue and Congo red dyes. *Bioresour. Technol.*, 191, 291–299, 2015.
48. Pardini, B., Kumar, R., Naccarati, A., Novotny, J., Prasad, R.B., Forsti, A., Bermejo, J.L., 5-Fluorouracil-based chemotherapy for colorectal cancer and MTHFR/MTRR genotypes. *Br. J. Clin. Pharmacol.*, 72, 1, 162, 2011.
49. Patel, J.J., Karve, M., Patel, N.K., Guar gum: a versatile material for pharmaceutical industries. *Int. J. Pharm. Pharm. Sci.*, 6, 8, 13–19, 2014.
50. Patience, G.S., *Experimental methods and instrumentation for chemical engineers*, Elsevier, 2017.
51. Patience, G.S., Experimental methods in chemical engineering: Preface. *Can. J. Chem. Eng.*, 96, 11, 2312–2316, 2018.
52. Patra, A.S., Ghorai, S., Sarkar, D., Das, R., Sarkar, S., Pal, S., Anionically functionalized guar gum embedded with silica nanoparticles: An efficient nanocomposite adsorbent for rapid adsorptive removal of toxic cationic dyes and metal ions. *Bioresour. Technol.*, 225, 367–376, 2017.
53. Poorna, K.S.V., Singh, A., Rathore, A., Kumar, A., Novel cross linked guar gum – g-poly (acrylate) porous superabsorbent hydrogels: Characterization and swelling behaviour in different environments. *Carbohydr. Polym.*, 149, 175–185, 2016.
54. Prabaharan, M., Chitosan derivatives as promising materials for controlled drug delivery. *J. Biomater. Appl.*, 23, 1, 5–36, 2008.
55. Prabaharan, M., Prospective of guar gum and its derivatives as controlled drug delivery systems. *Int. J. Biol. Macromol.*, 49, 2, 117–124, 2011.
56. Prajapati, S.S. and Apte, M., Gums and Mucilage as Multi-Functional Pharmaceutical Agent. *Int. J. Pharm. Res.*, 13, 2, 2021, (09752366).
57. Qu, Y., Chu, B.Y., Peng, J.R., Liao, J.F., Qi, T.T., Shi, K., Zhang, X.N., Wei, Y.Q., Qian, Z.Y., A biodegradable thermo-responsive hybrid hydrogel: Therapeutic

applications in preventing the post-operative recurrence of breast cancer. *NPG Asia Mater.*, 7, Article e207, 2015.
58. Rabinow, B.E., Nanosuspensions in drug delivery. *Nat. Rev. Drug Discov.*, 3, 9, 785–796, 2004.
59. Rai, V.K., Dwivedi, H., Yadav, N.P., Chanotiya, C.S., Saraf, S.A., Solubility enhancement of miconazole nitrate: binary and ternary mixture approach. *Drug Dev. Ind. Pharm.*, 40, 8, 1021–1029, 2014.
60. Rao, M.S., Kanatt, S.R., Chawla, S.P., Sharma, A., Chitosan and guar gum composite films: Preparation, physical, mechanical and antimicrobial properties. *Carbohydr. Polym.*, 82, 4, 1243–1247, 2010.
61. Reddy, T.T. and Tammishetti, S., Barium chloride crosslinked carboxymethyl guar gum beads for gastrointestinal drug delivery. *J. Appl. Polym. Sci.*, 82, 12, 3084–3000, 2001.
62. Rossman, G.R., Analytical methods for measuring water in nominally anhydrous minerals. *Rev. Mineral. Geochem.*, 62, 1, 1–28, 2006.
63. Saberi, B., Chockchaisawasdee, S., Golding, J.B., Scarlett, C.J., Stathopoulos, C.E., Characterization of pea starch-guar gum biocomposite edible films enriched by natural antimicrobial agents for active food packaging. *Food Bioprod. Process.*, 105, 51–63, 2017.
64. Saidin, N.M., Anuar, N.K., Affandi, M.M.M., Roles of polysaccharides in transdermal drug delivery system and future prospects. *J. Appl. Pharm. Sci.*, 8, 3, 141–157, 2018.
65. Sarmah, J.K., Mahanta, R., Bhattacharjee, S.K., Mahanta, R.K., Dey, A., Guha, P., Biswas, A., *In-vitro* cytotoxicity analysis of Tamoxifen citrate loaded cross-linked guar gum nanoparticles on jurkat (human T-cell leukemia) cell line. *J. Drug Deliv. Ther.*, 2, 2, 2012.
66. Shaikh, T. and Kumar, S.S., Pharmaceutical and pharmacological profile of guar gum an overview. *Int. J. Pharm. Pharm. Sci.*, 3, supplement 5, 38–40, 2011.
67. Sharma, A., Kaur, N., Sharma, S., Sharma, A., Rathore, M.S., Ajay, K., Mishra, N., Embelin-loaded guar gum microparticles for the management of ulcerative colitis. *J. Microencapsulation*, 35, 2, 181–191, 2018.
68. Sharma, G., Thakur, B., Naushad, M., Kumar, A., Stadler, F.J., Alfadul, S.M., Mola, G.T., Applications of nanocomposite hydrogels for biomedical engineering and environmental protection. *Environ. Chem. Lett.*, 16, 113–146.342, 2018.
69. Shenoy, M.A. and D'Melo, D.J., Synthesis and characterization of acryloyloxy guar gum. *J. Appl. Polym. Sci.*, 117, 148–154, 2010.
70. Shi, H.-Y. and Li, M.Z., New grafted polysaccharide based on O-carboxymethyl-O-hydroxypropyl guar gum and N-isopropylacrylamide: Synthesis and phase transition behaviour in aqueous media. *Carbohydr. Polym.*, 67, 337, 2007.
71. Singh, R.P., Biswal, D.R., Pal, S., Adhikary, P., Krishnamoorthy, S., Popular plastics and packaging. *Popular Plast. Packag.*, 83, 2006, June.

72. Singh, R.P., Nayak, B.R., Biswal, D.R., Tripathy, T., Banik, K., Biobased polymeric flocculants for industrial effluent treatment. *Mater. Res. Innov.*, 7, 4, 331–320, 2003.
73. Singh, R.P., Pal, S., Krishnamoorthy, S., Adhikary, P., Akbar, S., High-technology materials based on modified polysaccharides. *Pure Appl. Chem.*, 81, 3, 525–547, 2009.
74. Sinha, P., Srivastava, N., Rai, V.K., Mishra, R., Ajayakumar, P.V., Yadav, N.P., A novel approach for dermal controlled release of salicylic acid for improved anti-inflammatory action: Combination of hydrophilic-lipophilic balance and response surface methodology. *J. Drug Deliv. Sci. Technol.*, 52, 870–884, 2019.
75. Szopinski, D. and Luinstra, G.A., Viscoelastic properties of aqueous guar gum derivative solutions under large amplitude oscillatory shear (LAOS). *Carbohydr. Polym.*, 153, 312–319, 2016.
76. Slavin, J.L. and Greenberg, N.A., Partially hydrolyzed guar gum: clinical nutrition uses. *Nutrition*, 19, 6, 549–552, 2003.
77. Sood, A., Gupta, A., Agrawal, G., Recent advances in polysaccharides-based biomaterials for drug delivery and tissue engineering applications. *Carbohydr. Polym. Technol. Appl.*, 7, 100067, 2021.
78. Senapati, S., Mahanta, A.K., Kumar, S., Maiti, P., Controlled drug delivery vehicles for cancer treatment and their performance. *Signal Transduct. Target. Ther.*, 3, 1, 7, 2018.
79. Soppirnath, K.S. and Aminabhavi, T.M., Water transport and drug release study from cross-linked polyacrylamide grafted guar gum hydrogel microspheres for the controlled release application. *Eur. J. Pharm. Biopharm.*, 53, 1, 87–98, 2002.
80. Szopinski, D., Kulicke, W., Luinstra, G.A., Structure – property relationships of carboxymethyl hydroxypropyl guar gum in water and a hyperentanglement parameter. *Carbohydr. Polym.*, 119, 159–166, 2015.
81. Sung, H., Ferlay, J., Siegel, R. L., Laversanne, M., Soerjomataram, I., Jemal, A., Bray, F., Global cancer statistics 2020: GLOBOCAN estimates of incidence and mortality worldwide for 36 cancers in 185 countries. *CA Cancer J. Clin.*, 71, 3, 209–249, 2021.
82. Tang, R.-Z., Liu, Z.-Z., Gu, S.-S., Liu, X.-Q., Multiple local therapeutics based on nano-hydrogel composites in breast cancer treatment. *J. Mater. Chem. B*, 9, 1521, 2021.
83. Tain, LS., Lozano, E., Sáez, A.G., Leroi, A.M., Dietary regulation of hypodermal polyploidization in C. elegans. *BMC Dev. Biol.*, 8, 1, 28, 2008.
84. Theisen, C., Chemoprevention: what's in a name? *J. Natl. Cancer Inst.*, 93, 10, 743–743, 2001.
85. Thombare, N., Jha, U., Mishra, S., Siddiqui, M.Z., Guar gum as a promising starting material for diverse applications: A review. *Int. J. Biol. Macromol.*, 88, 361–372, 2016.

86. Tosco, T., Gastone, F., Sethi, R., Guar gum solutions for improved delivery of iron particles in porous media (Part 2): Iron transport tests and modeling in radial geometry. *J. Contam. Hydrol.*, 166, 34–51, 2014.
87. Tripathy, S. and Das, M.K., Guar Gum: Present Status and Applications. *J. Pharm. Sci. Innov.*, 4, 4, 24–28, 2013.
88. Vandamme, T.F., Lenourry, A., Charrueau, C., Chaumeil, J.C., The use of polysaccharides to target drugs to the colon. *Carbohydr. Polym.*, 48, 3, 219–231, 2002.
89. Vismara, E., Coletti, A., Valerio, A., Naggi, A., Urso, E., Torri, G., Anti-metastatic Semi-synthetic Sulfated Maltotriose C-C Linked Dimers. *Synthesis and Characterisation, Molecules*, 17, 9912–9930, 2012.
90. Von Aulock, F.W., Kennedy, B.M., Schipper, C.I., Castro, J.M., Martin, D.E., Oze, C., Tuffen, H., Advances in Fourier transform infrared spectroscopy of natural glasses: From sample preparation to data analysis. *Lithos*, 206, 52–64, 2014.
91. Venugopal, J., Prabhakaran, M.P., Zhang, Y., Low, S., Choon, A.T., Ramakrishna, S., Biomimetic hydroxyapatite-containing composite nano-fibrous substrates for bone tissue engineering. *Phil. Trans. R. Soc. A-Math. Phys. Eng. Sci.*, 368, 1917, 2065–2081, 2010.
92. Xiao, W. and Dong, L., Novel excellent property film Prepared from Methacryloyl chloride-graft-Guar Gum Matrixes, in: *Conference Location: Xian Ning*, pp. 1442–45, 2011.
93. Yadav, N., Francis, A.P., Priya, V.V., Patil, S., Mustaq, S., Khan, S.S., Mony, U., Polysaccharide-Drug Conjugates: A Tool for Enhanced Cancer Therapy. *Polymers*, 14, 950, 2022.
94. Yi, J. and Zhang, L., Biodegradable blend films based on two polysaccharide Derivatives and their use as ibuprofen-releasing matrices. *J. Appl. Polym. Sci.*, 103, 3553–9, 2007.
95. Zhang, J., Yuan, Y., Shen, J., Lin, S., Synthesis and characterization of chitosan grafted poly (N, N-dimethyl-N-methacryloxyethyl-N-(3-sulfopropyl) ammonium) initiated by ceric (IV) ion. *Eur. Polym. J.*, 39, 4, 847–850, 2003.
96. Zhang, L.M., Zhou, J.F., Hui, P.S., A comparative study on viscosity behavior of water-soluble chemically modified guar gum derivatives with different functional later Groups. *J. Sci. Food Agric.*, 85, 15, 2638–2644, 2005.
97. Zhuang, B., Chen, T., Xiao, Z., Jin, Y., Drug-loaded implantable surgical cavity-adaptive hydrogels for prevention of local tumor recurrence. *Int. J. Pharm.*, 577, 119048, 2020.

10

Agarose: Nanostructured Platforms for Drug Delivery in Cancer Treatment

Haleema Ahmad[1,2*] and Mohd Salik Usmani[3]

[1]Department of Radiotherapy, Jawaharlal Nehru Medical College, Aligarh Muslim University, Aligarh, Uttar Pradesh, India
[2]Department of Biochemistry, Jawaharlal Nehru Medical College, Aligarh Muslim University, Aligarh, Uttar Pradesh, India
[3]Department of Surgery, Jawaharlal Nehru Medical College, Aligarh Muslim University, Aligarh, Uttar Pradesh, India

Abstract

Agarose, a naturally occurring polysaccharide derived from agar, has gained significant attention as a nanostructured platform for drug delivery, particularly in the field of cancer treatment. Its unique properties, such as biocompatibility, non-toxicity, and the ability to form hydrogels, make it an ideal candidate for developing advanced drug delivery systems. This chapter delves into the various facets of agarose-based nanostructured platforms, emphasizing their potential to revolutionize cancer therapy. Agarose can form gels at low concentrations, coupled with its ease of functionalization, allowing for the creation of versatile drug delivery vehicles. These vehicles can encapsulate a wide range of therapeutic agents, including chemotherapeutic drugs, proteins, and nucleic acids. The encapsulation within agarose matrices not only enhances the stability and bioavailability of these drugs but also allows for their controlled and sustained release. This is advantageous in cancer treatment, where maintaining therapeutic drug levels within the tumor microenvironment is crucial for efficacy and minimizing systemic toxicity. One of the key advantages of agarose-based drug delivery systems is their configured physical and chemical properties. By changing factors such as the concentration of agarose and the degree of crosslinking, researchers can tailor the mechanical strength, porosity, and degradation rates of the resulting hydrogels. This customization enables the design of drug delivery platforms that can meet

**Corresponding author*: sheikhzaaraahmad@gmail.com

Luqman Jameel Rather, Showkat Ali Ganie and Mohammed A. Assiri (eds.) Polysaccharide Biomaterials in Cancer Research and Therapy: From Lab to Life, (301–338) © 2026 Scrivener Publishing LLC

the specific requirements of different types of cancer and therapeutic agents. The agarose nanostructures can be engineered to target cancer cells specifically, thus enhancing the precision of drug delivery. This can be achieved through surface modification by targeting ligands such as antibodies, peptides, or small molecules that recognize and bind to specific markers on cancer cells. Such targeted delivery minimizes the impact on healthy tissues and enhances the therapeutic index of the encapsulated drugs. Recent advancements in nanotechnology have also facilitated the development of multifunctional agarose-based platforms. The integration of magnetic nanoparticles within agarose hydrogels can enable magnetic resonance imaging (MRI)-guided drug delivery, providing a means to monitor and control the release of therapeutic agents in real time. Also, the incorporation of stimuli-responsive elements, such as pH-sensitive or thermoresponsive components, allows for the release of drugs in response to the specific conditions of the tumor microenvironment. Preclinical studies have demonstrated the efficacy of agarose-based drug delivery systems in various cancer models. These studies have shown improved tumor targeting, enhanced drug retention, and reduced side effects compared to conventional delivery methods. However, despite these promising results, challenges remain in translating these systems from the laboratory to clinical settings. Issues such as large-scale manufacturing, regulatory approval, and long-term biocompatibility need to be addressed to fully realize the potential of agarose-based nanostructures in cancer therapy. This chapter provides a comprehensive overview of the unique properties of agarose that contribute to its efficacy in drug delivery applications.

***Keywords*:** Agarose, drug delivery, cancer, biocompatible, targeted therapy

10.1 Introduction

Agarose is a linear polysaccharide derived primarily from the cell walls of red algae, notably from species such as Gelidium and Gracilaria [1]. Its primary chemical structure consists of repeating units of agarobiose, a disaccharide made up of D-galactose and 3,6-anhydro-L-galactopyranose [2]. These monosaccharides are connected by alternating α-(1→3) and β-(1→4) glycosidic bonds, forming the backbone of the agarose polymer. In terms of molecular composition, the D-galactose unit features a hydroxyl group at the C-4 position, which is linked to the anomeric carbon of the 3,6-anhydro-L-galactose [1, 2]. This anhydrous bridge in the L-galactose unit is a distinguishing feature that sets agarose apart from other polysaccharides. The general formula of agarose can be represented as (C12H18O9)n, where 'n' indicates the degree of polymerization, typically ranging from 800 to 1000 units. This extensive polymerization contributes to agarose's significant molecular weight and its gel-forming capabilities. In its solid state, agarose forms a double-helix structure stabilized by hydrogen bonds. These helices aggregate to create a three-dimensional network that can entrap water molecules, resulting in gel formation [3]. This gelation property is pivotal, as it allows agarose to form a semi-solid matrix capable of holding water and other molecules within its structure. The stability of this network is due to the hydrogen bonds and hydrophobic interactions between the helices, which make agarose gels thermally reversible. This means that the gel can transition between a liquid and solid state with temperature changes. Agarose contains several functional groups that contribute to its unique properties. The numerous hydroxyl groups on the galactose units facilitate extensive hydrogen bonding, which is essential for the gelation process. The 3,6-anhydro bridges introduce ether linkages that provide rigidity and contribute to the mechanical strength of the gel. The alternating glycosidic bonds offer the flexibility necessary for forming helical structures. The unique structural characteristics of agarose make it a vital material in various biochemical and molecular biology techniques. One of the most common uses of agarose is in gel electrophoresis, where agarose gels are employed to separate nucleic acids based on their size. The uniform pore size of the agarose gel matrix ensures consistent and reliable separation of DNA and RNA fragments [4]. Agarose gels are utilized in protein purification, chromatography, and immunodiffusion techniques.

Agarose, a polysaccharide derived from red algae, is renowned for its distinctive physical and chemical properties that make it indispensable in various scientific and industrial applications. Its primary structure consists of repeating units of agarobiose, composed of D-galactose and 3,6-anhydro-L-galactopyranose. These monosaccharides are connected through alternating α-(1→3) and β-(1→4) glycosidic bonds. This unique structure imparts agarose with its characteristic properties. Physically, agarose is a white or cream-white powder that is odorless and tasteless. It is highly soluble in hot water and forms a clear, firm gel upon cooling, a property that is exploited in various laboratory techniques. The gelation temperature of agarose is typically around 35–40°C, while its melting temperature is higher, around 85–95°C. This thermal hysteresis is a key feature, allowing agarose gels to remain solid at physiological temperatures while being easily melted when heated [4]. The gelation process is reversible, meaning that agarose can transition between gel and liquid states with temperature changes, which is advantageous for various experimental protocols. The gel strength of agarose is influenced by its concentration. At lower concentrations (0.5–2%), agarose forms soft gels, which are suitable for electrophoresis of large molecules like DNA. At higher concentrations, it forms stiffer gels, useful for applications requiring greater mechanical stability. The pore size of agarose gels is another critical physical property, which is inversely related to its concentration. Lower concentrations result in larger pores, allowing the separation of larger biomolecules, whereas higher concentrations create smaller pores for finer separations [4, 5].

Chemically, agarose is composed mainly of neutral sugars, with minimal presence of charged groups, which contributes to its low electroendosmosis (EEO). This property is particularly advantageous in performing electrophoresis, as it minimizes the movement of the gel matrix when the electric field is applied, resulting in sharper and more precise separation of molecules. The presence of 3,6-anhydro bridges in the L-galactose units adds rigidity to the polymer chain, enhancing the mechanical strength of the gels. Agarose is also notable for its inertness and lack of reactivity with biomolecules, which preserves the integrity of samples during experimental procedures. It is resistant to enzymatic degradation by most common glycosidases, ensuring stability in various biological assays. Agarose is non-toxic and biocompatible, apt for a wide range of biomedical applications that include cell culture and drug delivery systems [5, 6]. The clarity of agarose gels is another significant property, providing excellent visibility for the analysis of separated biomolecules, especially when stained with specific dyes. The high degree of purity in commercial agarose products ensures minimal interference from impurities, which is critical for sensitive analytical techniques.

10.2 Nanostructured Platforms for Drug Delivery

The manipulation of matter at the atomic and molecular level, or nanotechnology, is transforming medicine by offering cutting-edge approaches to illness detection, cure, and prevention. The main goal of nanotechnology in medicine is the creation of materials and tools at the nanoscale that have highly precise interactions with biological systems. Drug delivery systems, where nanoparticles are designed to transport medications directly to specified cells, are one of the most important uses [6]. This increases treatment efficacy and decreases negative effects. In disorders like cancer, where targeted delivery can greatly improve treatment outcomes, these nanoparticles can be engineered to overcome biological barriers and release therapeutic substances in a regulated manner. Diagnostic methods are being advanced using nanotechnology [7]. Early illness diagnosis is made possible by the extremely low quantities of biomarkers that can be detected by nanosensors and imaging agents. For example, the sensitivity and resolution of imaging modalities like fluorescence imaging and magnetic resonance imaging are being enhanced by quantum dots and magnetic nanoparticles, enabling the early detection of malignancies. It is essential to the field of regenerative medicine. Scaffolds that replicate the extracellular matrix and promote tissue growth and regeneration can be made using nanomaterials. These scaffolds present intriguing treatments for wounds and degenerative illnesses since they can be loaded with growth factors and stem cells to accelerate tissue regeneration and repair processes. The topic also includes the creation of nanoscale surgical instruments and apparatuses, which offer previously unheard-of levels of surgical precision. Minimally invasive surgery can be performed with nanoscale equipment, shortening recovery periods and enhancing patient outcomes [8]. Numerous benefits provided by nanostructured drug delivery devices greatly improve the effectiveness and safety of therapeutic interventions. Enhancing the bioavailability of medications is one of their main advantages. Drugs can be designed with nanoparticles to prevent them from degrading before they reach their intended location, delivering a larger concentration of the active ingredient exactly where it is needed [9]. When treating diseases like cancer, where traditional medicines frequently damage healthy tissues and have serious side effects, tailored delivery is especially helpful. Through mechanisms like the increased permeability and retention (EPR) effect, nanostructured systems can aggregate preferentially in tumor tissues, boosting therapeutic benefits while minimizing side effects. Drugs can be released gradually and under control with nanostructured drug delivery devices [10]. By lowering the frequency of dosage and enhancing patient compliance, this regulated release guarantees a constant therapeutic impact over protracted periods. To increase selectivity and lessen off-target effects, the surface of nanoparticles can also be altered with ligands or antibodies that bind to certain receptors on target cells. The adaptability of administration routes is an additional benefit. It is possible to construct nanoparticles for oral, injectable, transdermal, and inhaled administration routes, which provides versatility in treating a range of illnesses and enhances patient convenience. Nanoparticles' enormous surface area-to-volume ratio and compact size allow them to interact with biological membranes more easily, which improves their penetration and distribution throughout the body.

10.2.1 Types of Nanostructured Drug Delivery Platforms

Nanostructured drug delivery platforms encompass a diverse array of systems designed to improve the delivery, stability, and efficacy of therapeutic agents (Figure 10.1) [11]. The most well-known are nanoparticles, nanogels, and nanofibers; each has special benefits and uses in the medical industry. Nanoparticles are solid particles that range from 10 to 1000 nanometers (nm) in size. These particles are particularly effective for drug delivery due to their ability to encapsulate drugs, enhancing their stability and solubility [12]. Nanoparticles guarantee that an active ingredient is supplied at the exact location where it is needed by preventing medications from degrading before they reach their target. Drugs can be manipulated to release from nanoparticles, enhancing treatment pharmacokinetics and therapeutic results. Nanoparticles can be made from a variety of materials, including metals, lipids, and polymers [13]. Each material has unique features that are useful for applications. Lipid-based nanoparticles improve the bioavailability of poorly soluble medicines, whereas polymeric nanoparticles derived from biodegradable substances such as polylactic acid (PLA) or polylactic-co-glycolic acid (PLGA) offer controlled and prolonged drug release.

Nanogels are another important class of nanostructured drug delivery systems [14, 15]. These hydrogel particles, which are within the nanometer range, consist of a highly hydrated polymer network. This matrix offers a favorable environment for the prolonged release of medicinal substances

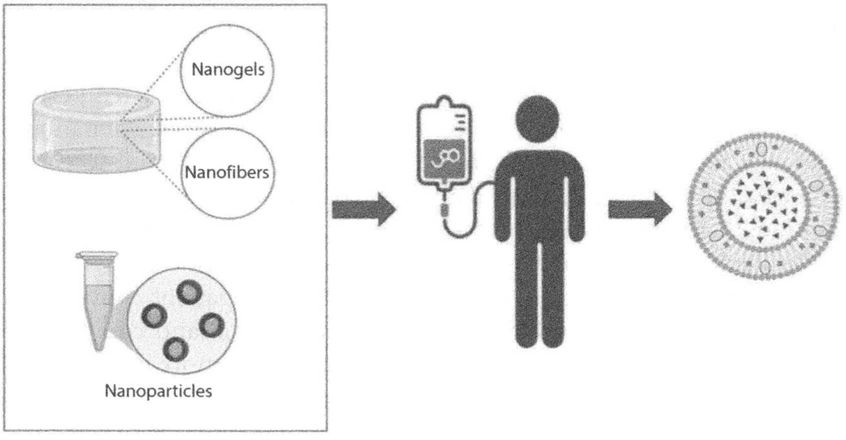

Figure 10.1 Illustration depicting types of nanostructured drug delivery platform.

and is perfect for drug loading. Because of their high-water content, nanogels are useful for a variety of medicinal applications, such as the transport of proteins, peptides, and nucleic acids, while also ensuring biocompatibility and minimizing toxicity. Additionally responsive to pH, temperature, and light, nanogels provide targeted and regulated medication release in certain tissues or cellular settings [14, 15]. By decreasing adverse effects and enhancing drug delivery precision, this responsiveness improves patient outcomes. Because of the versatility of nanogel production and functionalization, numerous therapeutic agents can be included, paving the way for combination therapy for difficult-to-treat disorders like cancer [15].

Nanofibers, with their fibrous structures produced by techniques such as electrospinning, represent a versatile platform for drug delivery and tissue engineering [16]. Through the process of electrospinning, fine fibers with a high surface area-to-volume ratio are drawn from a polymer solution using an electric field. Because of their large surface area and high drug-loading capacity, nanofibers are a great option for regulated and long-term drug administration [17]. Drugs can be engineered into nanofibers to release predictably, giving a continuous therapeutic impact. Since nanofibers' fibrous structure closely resembles the extracellular matrix, they are perfect scaffolds for wound healing and tissue regeneration.

10.3 Synthesis and Fabrication of Agarose-Based Nanostructures

The synthesis of agarose nanoparticles involves various techniques that harness the properties of agarose to make particles with specific sizes, shapes, and functionalities. Among the most prominent methods are solvent evaporation, nanoprecipitation, and emulsion techniques. Each method offers distinct advantages and can be tailored to produce agarose nanoparticles for diverse applications in drug delivery, bioimaging, and tissue engineering.

10.3.1 Methods of Agarose Nanoparticle Synthesis

Solvent evaporation is a widely used method for the synthesis of agarose nanoparticles [18]. In this technique, agarose is first dissolved in a suitable solvent, often an organic solvent that can dissolve agarose effectively. This agarose solution is then emulsified in a non-solvent, typically an aqueous phase that is immiscible with the organic solvent. The emulsification process is crucial as it creates a dispersion of small droplets of the agarose solution within the non-solvent. Once the emulsion is formed, the solvent is gradually evaporated, either under reduced pressure or by heating. As the solvent evaporates, the agarose molecules precipitate and coalesce to form solid nanoparticles. The size and morphology of the resulting nanoparticles can be controlled by adjusting parameters such as the concentration of agarose, the choice of solvent and non-solvent, the rate of solvent evaporation, and the emulsification conditions. This method is advantageous because it allows for the production of nanoparticles with a relatively uniform size distribution and high encapsulation efficiency of hydrophobic drugs or bioactive compounds.

Nanoprecipitation is another effective method for synthesizing agarose nanoparticles. This technique involves the rapid addition of an agarose solution into a non-solvent where agarose has poor solubility [18]. Typically, agarose is dissolved in a solvent such as dimethyl sulfoxide (DMSO) or acetone, which is then rapidly injected into an aqueous solution under stirring. The agarose precipitates out of the solution and forms nanoparticles when the agarose solution and non-solvent are mixed immediately, resulting in an abrupt shift in solubility. Several variables, including the amount of agarose in the solvent, the rate of addition, the kind of non-solvent, and the speed of mixing, affect the size and characteristics of the nanoparticles. Nanoprecipitation is particularly useful for producing nanoparticles with narrow size distributions and can be performed under mild conditions, preserving the bioactivity of sensitive therapeutic agents. This method is also relatively simple and scalable, making it suitable for large-scale production.

Emulsion techniques are versatile methods for agarose nanoparticle synthesis, involving the emulsification of an agarose solution in an immiscible liquid, followed by solidification to form nanoparticles [18]. In one common approach, an agarose solution is prepared by dissolving agarose in water at elevated temperatures. This hot agarose solution is then emulsified into an oil phase, typically using surfactants to stabilize the emulsion droplets. Upon cooling, the agarose solidifies within the droplets, forming solid nanoparticles. The solidification process can be facilitated by reducing the temperature or by adding a crosslinking agent that induces gelation. Emulsion techniques allow for the production of nanoparticles with controlled sizes, depending on the emulsification conditions such as the type and concentration of surfactants, the ratio of aqueous to oil phases, and the emulsification energy. These techniques enable the encapsulation of both hydrophilic and hydrophobic drugs, enhancing the versatility of the nanoparticles for various biomedical applications. Emulsion-based methods are also adaptable to producing composite nanoparticles by incorporating other materials, such as magnetic particles or fluorescent dyes, into the agarose matrix.

10.3.2 Hydrogel Formation and Crosslinking Techniques

Three-dimensional hydrophilic polymer networks, or hydrogels, can hold a lot of water or biological fluids. Crosslinking procedures play a major role in their creation and functionality by stabilizing their structure [19]. Crosslinking involves the creation of covalent or non-covalent bonds between polymer chains, transforming a liquid polymer solution into a solid or semi-solid gel. This process is crucial in determining the mechanical strength, porosity, and responsiveness of the hydrogel, which are essential for its various applications in biomedical engineering, drug delivery, and tissue engineering.

One of the most common methods for hydrogel formation is chemical crosslinking, which involves covalent bonding between polymer chains. This can be achieved through the use of crosslinking agents, such as glutaraldehyde, carbodiimides, or diisocyanates, which react with functional groups on the polymer chains to form stable links. Photopolymerization is an alternative method of chemical crosslinking in which light-sensitive initiators are exposed to UV or visible light and subsequently produce free radicals. The polymerization and crosslinking of monomers or pre-polymers with double bonds are subsequently started by these free radicals. Photopolymerization is very helpful for producing patterned or gradient hydrogels for sophisticated tissue engineering applications because it provides both spatial and temporal control over the gelation process.

Physical crosslinking, on the other hand, involves non-covalent interactions such as hydrogen bonding, ionic interactions, or hydrophobic interactions. One example of physical crosslinking is ionic gelation, where polymers with ionic groups are crosslinked through the addition of multivalent ions. For instance, alginate, a naturally derived polysaccharide, forms hydrogels when exposed to divalent cations like calcium ions. This method is advantageous for its simplicity and mild conditions, which are suitable for encapsulating sensitive biological molecules such as proteins and cells. Thermoresponsive hydrogels are another type of physically crosslinked hydrogels, which form gels upon temperature changes. Polymers like poly(N-isopropylacrylamide) (PNIPAAm) exhibit a lower critical solution temperature (LCST), above which they transition from a soluble state to a gel state [20]. This property can be used for controlled drug release and injectable hydrogel systems.

Enzymatic crosslinking is another method for creating hydrogels, in which enzymes catalyze the creation of covalent links between polymer strands. For instance, in physiological settings, horseradish peroxidase (HRP) can catalyze the crosslinking of phenolic compounds with hydrogen peroxide, resulting in the formation of hydrogels. Because of its specificity and biocompatibility, this technique is perfect for *in situ* gel creation inside the body, which is useful for processes like tissue regeneration and wound healing. Another interesting process for the production of hydrogels is self-assembly, in which certain chemical interactions cause amphiphilic peptides or block copolymers to spontaneously arrange into nanostructures. The sequence or composition of the building elements of these self-assembling hydrogels can be changed to precisely control the gel's properties. Hydrogels that self-assemble show great promise in constructing biomimetic environments for tissue engineering and cell culture [19, 20]. Because of its great efficiency and specificity, click chemistry has become a potent method for hydrogel creation in recent years. Under mild conditions, covalent crosslinks can be formed by click reactions, such as thiol-ene interactions or azide-alkyne cycloaddition. This method enables the production of multifunctional hydrogels with customized characteristics as well as the integration of bioactive compounds.

10.3.3 Characterization of Agarose Nanostructures

Characterization of agarose nanostructures is crucial for understanding their morphology, size distribution, surface properties, and stability, all of which are vital for their performance in various applications. Several advanced techniques are employed to provide detailed insights into these characteristics, with transmission electron microscopy (TEM), scanning electron microscopy (SEM), and dynamic light scattering (DLS) being most used. TEM is a tool used for the high-resolution imaging of agarose nanoparticles. TEM works by transmitting a beam of electrons through a very thin sample and capturing the interaction of electrons as they pass through the sample [21]. This technique provides images with extremely high resolution, often at the atomic or molecular level, allowing researchers to observe the fine details of nanoparticle morphology and size. For agarose nanostructures, TEM can reveal the precise shape and internal structure of the particles, including any core-shell formations or encapsulated materials. The high-resolution images obtained from TEM are crucial for verifying the uniformity of the nanoparticles, identifying any structural anomalies, and confirming successful synthesis. TEM can also be used to perform electron diffraction studies, which provide information about the crystalline structure of the nanoparticles, aiding in the understanding of their physical properties [22].

SEM gives detailed surface imaging and structural analysis of agarose nanostructures. A concentrated electron beam is scanned across a sample's surface by SEM, which then detects the secondary electrons that are released, revealing details about the sample's composition and topography [23]. SEM is particularly useful for examining the surface morphology and texture of agarose nanoparticles, as it provides three-dimensional-like images with a high depth of field. This technique is essential for analyzing the surface roughness, porosity, and overall shape of the nanoparticles. Additionally, elemental analysis can be obtained using SEM in conjunction with energy-dispersive X-ray spectroscopy (EDS), which can assist in verifying the composition of the nanoparticles and identifying any contaminants or surface alterations [23]. SEM is a vital tool for determining the homogeneity and distribution of nanoparticle populations because of its speedy imaging capabilities over wide sample areas.

A potent method for determining the particle size distribution and stability of agarose nanoparticles in suspension is dynamic light scattering (DLS). DLS examines how particles in a liquid suspension scatter laser light, with the scattered light's intensity varying as a result of the particles' Brownian motion [23]. By measuring these fluctuations, DLS provides information on the hydrodynamic diameter of the nanoparticles, which is an effective size that includes the particle and its surrounding solvation layer. This technique is particularly advantageous for its ability to measure particle sizes in the submicron range quickly and with high sensitivity. DLS can also provide insights into the polydispersity index (PDI), indicating the uniformity of the nanoparticle sizes in a sample [17]. A low PDI suggests a uniform size distribution, which is often desirable for consistent performance in applications. DLS can be used to monitor the stability of nanoparticle suspensions over time by measuring changes in size distribution, which may indicate aggregation or degradation.

10.4 Functionalization and Modification of Agarose Nanostructures

10.4.1 Surface Modification for Targeted Drug Delivery

Enhancing the functioning of agarose nanostructures for targeted drug delivery applications requires surface modification [24]. Through the functionalization of nanoparticles' surfaces with ligands or targeting moieties, scientists can enhance their capacity to bind to target cells or tissues with greater selectivity, improving drug delivery efficiency while reducing off-target effects. Agarose nanostructures can now be surface-modified for targeted drug administration using a variety of techniques, such as conjugating targeting ligands, adding stimuli-responsive moieties, and applying bio-orthogonal chemistry [25]. The conjugation of targeted ligands onto the surface of agarose nanoparticles is one method of surface modification. Antibodies, peptides, and aptamers are examples of targeting ligands that can identify and attach to receptors or biomarkers that are overexpressed on the surface of sick cells or tissues. Researchers can improve the selectivity and affinity of agarose nanoparticles for target cells, leading to an increase in the effectiveness of drug administration, by affixing targeting ligands to their surface. For instance, agarose nanoparticles' surface can be coupled with antibodies against cancer-specific antigens to allow for the targeted delivery of anticancer medications to tumor cells while reducing systemic toxicity. Like this, targeted drug delivery to sick tissues, such as inflamed or infected regions, can be facilitated by peptides or aptamers that have a high affinity for cell surface receptors. Adding stimuli-responsive moieties to the surface of agarose nanoparticles is an additional method of surface modification. Materials that are stimulus-responsive change chemically or experience structural changes in response to outside stimuli like pH, temperature, or enzyme activity. Researchers can create drug delivery systems that react to certain bodily cues by adding stimuli-responsive moieties to the surface of agarose nanoparticles [24, 25]. This allows for the regulated release of therapeutic drugs to specific target areas. For instance, the surface of agarose nanoparticles can be linked to pH-responsive polymers, like poly(acrylic acid) or poly(histidine), to allow for selective drug release in acidic conditions, like those seen in tumor tissues or inflammatory areas. Analogously, temperature-sensitive polymers, like poly(N-isopropyl acrylamide), can be utilized to create agarose nanoparticles that release medications in reaction to temperature variations, including those brought on by fever or inflammation.

Bio-orthogonal chemistry techniques offer a versatile approach to surface modification of agarose nanostructures for targeted drug delivery [26]. Bio-orthogonal chemistry refers to chemical reactions that can proceed selectively in biological environments without interfering with endogenous biological processes [26]. By exploiting bio-orthogonal reactions, researchers can functionalize the surface of agarose nanoparticles with a wide range of molecules, including fluorescent dyes, imaging agents, or therapeutic payloads, while minimizing non-specific interactions with biological components. High efficiency and specificity can be achieved by conjugating bioactive compounds onto the surface of agarose nanoparticles using click chemistry reactions, such as thiol-ene coupling or azide-alkyne cycloaddition. This makes it possible to precisely regulate the activity and makeup of agarose nanoparticles for applications involving targeted drug delivery.

10.4.2 Encapsulation Techniques for Drug Loading

The effective loading of medications into agarose nanostructures, which allows for precise control over drug release kinetics and improves therapeutic efficacy, is made possible *via* encapsulation techniques [27]. These technologies include a variety of approaches designed to ensnare medications either inside or on the exterior of agarose nanoparticles, guaranteeing their stability and precise delivery to desired locations within the body. Numerous encapsulation techniques have been discovered, with distinct benefits and uses in drug delivery, including chemical conjugation, physical encapsulation, and electrostatic interactions. One of the easiest and most popular methods for putting medications into agarose nanostructures is physical encapsulation [28]. This method involves simply dispersing pharmaceuticals in a solution containing agarose polymers, which then use emulsion processes, solvent evaporation, or nanoprecipitation to self-assemble into nanoparticles. Drugs are entrapped in the polymer matrix during the production of agarose nanoparticles *via* non-covalent interactions including hydrophobic or hydrogen bonding. The simplicity, adaptability, and capacity of this approach to encapsulate a variety of therapeutic molecules including hydrophilic, hydrophobic, and amphiphilic compounds make it beneficial. The effective therapy requires optimizing formulations, as drugs and the agarose matrix impact loading efficiency and release kinetics.

Chemical conjugation, which involves the covalent attachment of pharmaceuticals to polymer chains through chemical processes, provides an alternate method for encasing drugs within agarose nanostructures [29]. Reactive groups, including amino, carboxyl, or thiol groups, are used in this approach to functionalize pharmaceuticals. These groups can then react with other functional groups within the agarose matrix or on its surface. For instance, amide bonds can be formed to conjugate pharmaceuticals with amino groups to carboxyl-functionalized agarose polymers, resulting in stable drug–polymer conjugates that can self-assemble into nanoparticles. Precise control over the loading capacity and release kinetics of pharmaceuticals can be achieved through chemical conjugation, enabling customized drug delivery systems with improved stability and bioavailability.

With this method, agarose nanoparticles can have extra functions added to their surface, such as targeting ligands or imaging agents, which can further improve their therapeutic potential for certain uses. Another efficient way to encapsulate medications into agarose nanostructures is through electrostatic interactions, which work especially well for charged or polar drug molecules. This method creates drug-loaded nanoparticles by complexing medicines with molecules or polymers that have opposing charges, like surfactants or polyelectrolytes, through electrostatic interactions. For example, electrostatic attraction can be used to combine positively charged medicines with negatively charged agarose polymers, which can then form stable nanoparticles through coacervation or self-assembly [29]. Due to its many benefits, including high loading efficiency, superior stability, and adjustable release kinetics, electrostatic encapsulation is a viable delivery method for a variety of therapies, including peptides, small molecules, and nucleic acids.

10.4.3 Release Mechanisms and Kinetics

The precise release of therapeutic drugs from agarose nanostructures is regulated by release mechanisms and kinetics, which are essential components of drug delivery systems. Comprehending these mechanisms plays a pivotal role in formulating drug delivery systems including customized release profiles, which provide accurate regulation of drug release rates and durations to attain ideal therapeutic results [30]. Drug release from agarose nanostructures is regulated by several release mechanisms and kinetics, such as stimulus-responsive release, degradation-controlled release, and diffusion-controlled release [31].

Diffusion-controlled release is one of the most common mechanisms governing drug release from agarose nanostructures. In this mechanism, drugs are released from the nanostructures by diffusion through the polymer matrix or along the surface of the nanoparticles [32]. As the nanostructures come into contact with the surrounding biological environment, the concentration gradient between the interior and exterior of the nanoparticles drives the diffusion of drugs out of the matrix. The hydrophilicity/hydrophobicity of the drug molecules, the size and porosity of the nanostructures, and the viscosity of the surrounding media are some of the parameters that affect the rate of drug release. Diffusion-controlled release typically follows Fick's law of diffusion and exhibits sustained release kinetics, where the release rate decreases over time as the concentration gradient diminishes. This mechanism is advantageous for delivering hydrophobic drugs or large molecules that cannot easily diffuse through biological barriers [31].

Degradation-controlled release is another important mechanism that governs drug release from agarose nanostructures, particularly for biodegradable polymers. In this mechanism, the polymer matrix undergoes degradation or erosion over time, releasing encapsulated drugs. Drugs can seep out of the matrix due to the nanostructures' impaired integrity caused by the degradation of the polymer. The polymer's degradation kinetics, influenced by the polymer's molecular weight, crosslinking density, and chemical composition, dictate the drug release rate. Degradation-controlled release minimizes the impacts of burst release while permitting continuous and regulated release of medicines, making it a useful method for administering medication over long periods [32]. When administering bioactive compounds or medications with short half-lives that need to be continuously administered, this technique is especially helpful.

Drugs can be released from agarose nanostructures on-demand or triggered in response to particular environmental stimuli thanks to a flexible technique called stimulus-responsive release. Drugs that are encapsulated are released by stimuli-responsive materials, such as pH-sensitive polymers, temperature-sensitive polymers, or enzyme-responsive polymers, which undergo conformational changes or chemical reactions in response to external stimuli. To release pharmaceuticals, pH-sensitive agarose nanostructures, for instance, can be engineered to swell or change structurally in acidic environments, including tumor tissues or inflammatory areas. Drugs can also be released by engineering temperature-sensitive agarose nanostructures to go through phase or sol–gel transitions in response to temperature variations. Stimulus-responsive release reduces systemic side effects and increases therapeutic efficacy by providing precise control over drug release kinetics and enabling the targeted distribution of medicines to specific locations inside the body.

10.5 Mechanisms of Drug Delivery in Cancer Treatment

Drug delivery systems are critical in evaluating the effectiveness and specificity of therapeutic interventions in the treatment of cancer. Active targeting and passive targeting are the two main drug delivery techniques, each with unique benefits and methods for getting anticancer drugs into tumor tissues (Table 10.1).

Table 10.1 Summary of different mechanisms of drug delivery.

Component	Features	Methods
Passive vs. active targeting	Strategies for targeting drugs to specific tissues or cells	Passive targeting (EPR effect), active targeting (ligand–receptor interactions)
EPR effect on tumor targeting	Explains the enhanced permeability and retention (EPR) effect in targeting tumors	Tumor vasculature permeability, retention in tumor tissues
Cellular uptake and intracellular trafficking	Mechanisms by which drugs enter cells and their subsequent intracellular movement	Endocytosis, lysosomal degradation, cytoplasmic trafficking

10.5.1 Passive vs. Active Targeting

Passive targeting uses the intrinsic features of tumors—such as leaky vasculature and poor lymphatic drainage—to increase the amount of medication that accumulates in tumor tissues. Tumors frequently have aberrant blood arteries with faulty endothelial cell connections, which increases vascular permeability and allows macromolecules to seep into the interstitium around the tumor [33]. Through passive diffusion, this phenomenon—known as the increased permeability and retention, or EPR, effect—allows macromolecular medications and nanoparticles to collect preferentially within tumor tissues. Because lymphatic drainage is frequently impaired in tumors, medications are often retained in the tumor microenvironment for extended periods. By making use of these characteristics of tumors, passive targeting minimizes drug exposure to healthy tissues while achieving a selective buildup of medication within malignant tissues. Passive targeting by itself, however, could not be effective or specific enough, especially in cancers that are heterogeneous and have varying vascular permeability.

Active targeting involves conjugating targeting ligands or antibodies to the drug carrier surface to enhance specificity for cancer cells. Ligands such as aptamers, peptides, and antibodies recognize and bind to overexpressed antigens or receptors on cancer cells. This allows drug-loaded carriers to be selectively absorbed into tumor tissues. Active targeting allows for the exact localization of therapeutic agents within cancer cells by conjugating targeting ligands to drug carriers [33]. This maximizes therapeutic efficacy while limiting off-target effects on healthy tissues. The drawbacks of passive targeting, such as heterogeneity in the tumor vasculature and variations in the EPR effect between tumor types, can be addressed by active targeting. However, to guarantee effective binding, internalization, and transport of the therapeutic payload to cancer cells, active targeting techniques necessitate careful selection of targeting ligands and optimization of carrier features.

10.5.2 EPR Effect on Tumor Targeting

The phenomenon known as the enhanced permeability and retention (EPR) effect has completely changed the way cancer drugs are delivered by providing a way for therapeutic chemicals to accumulate preferentially inside tumor tissues [34]. Designing nanoparticle-based drug delivery systems that take advantage of the special features of tumor vasculature and microenvironment to increase the effectiveness of anticancer treatments requires an understanding of the EPR effect. Increased vascular permeability and leakiness are caused by aberrant blood arteries with abnormalities in endothelial cell connections that are characteristic of tumors. The unchecked growth of cancer cells drives fast angiogenesis, which results in this aberrant vasculature. Tumor blood vessels therefore differ from normal blood vessels both physically and functionally, displaying fenestrations, gaps, and discontinuities in the endothelium lining. Because the tumor interstitium is a more effective place for macromolecules, nanoparticles, and drug carriers to extravasate from the bloodstream than healthy tissues, these vascular anomalies contribute to the EPR effect [34].

Through a process called extravasation, the leaky vasculature of tumors makes it easier for macromolecular medications and nanoparticles to passively accumulate within tumor tissues. Because of malfunctioning lymphatic vessels, nanoparticles in the tumor interstitium experience decreased lymphatic outflow, which prolongs their retention in the tumor microenvironment. The retention feature of the EPR effect is the term used to describe this phenomenon. The EPR effect, which minimizes exposure to healthy tissues and allows for the targeted delivery of therapeutic drugs to cancer cells, is the result of improved extravasation and retention of nanoparticles within tumor tissues [35]. The EPR effect has important ramifications for the administration of cancer drugs because it justifies the creation of formulations based on nanoparticles that take advantage of vascular anomalies unique to individual tumors.

To improve their circulation time, stability, and selectivity for tumor tissues, nanoparticles can be designed to incorporate chemotherapeutic medicines, imaging agents, or nucleic acids. They can also be changed with surface coatings or targeting ligands. When compared to traditional chemotherapy, nanoparticle-based drug delivery systems can reach higher drug concentrations within tumors by making use of the EPR effect. This leads to better therapeutic outcomes and less systemic toxicity. The therapeutic translation of the EPR effect has encountered difficulties despite its potential benefits because of the poor predictability of nanoparticle accumulation within tumors and interpatient variations in tumor vasculature. The effectiveness of drug delivery systems that target the EPR effect can be influenced by the heterogeneity of the tumor vasculature and the presence of stromal components, such as immune cells and fibroblasts [35]. Optimizing the size, shape, surface charge, and surface functionalization of nanoparticles to increase tumor penetration and cellular uptake is one way to optimize the EPR effect and get beyond these obstacles. Combination medicines can increase the EPR impact and improve therapeutic outcomes by targeting both cancer cells and the tumor vasculature.

10.5.3 Cellular Uptake and Intracellular Trafficking

The effective delivery of therapeutic drugs to specific areas within cells by nanoparticle-based drug delivery systems is contingent upon the processes of cellular uptake and intracellular trafficking. Optimizing the design of nanoparticles and increasing their therapeutic efficacy in cancer treatment and other biomedical applications require an understanding of the principles underlying cellular uptake and intracellular trafficking [36]. Nanoparticles can enter cells *via* several different routes, such as passive diffusion, receptor-mediated endocytosis, and endocytosis. Particle size and concentration gradients cause passive diffusion, which is the direct penetration of nanoparticles across the cell membrane. Nevertheless, this process is restricted to hydrophobic compounds and tiny nanoparticles.

In contrast, endocytosis is a tightly controlled process by which cells create vesicles out of the plasma membrane to absorb external molecules. There are various forms of endocytosis, each with unique requirements and mechanisms, including as macropinocytosis, caveolae-mediated endocytosis, and clathrin-mediated endocytosis. The process of receptor-mediated endocytosis entails the attachment of nanoparticle ligands to particular cell surface receptors, which then facilitates the internalization of the particles through receptor-mediated pathways. This technique improves the cellular absorption efficiency of nanoparticles by enabling their selective administration to particular cell types. After internalization, nanoparticles travel within cells *via* the endosomal–lysosomal pathway, where they come into contact with different cell compartments and either degrade or release their cargo [36]. Nuclear localization signals, for instance, can be functionalized on nanoparticles so they can target the nucleus and deliver nucleic acid-based treatments, such as siRNA or gene editing tools, to modify gene expression. Similarly, treatments for illnesses involving protein folding or mitochondrial dysfunction can be delivered using nanoparticles that have targeting ligands for the endoplasmic reticulum or mitochondria, respectively. Designing nanoparticles with improved subcellular targeting and therapeutic efficacy for a range of disorders is made possible by an understanding of the intracellular trafficking pathways of these particles.

10.6 Applications of Agarose Nanostructures in Cancer Therapy

10.6.1 Chemotherapeutic Drug Delivery

Agarose nanostructures, with their special benefits like biocompatibility, adjustable characteristics, and easy surface functionalization, have emerged as attractive platforms for the administration of chemotherapeutic medicines in cancer therapy [37]. Researchers can get around some of the drawbacks of traditional chemotherapy, such as low solubility, non-specific distribution, and systemic toxicity, by encasing chemotherapeutic chemicals inside agarose nanoparticles. Several approaches have been devised to maximize the therapeutic efficiency of chemotherapeutic medications while avoiding adverse effects by taking advantage of the features of agarose nanostructures for targeted and controlled administration. Agarose nanostructures have several benefits, including minimal cytotoxicity and biocompatibility, which make them effective vehicles for delivering chemotherapy medications to cancerous cells. Seaweed naturally contains agarose, a polymer that is frequently employed in biomedical applications because it is immunogenicity-free, biodegradable, and inert. Hydrophobic and hydrophilic chemotherapeutic medicines can be easily encapsulated in agarose nanoparticles using processes like solvent evaporation, nanoprecipitation, or emulsion techniques. Because agarose nanostructures are biocompatible, there is less chance of harm to healthy tissues, which makes them perfect for systemic delivery of chemotherapeutic drugs [37].

Agarose nanostructures provide precise regulation of drug release kinetics and improved therapeutic efficacy by providing chances for the regulated and sustained release of chemotherapeutic medicines. The customizable features of agarose matrices allow the construction of drug delivery systems with customized release profiles, while the porous nature of agarose nanoparticles facilitates the effective loading and encapsulation of pharmaceuticals [38]. Researchers can optimize the pharmacokinetics and pharmacodynamics of chemotherapeutic drugs for cancer therapy by controlling the rate and duration of drug release by the manipulation of agarose nanoparticles' size, shape, porosity, and surface chemistry. To maximize therapeutic results and patient compliance, controlled-release formulations can decrease systemic toxicity, decrease dosage frequency, and increase drug bioavailability. Agarose nanostructures' adaptable surface chemistry makes it simple to functionalize them with stimuli-responsive moieties, targeting ligands, or imaging agents for improved tumor targeting and precision medicine. By adding targeting ligands, such as peptides, aptamers, or antibodies, to the surface of agarose nanoparticles, it becomes possible to selectively bind to receptors or biomarkers that are overexpressed on the surface of cancer cells. This enables the targeted delivery of chemotherapy drugs to tumor tissues while protecting healthy cells. It is possible to design stimuli-responsive agarose nanoparticles that will react to stimuli found in the tumor microenvironment, such as pH, temperature, or enzyme activity. This would enhance the effectiveness of treatment by causing site-specific drug release.

10.6.2 Gene Therapy and RNAi Delivery

Agarose nanostructures provide flexible platforms for the targeted and effective delivery of nucleic acid-based therapies to cancer cells. They have demonstrated enormous promise in the fields of gene therapy and RNA interference (RNAi) delivery [39]. Gene therapy employs nucleic acids, such as DNA or RNA, to target cells to modify gene expression or correct genetic defects; on the other hand, RNA interference (RNAi) therapy uses small RNA molecules, such as microRNA (miRNA) or small interfering RNA (siRNA), to silence particular genes implicated in the development of cancer. Agarose nanostructures are attractive vehicles for overcoming the difficulties associated with nucleic acid delivery because of their adjustable characteristics, ease of surface functionalization, and biocompatibility, which are all beneficial for gene therapy and RNAi administration [40]. The biocompatibility and low cytotoxicity of agarose nanostructures are important features in gene therapy and RNAi administration, as they guarantee the effectiveness and safety of nucleic acid delivery systems. Seaweed is the natural source of agarose, a polysaccharide that is recognized for its inertness, biodegradability, and lack of immunogenicity. Nucleic acids can be encapsulated in agarose nanoparticles without sacrificing their stability or activity using gentle and friendly manufacturing methods such as solvent evaporation or nanoprecipitation. Agarose nanostructures are biocompatible, reducing harm to healthy tissues and making them ideal for delivering nucleic acid therapies to cancer cells.

Agarose nanostructures provide options for nucleic acid treatments to be delivered in a regulated and targeted manner, allowing for precise gene expression modification and improved therapeutic efficacy. Agarose nanoparticles' porosity structure makes it possible to load and encapsulate nucleic acids efficiently, shielding them from deterioration and promoting intracellular transport. Nucleic acid delivery systems with customized release profiles and cellular absorption methods can be designed thanks to the agarose matrix's variable size, shape, porosity, and surface chemistry. Researchers can achieve selective binding to specific receptors or biomarkers overexpressed on the surface of cancer cells by modifying the surface of agarose nanoparticles with targeting ligands, such as peptides, antibodies, or aptamers. This allows for the targeted delivery of nucleic acid therapeutics to tumor tissues while sparing healthy cells [40]. The ability to incorporate stimuli-responsive moieties, such as pH-sensitive polymers or light-sensitive molecules, into agarose nanostructures provides for the site-specific release of nucleic acid therapeutics in response to environmental cues within the tumor microenvironment. It is possible to design stimuli-responsive agarose nanoparticles that, in reaction to variations in pH, temperature, or enzyme activity, will undergo structural changes or initiate intracellular signaling pathways and release nucleic acids into cancer cells under regulated conditions. Agarose-based delivery systems have potential for clinical applications in gene therapy and RNAi-based cancer therapy because of their spatiotemporal control over nucleic acid delivery, which increases therapeutic efficacy and decreases off-target effects.

10.6.3 Photothermal and Photodynamic Therapy

Photothermal therapy (PTT) and photodynamic therapy (PDT) are emerging modalities in cancer treatment that utilize light-responsive agents to induce localized cytotoxic effects within tumor tissues. Agarose nanostructures have recently gained attention as promising carriers for photothermal and photodynamic agents, offering unique advantages such as biocompatibility, tunable properties, and facile surface functionalization. By incorporating photothermal or photosensitizing agents into agarose nanoparticles, researchers can develop targeted delivery systems for PTT and PDT, enabling precise and efficient cancer therapy while minimizing negative impacts [41]. Photothermal therapy works by the conversion of light energy into heat by photothermal agents, leading to localized hyperthermia and selective ablation of tumor cells. Agarose nanostructures can serve as carriers for photothermal agents, such as gold nanoparticles, carbon nanotubes, or graphene oxide, which possess strong light-absorbing properties and efficient photothermal conversion. The stability, biocompatibility, and tumor-targeting capacity of agarose nanoparticles can be improved by researchers to facilitate efficient delivery of photothermal medicines to tumor tissues. Agarose-based nanocomposites sustain localized thermal damage to cancer cells while protecting surrounding healthy tissues from near-infrared (NIR) laser irradiation. Precise control over the size, form, and surface chemistry of nanoparticles is made possible by the tunable characteristics of agarose matrices, which maximizes their photothermal conversion efficiency and PTT therapeutic efficacy [42].

On the other hand, photodynamic therapy depends on photosensitizing drugs producing reactive oxygen species (ROS) in the presence of light, which causes oxidative damage and cell death (Table 10.2). Photosensitizing compounds with potent light-absorbing and ROS-generating qualities, like phthalocyanines, chlorins, and porphyrins, can be encapsulated in agarose nanostructures and used as carriers. Researchers can prevent photosensitizing drugs from degrading too soon and improve their tumor-targeting capacity by encasing them in agarose nanoparticles, which makes it

Table 10.2 Summary of the applications of drug delivery in cancer therapy.

Component	Features	Methods
Chemotherapeutic drug delivery	Use of agarose nanostructures to deliver chemotherapy agents specifically to cancer cells	Doxorubicin-loaded nanostructures, targeted delivery systems
Gene therapy and RNAi delivery	Application of agarose nanostructures in delivering genetic material or RNA interference molecules	siRNA encapsulation, DNA plasmid delivery
Photothermal and photodynamic therapy	Use of agarose nanostructures in therapies that utilize light to treat cancer	Photothermal agents, photodynamic agents

possible to transport them to cancer cells effectively. Agarose-based nanocomposites produce ROS in response to specific wavelengths of light, which causes tumor cells to undergo apoptosis or necrosis while causing the least amount of damage to the surrounding healthy tissues [41, 42]. Because of the adaptable surface chemistry of agarose nanostructures, targeting ligands or stimuli-responsive moieties can be included to enable site-specific delivery and controlled release of photosensitizing drugs, which can improve therapeutic efficacy.

10.7 *In Vitro* and *In Vivo* Studies

10.7.1 Cell Culture Studies and Cytotoxicity Assays

Evaluation of new treatments and drug delivery systems, such as agarose nanostructures, for possible use in cancer therapy, depends heavily on cell culture research and cytotoxicity assays [43]. These investigations offer important information about the safety, effectiveness, and biocompatibility of nanoparticles, which can assist in direct future research and development of these materials for use in *in vivo* applications. In cell culture studies, cancer cells are cultured *in vitro* and exposed to agarose nanostructures to evaluate their effects on cell viability, proliferation, and morphology. These studies often utilize a variety of cancer cell lines representing different types of cancer, allowing researchers to assess the broad applicability of agarose-based drug delivery systems. Cell culture studies typically involve treating cancer cells with varying concentrations of agarose nanoparticles and assessing their cytotoxic effects using assays such as the MTT assay, which measures cell viability, or the trypan blue exclusion assay, which assesses cell membrane integrity. These assays provide quantitative data on the cytotoxicity of agarose nanoparticles and help to determine their optimal concentration and formulation for further evaluation.

Cell culture studies enable researchers to investigate the mechanisms underlying the cytotoxic effects of agarose nanoparticles, including their cellular uptake, intracellular trafficking, and interactions with cellular organelles and signaling pathways. Techniques such as confocal microscopy, flow cytometry, and immunofluorescence staining allow for visualization and quantification of nanoparticle uptake, subcellular localization, and intracellular fate within cancer cells. By elucidating the mechanisms of action of agarose nanoparticles, researchers can gain insights into their mode of cytotoxicity and identify potential targets for improving their therapeutic efficacy and specificity [44]. These studies evaluate the effects of nanoparticles on cell morphology, adhesion, migration, and apoptosis, and their potential to induce inflammatory responses or DNA damage. Through longitudinal monitoring of cellular reactions to agarose nanoparticles, scientists can detect unfavorable outcomes and fine-tune nanoparticle compositions to reduce toxicity and enhance therapeutic effectiveness.

10.7.2 Animal Models for Cancer Treatment

Animal models are indispensable tools for preclinical evaluation of novel cancer therapeutics, including drug delivery systems based on agarose nanostructures. These models provide important information on the pharmacokinetics, biodistribution, efficacy, and safety of therapeutic agents in a complex biological system that more closely mimics human physiology and pathology than *in vitro* models [45]. Utilizing animal models for cancer treatment allows researchers to assess the therapeutic potential of agarose nanostructures in a dynamic and physiologically relevant environment, providing critical data for translational research and clinical development. There are several animal models used in cancer research, and each has benefits and drawbacks. In xenograft models, immunocompromised mice are implanted with human cancer cells, enabling the assessment of tumor growth, metastasis, and therapeutic response. By implanting cancer cells into an animal's anatomically precise location, orthotopic models enable the evaluation of tumor growth and invasion in a tissue-specific setting. Through the alteration of mouse genes, spontaneous or inducible tumors can be developed in genetically engineered mouse models (GEMMs), which offer valuable insights into the initiation, development, and response to therapy of malignancies.

Tumor heterogeneity and personalized medicine techniques can be studied using patient-derived xenograft (PDX) models, which entail transplanting tumor samples from patients into immunodeficient mice. Animal models for cancer treatment serve several key purposes in evaluating agarose nanostructures and other drug delivery systems. Firstly, these models allow researchers to assess the pharmacokinetics and biodistribution of nanoparticles following administration, providing insights into their systemic circulation, tissue accumulation, and clearance pathways [45]. Nanoparticle distribution and tumor targeting can be monitored non-invasively *in vivo* by methods including magnetic resonance imaging (MRI), fluorescence imaging, and positron emission tomography (PET). This allows for improved efficacy and specificity when optimizing nanoparticle formulations. Second, *in vivo* assessments of the safety and therapeutic effectiveness of agarose nanostructures are possible thanks to animal models. Researchers can evaluate the efficacy of drug delivery systems based on nanoparticles in treating cancer by measuring tumor growth suppression, metastasis prevention, and overall survival in animal models. Animal models enable the assessment of potential adverse effects and toxicity associated with nanoparticle administration, informing decisions regarding dosage, formulation, and route of administration for clinical translation. Animal models provide important information into the mechanisms of action underlying the anticancer effects of agarose nanostructures. By investigating cellular and molecular changes within tumors following nanoparticle treatment, researchers can elucidate the pathways involved in nanoparticle uptake, intracellular trafficking, and cytotoxicity, as well as the host immune response to nanoparticle administration. These mechanistic insights are essential for optimizing nanoparticle formulations and developing combination therapies that enhance therapeutic efficacy and overcome drug resistance in cancer treatment.

10.7.3 Biodistribution and Pharmacokinetics

Drug delivery systems, like agarose nanostructures, have biodistribution and pharmacokinetics that must be understood to evaluate their safety, efficacy, and potential for clinical application in cancer therapy. While pharmacokinetics studies the absorption, distribution, metabolism, and excretion (ADME) of nanoparticles over time, biodistribution describes the distribution of nanoparticles within the body after delivery [46]. Analyzing agarose nanostructures' biodistribution and pharmacokinetics in preclinical models offers important information on how they behave *in vivo*, which helps with optimization and clinical application translation.

The goal of biodistribution studies is to ascertain how nanoparticles are distributed after injection across different tissues, organs, and biological fluids. These studies usually entail real-time tracking of the location and accumulation of nanoparticles using imaging techniques such as magnetic resonance imaging (MRI), positron emission tomography (PET), single-photon emission computed tomography (SPECT), and fluorescence imaging. Through the application of contrast chemicals or imaging probes, researchers can track the biodistribution and tissue-targeting specificity of nanoparticles over time. By offering important insights into the systemic circulation, tissue accumulation, and clearance pathways of agarose nanostructures, biodistribution studies aid in the formulation and dosage optimization of these drugs for increased therapeutic efficacy and decreased off-target effects [46]. The quantitative measurement of nanoparticle content in biological samples, including blood, plasma, urine, and tissues, over some time after delivery is known as pharmacokinetic research. The objective of these investigations is to describe the pharmacokinetic characteristics of nanoparticles, including area under the curve (AUC), half-life ($t\frac{1}{2}$), clearance (CL), and volume of distribution (Vd), as well as their absorption, distribution, metabolism, and excretion inside the body. Pharmacokinetic studies shed light on the agarose nanostructures' systemic exposure, circulation, and elimination kinetics. This information is useful for determining dosage schedules, delivery methods, and therapeutic monitoring in clinical settings. Researchers can evaluate the stability and biocompatibility of agarose nanostructures in biological fluids and tissues by use of pharmacokinetic experiments. Through the longitudinal assessment of nanoparticle breakdown, metabolism, and clearance, scientists can assess the possibility of systemic toxicity, immunogenicity, and long-term unfavorable consequences linked to the administration of nanoparticles. The optimization of nanoparticle formulations for better pharmacokinetic profiles and therapeutic results is made possible by pharmacokinetic studies, which shed light on the variables such as particle size, surface charge, surface chemistry, and surface modification that affect nanoparticle behavior *in vivo*.

10.8 Clinical Translation and Challenges

The creation of agarose nanostructures for cancer therapy has substantial obstacles in moving from preclinical investigations to clinical translation. Preclinical research on agarose-based drug delivery systems in animal models offers important insights into their safety, efficacy, and viability; however, transferring these discoveries into clinical settings necessitates careful consideration of several factors, including regulatory approval, scalability, biocompatibility, and clinical validation [47]. The acquisition of regulatory permission for agarose nanostructures as therapeutic agents for cancer treatment is a major obstacle in the preclinical to clinical transition process. Before commencing clinical trials, regulatory bodies such as the European Medicines Agency (EMA) in Europe and the Food and Drug Administration (FDA) in the United States require substantial preclinical data proving the quality, safety, and efficacy of a treatment. To analyze potential side effects and long-term safety profiles of agarose nanostructures in animal models, this includes thorough pharmacokinetic and biodistribution investigations in addition to toxicological evaluations. Meeting regulatory requirements for clinical translation necessitates robust preclinical evidence supporting the therapeutic potential and safety of agarose-based drug delivery systems, which can be time-consuming and resource-intensive [47]. The scalability and reproducibility of manufacturing processes for agarose nanostructures pose significant challenges in transitioning from preclinical studies to clinical applications. While laboratory-scale synthesis methods may be suitable for preclinical research, scaling up production to meet clinical demand requires optimization of manufacturing processes, quality control measures, and regulatory compliance with good manufacturing practices (GMP). Ensuring batch-to-batch consistency, purity, and sterility of agarose nanostructures is essential for maintaining product quality and safety in clinical settings. The cost-effectiveness and scalability of manufacturing processes are critical considerations for the commercialization and widespread adoption of agarose-based drug delivery systems in clinical practice.

Addressing issues with agarose nanostructures' biocompatibility, immunogenicity, and long-term safety in human beings is another difficulty in the preclinical to clinical transition process. Preclinical research in animal models offers important insights into the safety and biocompatibility characteristics of nanoparticles; however, phase I, II, and III clinical trials are necessary for rigorous clinical validation before these findings can be applied to people [48]. Clinical trials are crucial for determining possible side effects and maximizing treatment plans, as well as for assessing the pharmacokinetics, biodistribution, safety, and effectiveness of agarose-based drug delivery systems in human patients. To ensure patient safety and regulatory approval, concerns regarding immunogenicity, potential off-target effects, and long-term biocompatibility of agarose nanostructures in clinical settings must be addressed.

A key factor in the clinical application of agarose nanostructures for cancer treatment is regulatory considerations. The development, testing, and approval of novel therapeutics, including drug delivery systems based on agarose nanostructures, are subject to strict guidelines and requirements set by regulatory agencies, such as the European Medicines Agency (EMA) in Europe and the Food and Drug Administration (FDA) in the United States. Demonstrating the safety and efficacy of agarose nanostructures through preclinical research carried out by regulatory requirements is one of the most important regulatory factors in the clinical translation of these materials. Comprehensive data on the pharmacokinetics, biodistribution, toxicology, and biocompatibility of agarose nanostructures in animal models, along with proof of their therapeutic efficacy in pertinent disease models like orthotopic tumor models or cancer xenografts, must be provided by preclinical studies [47, 48]. The planning and execution of clinical trials assessing the efficacy, safety, and tolerability of agarose-based drug delivery systems in human patients are among the regulatory issues.

Phase I studies are used to examine safety and pharmacokinetics; phase II trials are used to assess preliminary efficacy; and phase III trials are used to establish efficacy and safety in larger patient groups. Clinical trials are carried out in stages [48]. Regulatory bodies verify that clinical trial protocols, research endpoints, patient recruiting standards, and data collection methods are compliant with regulations and adhere to ethical and scientific standards.

10.9 Scalability and Regulatory Challenges

The clinical translation of agarose nanostructures for cancer therapy is a complex process that faces significant challenges in scalability, regulatory compliance, and clinical validation. Addressing these issues is essential to transition these innovative drug delivery systems from preclinical research to real-world clinical applications. Scaling up the production of agarose nanostructures from laboratory settings to clinical manufacturing requires optimizing processes to achieve consistency, efficiency, and quality. Laboratory-scale synthesis methods are often unsuitable for large-scale production due to limitations in capacity, throughput, and reproducibility. Small variations in reaction conditions, such as temperature, pH, or agitation, can significantly alter nanoparticle properties, posing challenges for batch-to-batch consistency. Moreover, downstream processes such as purification, formulation, and sterilization must be adapted to accommodate larger production volumes without compromising product quality. To overcome these challenges, scalable and automated production systems need to be developed, incorporating advancements in biomanufacturing technologies. Employing high-throughput synthesis techniques, such as microfluidics, and integrating real-time quality control measures can improve reproducibility and efficiency. Additionally, adopting modular and flexible manufacturing systems can streamline production workflows, enabling rapid adaptation to different scales and formulations.

Navigating the regulatory landscape for agarose nanostructures is another critical hurdle in their clinical translation. Regulatory agencies such as the FDA and EMA require comprehensive preclinical data demonstrating the safety, efficacy, and quality of these systems before they can proceed to clinical trials. This includes detailed studies on pharmacokinetics, biodistribution, toxicology, and biocompatibility. Meeting these requirements can be resource-intensive and time-consuming, posing significant challenges for researchers and developers. Strategies to address regulatory challenges include engaging with regulatory bodies early in the development process to align preclinical study designs with regulatory expectations. Establishing robust documentation and quality management systems ensures compliance with Good Laboratory Practices (GLP) and Good Manufacturing Practices (GMP). Leveraging regulatory science to develop novel testing protocols tailored to the unique properties of agarose nanostructures can also help streamline the approval process.

A critical aspect of clinical translation is ensuring that agarose nanostructures are biocompatible, non-immunogenic, and safe for long-term use in humans. Preclinical studies provide valuable insights, but human clinical trials (phases I–III) are essential for thorough validation. These trials evaluate safety, pharmacokinetics, and efficacy in progressively larger patient cohorts. To mitigate immunogenicity and off-target effects, surface modification of agarose nanostructures with inert or biomimetic coatings can be employed. Designing nanoparticles with tailored release profiles and targeting ligands minimizes exposure to non-target tissues, reducing potential side effects. Advanced modeling techniques and predictive analytics can aid in anticipating long-term safety concerns, allowing for proactive risk management.

- ➢ **Collaborative efforts**: Partnerships between academic researchers, industry, and regulatory agencies can facilitate the translation process by pooling expertise, resources, and funding.
- ➢ **Innovative manufacturing solutions**: Adopting advanced manufacturing technologies, such as 3D bioprinting and continuous flow reactors, can enhance scalability and efficiency.
- ➢ **Regulatory innovations**: Advocating for adaptive regulatory frameworks that accommodate emerging technologies, such as nanomedicine, can help streamline approval processes.
- ➢ **Enhanced preclinical models**: Using advanced *in vitro* and *in vivo* models that closely mimic human physiology can improve the predictive accuracy of preclinical studies.
- ➢ **Public–private partnerships**: Encouraging collaborations between government agencies and private entities can provide the necessary support for navigating regulatory and manufacturing challenges.

10.10 Future Directions and Emerging Trends

Future directions in the design of agarose nanostructures for cancer therapy are poised to capitalize on recent advances in nanotechnology, materials science, and biomedical engineering to enhance the therapeutic efficacy, specificity, and safety of drug delivery systems. Emerging trends in agarose nanostructure design are focused on overcoming existing limitations and harnessing the unique properties of agarose matrices to develop innovative solutions for targeted drug delivery, combination therapies, and personalized medicine approaches. One key direction in agarose nanostructure design is the development of multifunctional nanoparticles capable of delivering multiple therapeutic agents simultaneously. By incorporating synergistic combinations of chemotherapeutic drugs, targeted therapies, and immunomodulators within agarose nanostructures, researchers can enhance therapeutic efficacy, overcome drug resistance, and minimize off-target effects. Multifunctional nanoparticles can be engineered to target specific molecular pathways, cellular receptors, or microenvironments within tumors, enabling precise modulation of tumor biology and immune responses for personalized cancer therapy. Another emerging trend is the integration of stimuli-responsive and on-demand drug release mechanisms into agarose nanostructures. By incorporating stimuli-sensitive polymers, light-responsive molecules, or enzymatically cleavable linkers within agarose matrices, researchers can design nanoparticles capable of responding to external stimuli or endogenous signals within the tumor microenvironment to trigger site-specific drug release. Stimuli-responsive agarose nanostructures enable spatiotemporal control over drug delivery, allowing for tailored treatment regimens and minimization of systemic toxicity. The creation of patient-specific agarose nanostructures that are customized to each patient's unique tumor biology and genetic profile is being fueled by the emergence of precision medicine and personalized oncology. Through the integration of genomic, proteomic, and imaging data into the design of nanoparticles, researchers can create drug delivery systems that are tailored to target certain tumor subtypes, molecular signatures, or therapy responses in patients. By more precisely and specifically targeting tumors, personalized agarose nanostructures have the potential to enhance treatment outcomes, minimize side effects, and slow the emergence of drug resistance.

Combination treatments are a promising method for cancer treatment that aims to overcome medication resistance, maximize side effects, and improve efficacy. They involve the simultaneous or sequential administration of numerous therapeutic drugs. Combination therapy can be flexibly delivered to tumor areas using agarose nanostructures, which facilitate the co-administration of immunomodulators, targeted medicines, chemotherapeutic medications, and imaging contrast agents. Combination therapy given using agarose nanostructures has the advantage of being able to target numerous pathways or cellular processes involved in the evolution of cancer at the same time. By co-encapsulating synergistic combinations of therapeutics within agarose nanoparticles, researchers can achieve additive or synergistic effects, leading to enhanced tumor cell killing and improved therapeutic outcomes. For example, combining chemotherapeutic drugs with targeted agents that inhibit specific signaling pathways or immunomodulatory agents that enhance antitumor immune responses can overcome mechanisms of drug resistance and enhance treatment efficacy.

Agarose nanostructures can be designed to provide for both temporal and spatial control over drug release, which makes it easier to administer various therapeutic agents one after the other in order to maximize treatment plans. Researchers can create nanoparticles that release therapeutic payloads in response to certain cues within the tumor microenvironment, such as pH, temperature, or enzyme activity, by combining stimuli-responsive polymers or triggerable drug release mechanisms into agarose matrices. Therapeutics can be delivered sequentially to maximize therapeutic efficacy and minimize off-target effects while enabling customized treatment plans. Combination treatments made possible by agarose nanostructures have the potential to revolutionize personalized medicine by addressing the unique traits of each patient as well as the biology of their tumors. By integrating genomic, proteomic, and imaging data into nanoparticle design, researchers can develop patient-specific combination therapies optimized for specific tumor subtypes, molecular signatures, or treatment responses. Personalized combination therapies offer the potential to improve treatment outcomes, reduce adverse effects, and minimize the development of drug resistance by targeting tumors with greater precision and specificity. The revolutionary fields of precision oncology and personalized medicine seek to customize therapeutic strategies to the unique characteristics of each patient as well as the biology and genetic makeup of their tumors. Agarose nanostructures, which allow for targeted drug delivery, imaging, and therapy monitoring according to the individual needs of each patient, hold great potential for improving precision oncology and customized medicine.

Agarose nanostructures play an important part in enabling precision oncology approaches that aim to identify and target specific molecular aberrations driving cancer progression. By incorporating imaging contrast agents or targeting ligands within agarose nanoparticles, researchers can develop diagnostic and therapeutic platforms capable of detecting tumor biomarkers, monitoring treatment responses, and guiding therapeutic interventions in real time. Precision oncology strategies, such as companion diagnostics and theranostics, leverage the capabilities of agarose nanostructures to deliver personalized treatments based on individual patient characteristics and disease biology. Theranostic nanoparticles, for example, combine diagnostic and therapeutic functionalities within a single platform, allowing for non-invasive imaging of tumors and targeted delivery of therapeutic agents to tumor sites. Non-invasive imaging techniques facilitated by agarose nanostructures enable clinicians to assess treatment responses, detect early signs of disease recurrence, and adjust therapeutic regimens, accordingly, optimizing patient care and outcomes.

Another promising area is the application of artificial intelligence (AI) in designing personalized drug delivery systems. AI algorithms can analyze vast amounts of patient data, including genetic profiles, tumor microenvironment characteristics, and treatment history, to tailor agarose-based delivery platforms for optimized efficacy and minimal side effects. Machine-learning models can predict drug release kinetics and optimize the nanostructure of agarose carriers for specific therapeutic needs, significantly enhancing the precision and effectiveness of cancer treatments. Another exciting trend is the integration of agarose-based platforms with immunotherapy and CRISPR-based gene-editing technologies. CRISPR-based technologies offer unprecedented precision in genetic modifications, and agarose nanostructures can serve as efficient vehicles for delivering CRISPR-Cas9 components to cancer cells. This integration opens new possibilities for targeted genome editing to correct mutations or sensitize cancer cells to other treatments. Together, these innovations represent a transformative approach to cancer therapy, pushing the boundaries of personalized and precision medicine.

10.11 Conclusion

Agarose nanostructures represent a versatile and highly promising platform for drug delivery in cancer treatment, offering numerous advantages that address the complex challenges of oncology. This chapter has examined the synthesis, characterization, and applications of agarose-based drug delivery systems, highlighting their potential to revolutionize cancer therapy.

As a biocompatible and biodegradable polysaccharide, agarose provides an ideal matrix for nanoparticle formulation due to its tunable properties, ease of surface modification, and controlled drug release capabilities. Researchers can precisely engineer the size, shape, and surface chemistry of agarose nanostructures using techniques such as solvent evaporation, nanoprecipitation, and emulsion methods. Advanced characterization tools, including DLS, SEM, and TEM, enable a deeper understanding of nanoparticle morphology, size distribution, and stability, optimizing their design for therapeutic use. Agarose-based nanostructures show great potential to overcome critical challenges in cancer treatment, such as drug resistance, off-target effects, and systemic toxicity. By encapsulating a wide range of therapeutic agents such as chemotherapeutics, targeted drugs, immunomodulators, and imaging agents, agarose matrices enable the development of multifunctional nanoparticles capable of precise drug delivery, combination therapies, and theranostic applications. Their ability to provide controlled, stimuli-responsive, and on-demand drug release ensures that medications are delivered in a targeted manner, minimizing side effects and enabling personalized treatment strategies.

The adaptability of agarose nanostructures opens doors to personalized medicine and precision oncology. By integrating data from genomics, proteomics, and advanced imaging into the design of these nanoparticles, researchers can create patient-specific drug delivery systems optimized for unique tumor subtypes and molecular profiles. This approach enhances treatment efficacy, reduces adverse effects, and helps mitigate the development of drug resistance, ultimately improving the overall quality of life for cancer patients. Agarose nanostructures offer a transformative potential for cancer therapy due to their biocompatibility, tunable properties, and multifunctional capabilities. Continued research and innovation in this field are expected to accelerate the clinical translation of agarose-based delivery systems, paving the way for groundbreaking advancements in precision oncology. These developments promise not only to improve treatment outcomes but also to redefine how cancer care is delivered, offering hope for a future of more effective, tailored, and patient-centered therapies.

AI disclosure statement: The author acknowledges the use of AI-based tools for minor language editing or grammatical correction. However, all intellectual contributions, analyses, and conclusions presented in this chapter are entirely the author's own.

References

1. Padmesh, S. and Singh, A., Agars: Properties and applications, in: *Polysaccharides: Properties and Applications*, vol. 17, pp. 75–93, 2021 May.
2. Lee, W.K., Lim, Y.Y., Leow, A.T., Namasivayam, P., Abdullah, J.O., Ho, C.L., Biosynthesis of agar in red seaweeds: A review. *Carbohydr. Polym.*, 164, 23–30, 2017 May 15.
3. Normand, V., Lootens, D.L., Amici, E., Plucknett, K.P., Aymard, P., New insight into agarose gel mechanical properties. *Biomacromolecules*, 1, 4, 730–8, 2000 Dec 12.
4. Pandya, Y.H., Bakshi, M., Sharma, A., Pandya, H., Pandya, H., Agar-agar extraction, structural properties and applications: A review. *Pharma Innov. J.*, 6, 1151–7, 2022.
5. Elmowafy, M. and Al-Sanea, M.M., Nanostructured lipid carriers (NLCs) as drug delivery platform: Advances in formulation and delivery strategies. *Saudi Pharm. J.*, 29, 9, 999–1012, 2021 Sep 1.
6. Tay, A. and Melosh, N., Nanostructured materials for intracellular cargo delivery. *Acc. Chem. Res.*, 52, 9, 2462–71, 2019 Aug 29.
7. Ouyang, J., Xie, A., Zhou, J., Liu, R., Wang, L., Liu, H., Kong, N., Tao, W., Minimally invasive nanomedicine: nanotechnology in photo-/ultrasound-/radiation-/magnetism-mediated therapy and imaging. *Chem. Soc. Rev.*, 51, 12, 4996–5041, 2022.
8. Blanco, E., Shen, H., Ferrari, M., Principles of nanoparticle design for overcoming biological barriers to drug delivery. *Nat. Biotechnol.*, 33, 9, 941–51, 2015 Sep.
9. Petros, R.A. and DeSimone, J.M., Strategies in the design of nanoparticles for therapeutic applications. *Nat. Rev. Drug Discov.*, 9, 8, 615–27, 2010 Aug.
10. Mahfuz, A.M., Hossain, M.K., Khan, M.I., Hossain, I., Anik, M.I., *Smart drug-delivery nanostructured systems for cancer therapy*, Elsevier, Amsterdam, The Netherlands, 2022 Oct 7.
11. Mohanraj, V.J. and Chen, Y.J., Nanoparticles-a review. *Trop. J. Pharm. Res.*, 5, 1, 561–73, 2006.
12. Vargas-Molinero, H.Y., Serrano-Medina, A., Palomino-Vizcaino, K., López-Maldonado, E.A., Villarreal-Gómez, L.J., Pérez-González, G.L., Cornejo-Bravo, J.M., Hybrid systems of nanofibers and polymeric nanoparticles for biological application and delivery systems. *Micromachines*, 14, 1, 208, 2023 Jan 14.
13. Grimaudo, M.A., Concheiro, A., Alvarez-Lorenzo, C., Nanogels for regenerative medicine. *J. Control. Release*, 313, 148–60, 2019 Nov 10.
14. Yallapu, M.M., Jaggi, M., Chauhan, S.C., Design and engineering of nanogels for cancer treatment. *Drug Discov. Today*, 16, 9–10, 457–63, 2011 May 1.
15. Yilmaz, E. and Soylak, M., Nanotechnological Developments in Nanofiber-Based Membranes Used for Water Treatment Applications. *Environ. Nanotechnol.*, 5, 205–59, 2021.

16. Leung, V. and Ko, F., Biomedical applications of nanofibers. *Polym. Adv. Technol.*, 22, 3, 350–65, 2011 Mar.
17. Yazdi, M.K., Taghizadeh, A., Taghizadeh, M., Stadler, F.J., Farokhi, M., Mottaghitalab, F., Zarrintaj, P., Ramsey, J.D., Seidi, F., Saeb, M.R., Mozafari, M., Agarose-based biomaterials for advanced drug delivery. *J. Control. Release*, 326, 523–43, 2020 Oct 10.
18. Lee, K.Y., Kong, H.J., Larson, R.G., Mooney, D.J., Hydrogel formation *via* cell crosslinking. *Adv. Mater.*, 15, 21, 1828–32, 2003 Nov 4.
19. Braun, G.A., Ary, B.E., Dear, A.J., Rohn, M.C., Payson, A.M., Lee, D.S., Parry, R.C., Friedman, C., Knowles, T.P., Linse, S., Åkerfeldt, K.S., On the mechanism of self-assembly by a hydrogel-forming peptide. *Biomacromolecules*, 21, 12, 4781–94, 2020 Nov 10.
20. Burghardt, R.C. and Droleskey, R., Transmission electron microscopy. *Curr. Protoc. Microbiol.*, 3, 1, 2B–1, 2006 Dec.
21. Tang, C.Y. and Yang, Z., Transmission electron microscopy (TEM), in: *Membrane Characterization*, pp. 145–159, Elsevier, 2017 Jan 1.
22. Mohammed, A. and Abdullah, A., Scanning electron microscopy (SEM): A review, in: *Proceedings of the 2018 International Conference on Hydraulics and Pneumatics—HERVEX*, Băile Govora, Romania, 2018 Nov 7, vol. 2018, pp. 7–9.
23. Stetefeld, J., McKenna, S.A., Patel, T.R., Dynamic light scattering: a practical guide and applications in biomedical sciences. *Biophys. Rev.*, 8, 409–27, 2016 Dec.
24. Zarrintaj, P., Manouchehri, S., Ahmadi, Z., Saeb, M.R., Urbanska, A.M., Kaplan, D.L., Mozafari, M., Agarose-based biomaterials for tissue engineering. *Carbohydr. Polym.*, 187, 66–84, 2018 May 1.
25. Scinto, S.L., Bilodeau, D.A., Hincapie, R., Lee, W., Nguyen, S.S., Xu, M., Am Ende, C.W., Finn, M.G., Lang, K., Lin, Q., Pezacki, J.P., Bioorthogonal chemistry. *Nat. Rev. Methods Primers*, 1, 1, 30, 2021 Apr 15.
26. Rivas, C.J., Tarhini, M., Badri, W., Miladi, K., Greige-Gerges, H., Nazari, Q.A., Rodríguez, S.A., Román, RA., Fessi, H., Elaissari, A., Nanoprecipitation process: From encapsulation to drug delivery. *Int. J. Pharm.*, 532, 1, 66–81, 2017 Oct 30.
27. Kumari, A., Singla, R., Guliani, A., Yadav, S.K., Nanoencapsulation for drug delivery. *EXCLI J.*, 13, 265, 2014.
28. Tran, T.T. and Tran, P.H., Nanoconjugation and encapsulation strategies for improving drug delivery and therapeutic efficacy of poorly water-soluble drugs. *Pharmaceutics*, 11, 7, 325, 2019 Jul 10.
29. Kamaly, N., Yameen, B., Wu, J., Farokhzad, O.C., Degradable controlled-release polymers and polymeric nanoparticles: mechanisms of controlling drug release. *Chem. Rev.*, 116, 4, 2602–63, 2016 Feb 24.
30. Gil, C.J., Li, L., Hwang, B., Cadena, M., Theus, A.S., Finamore, T.A., Bauser-Heaton, H., Mahmoudi, M., Roeder, R.K., Serpooshan, V., Tissue engineered

drug delivery vehicles: Methods to monitor and regulate the release behavior. *J. Control. Release*, 349, 143–55, 2022 Sep 1.
31. Bayer, I.S., Controlled drug release from nanoengineered polysaccharides. *Pharmaceutics*, 15, 5, 1364, 2023 Apr 28.
32. Chen, Z., Kankala, R.K., Yang, Z., Li, W., Xie, S., Li, H., Chen, A.Z., Zou, L., Antibody-based drug delivery systems for cancer therapy: Mechanisms, challenges, and prospects. *Theranostics*, 12, 8, 3719, 2022.
33. Subhan, M.A., Yalamarty, S.S., Filipczak, N., Parveen, F., Torchilin, V.P., Recent advances in tumor targeting *via* EPR effect for cancer treatment. *J. Pers. Med.*, 11, 6, 571, 2021 Jun 18.
34. Shi, Y., van der Meel, R., Chen, X., Lammers, T., The EPR effect and beyond: Strategies to improve tumor targeting and cancer nanomedicine treatment efficacy. *Theranostics*, 10, 17, 7921, 2020.
35. Foroozandeh, P. and Aziz, A.A., Insight into cellular uptake and intracellular trafficking of nanoparticles. *Nanoscale Res. Lett.*, 13, 1, 339, 2018 Dec.
36. Raavé, R., van Kuppevelt, T.H., Daamen, W.F., Chemotherapeutic drug delivery by tumoral extracellular matrix targeting. *J. Control. Release*, 274, 1–8, 2018 Mar 28.
37. Kumari, P., Ghosh, B., Biswas, S., Nanocarriers for cancer-targeted drug delivery. *J. Drug Target.*, 24, 3, 179–91, 2016 Mar 15.
38. Caplen, N.J., RNAi as a gene therapy approach. *Expert Opin. Biol. Ther.*, 3, 4, 575–86, 2003 Jul 1.
39. Xin, Y., Huang, M., Guo, W.W., Huang, Q., Zhang, L.Z., Jiang, G., Nano-based delivery of RNAi in cancer therapy. *Mol. Cancer*, 16, 1–9, 2017 Dec.
40. Shibu, E.S., Hamada, M., Murase, N., Biju, V., Nanomaterials formulations for photothermal and photodynamic therapy of cancer. *J. Photochem. Photobiol., C*, 15, 53–72, 2013 Jun 1.
41. Kadkhoda, J., Tarighatnia, A., Barar, J., Aghanejad, A., Davaran, S., Recent advances and trends in nanoparticles based photothermal and photodynamic therapy. *Photodiagn. Photodyn. Ther.*, 37, 102697, 2022 Mar 1.
42. Eastman, A., Improving anticancer drug development begins with cell culture: misinformation perpetrated by the misuse of cytotoxicity assays. *Oncotarget*, 8, 5, 8854, 2017 Jan 1.
43. Aslantürk ÖS. *In vitro* cytotoxicity and cell viability assays: principles, advantages, and disadvantages, in: *Genotoxicity-A predictable risk to our actual world*, vol. 2, pp. 64–80, 2018 Jul 11.
44. Ruggeri, B.A., Camp, F., Miknyoczki, S., Animal models of disease: pre-clinical animal models of cancer and their applications and utility in drug discovery. *Biochem. Pharmacol.*, 87, 1, 150–61, 2014 Jan 1.
45. Chiari-Andréo, B.G., Abucafy, M.P., Manaia, E.B., da Silva, B.L., Rissi, N.C., Oshiro-Junior, J.A., Chiavacci, L.A., Drug delivery using theranostics: an overview of its use, advantages and safety assessment. *Curr. Nanosci.*, 16, 1, 3–14, 2020 Jan 1.

46. Younis, M.A., Tawfeek, H.M., Abdellatif, A.A., Abdel-Aleem, J.A., Harashima, H., Clinical translation of nanomedicines: Challenges, opportunities, and keys. *Adv. Drug Deliv. Rev.*, 181, 114083, 2022 Feb 1.
47. Gawne, P.J., Ferreira, M., Papaluca, M., Grimm, J., Decuzzi, P., New opportunities and old challenges in the clinical translation of nanotheranostics. *Nat. Rev. Mater.*, 8, 12, 783–98, 2023 Dec.
48. Nabil, G., Bhise, K., Sau, S., Atef, M., El-Banna, H.A., Iyer, A.K., Nano-engineered delivery systems for cancer imaging and therapy: Recent advances, future direction and patent evaluation. *Drug Discov. Today*, 24, 2, 462–91, 2019 Feb 1.

11

Pectin: Chemical Functionalization for Targeted Cancer Treatment

Shazia Shahen Mir[1], Shahnawaz Ahmad Bhat[2,3], Md. Saddam[3], Zeenat Islam[4] and Luqman Jameel Rather[5*]

[1]Laboratory Medicine Department, Faculty of Applied Medical Sciences, Al Baha University, Al Baha, Saudi Arabia
[2]Department of Chemistry, Jamia Millia Islamia, New Delhi, India
[3]Central Ayurveda Research Institute, Jhansi, (U.P.), India
[4]Advanced Research Laboratory, Department of Zoology, School of Life Sciences, University of Kashmir, Srinagar, Jammu & Kashmir, India
[5]College of Sericulture, Textile and Biomass Science, Southwest University, Chongqing, P.R. China

Abstract

Pectin, a natural polysaccharide derived from plant cell walls, has emerged as a versatile and biocompatible material for developing advanced drug delivery systems in targeted cancer therapy. The distinctive structural characteristics of pectin, including its galacturonic acid-dominant backbone and reactive functional groups, enable significant chemical changes to improve its stability, specificity, and therapeutic effectiveness. Pectin-based nanoparticles demonstrate pH sensitivity, substantial drug-loading capacity, and stimuli-responsive characteristics, rendering them suitable for the targeted delivery of chemotherapeutic drugs to the tumor microenvironment. By integrating specific ligands or hybridizing with alternative polymers and nanomaterials, these systems may further alter the tumor microenvironment, trigger apoptosis, and surmount treatment resistance. Pectin-based nanoparticles have shown potential in multimodal treatment approaches, including chemo-photothermal and chemo-radiotherapy, as well as in theranostic applications that combine diagnostic and therapeutic capabilities. Notwithstanding obstacles including stability, scalability, and tumor heterogeneity, progress in AI-driven design, hybrid material systems, and clinical translation

Corresponding author: luqmanjamel123@gmail.com

Luqman Jameel Rather, Showkat Ali Ganie and Mohammed A. Assiri (eds.) Polysaccharide Biomaterials in Cancer Research and Therapy: From Lab to Life, (339–364) © 2026 Scrivener Publishing LLC

methodologies is mitigating these issues. Pectin nanoparticles provide significant promise to transform precision oncology by providing safer, more effective, and customized cancer therapies.

***Keywords*:** Pectin nanoparticles, targeted cancer therapy, chemical functionalization, stimuli-responsive drug delivery, tumor microenvironment targeting

11.1 Introduction

Pectin, a complex anionic polysaccharide predominantly extracted from the cell wall of fruits and vegetables, has gathered significant attention in biomedical research owing to its distinctive structural properties and versatile functionalization potential [1]. As a biopolymer, it features a backbone rich in galacturonic acid, along with numerous hydroxyl (-OH) and carboxyl (-COOH) groups that enable specific chemical modifications for specialized applications [2]. Pectin is esteemed for its biocompatibility, biodegradability, and low toxicity, rendering it an optimal candidate for the development of drug delivery and other therapeutic systems [3]. The utilization of pectin-based systems in cancer therapy has proliferated swiftly, propelled by the demand for safer and more effective therapeutic options [4]. Pectin possesses inherent pH-responsive characteristics, rendering it particularly effective for the targeted delivery of chemotherapeutic drugs to the acidic tumor microenvironment [5]. This targeted release reduces systemic toxicity and improves medication efficacy. Moreover, pectin's capacity to create hydrogels, nanoparticles, and other nanoscale structures offers a flexible platform for encapsulating pharmaceuticals, biologics, and imaging agents [6].

Pectin, in addition to serving as a drug carrier, has exhibited direct biological effects that enhance its anticancer potential [7]. Pectin and its derivatives have demonstrated the ability to induce apoptosis, suppress cancer cell proliferation, and alter tumor microenvironments. Modified pectin can inhibit galectin-3, a protein associated with cancer progression and metastasis, therefore diminishing tumor growth and dissemination [8]. Moreover, pectin's engagement with reactive oxygen species (ROS) pathways might exacerbate oxidative stress in cancer cells, resulting in their demise while preserving normal cells [9]. Chemical functionalization has expanded the applications of pectin in targeted cancer therapy. Attaching hydrophobic moieties or ligands, such as antibodies or peptides, to pectin nanoparticles can increase their stability, bioavailability, and tumor specificity [10]. These functionalized nanoparticles can be designed to react to specific stimuli in the tumor microenvironment, including pH, temperature, or enzyme activity, so ensuring targeted drug release at the intended location [11, 12]. Moreover, the amalgamation of pectin with other polymers, metals, or nanomaterials has produced hybrid systems endowed with multifunctional properties, including integrated drug transport, imaging, and therapeutic effects [13].

Recent advancements in nanotechnology have enabled the application of pectin in multimodal cancer therapies [14]. Pectin-based systems have been utilized for the co-delivery of several medicines, facilitating synergistic therapeutic effects and addressing drug resistance [15]. They have also been included into photothermal treatment (PTT), photodynamic therapy (PDT), and radiation modalities, offering supplementary mechanisms for tumor elimination [16]. Notwithstanding its considerable benefits, the advancement of pectin-based systems for cancer treatment presents hurdles [17]. Challenges that must be overcome for clinical translation include storage stability, scalability for large-scale production, and regulatory obstacles [18]. Nonetheless, current investigations into sophisticated fabrication methods, including microfluidics, and computational technologies such as artificial intelligence (AI) are facilitating the resolution of these challenges [19]. This chapter examines the structural and chemical properties of pectin that render it a significant material for cancer nanomedicine. It further examines the diverse functionalization procedures utilized to augment its therapeutic efficacy and its implications in targeted cancer treatment. Ultimately, it examines the processes *via* which pectin-based systems demonstrate their anticancer properties and offers perspectives on the problems and future trajectories of this intriguing domain.

11.2 Structure and Chemistry of Pectin

Pectin is a complex polysaccharide widely found in the cell walls of plants, particularly in fruits and vegetables, where it plays an essential role in structural integrity and intercellular adhesion. Its unique chemical composition, structural diversity, and abundance of reactive functional groups make it a versatile material for biomedical applications, including cancer therapy [20]. Pectin is composed of α-(1→4)-linked D-galacturonic acid (GalA) residues with partially methyl-esterified or fully de-esterified and its structure is characterized by three chemically distinct regions:

homogalacturonan (HG), rhamnogalacturonan-I (RG-I), and rhamnogalacturonan-II (RG-II). The homogalacturonan region, a linear chain of GalA units, constitutes the backbone of pectin, while RG-I and RG-II regions include branched or substituted domains with diverse sugar compositions [21]. Variations in these regions contribute to pectin's structural heterogeneity and functional properties (Figure 11.1) [22, 23]. The degree of esterification (DE) of GalA residues is a crucial factor that influences the physicochemical properties of pectin [24]. High methoxyl pectin (HMP) with a degree of esterification of greater than 50% forms hydrogels in the presence of sugar under acidic conditions, whereas low methoxyl pectin (LMP) with the same degree of esterification forms ionic crosslinked gels with divalent cations (calcium) [25]. This "egg-box" model of crosslinking makes LMP particularly suitable for applications requiring stable networks, such as drug delivery systems (Figure 11.2) [26]. Furthermore, the structural characteristics of pectin differ markedly depending on its origin. Pectins sourced from apples and citrus fruits are abundant in homogalacturonan, rendering them appropriate for pharmaceutical applications due to their uniformity and purity, whereas sugar beet pectin, characterized by a high RG-I content, demonstrates enhanced hydrophilicity and flexibility in formulations [20, 27]. Pectin's functionality in biomedical applications

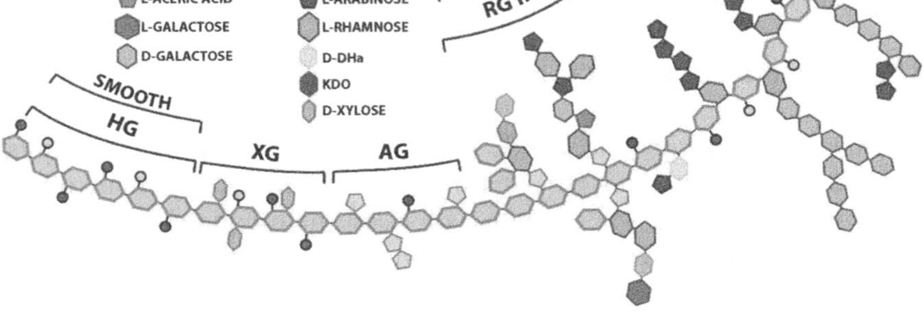

Figure 11.1 Schematic structure of pectin showing the homogalacturonan (HG), xylogalacturonan (XG), apiogalacturonan (AG), rhamnogalacturonan II (RG-II), and rhamnogalacturonan I (RG-i) regions [23].

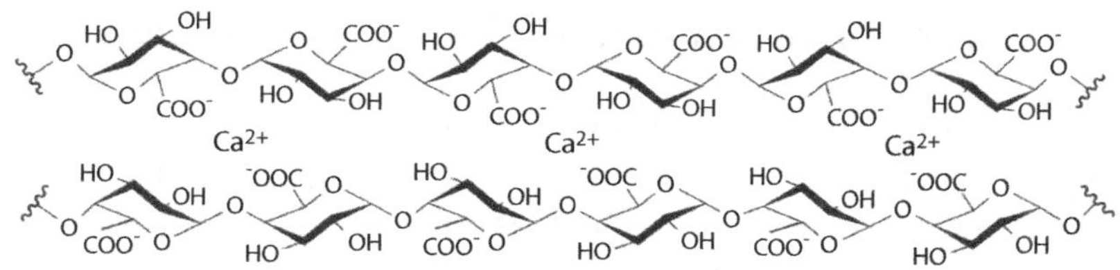

Figure 11.2 Illustration of the "egg-box" model depicting ionic crosslinking of pectin with calcium ions [29].

is attributed to the presence of enormous amounts of functional reactive groups such as carboxyl (-COOH), hydroxyl (-OH), and ester (-$COOCH_3$) groups [7, 10, 28].

Carboxyl groups play a crucial role in ionic crosslinking with calcium ions, enabling the formation of nanoparticles and hydrogels. Hydroxyl groups serve as attachment sites for hydrophilic and hydrophobic modifications, allowing enhancements in solubility, stability, and drug encapsulation. Meanwhile, ester groups contribute to pectin's gelation properties and can be enzymatically or chemically modified to adjust its behavior under specific conditions [23]. These properties allow pectin to be tailored into nanoparticles, nanogels, and in other drug delivery systems with characteristic modifications enabling precise control over size, stability, and kinetic release profiles [28]. The inherent properties of pectin make it particularly suitable for cancer therapy applications. Its ability to form stable nanoparticles through ionic crosslinking mechanism allows for efficient encapsulation and sustained release of hydrophilic drugs [4]. Chemical modifications further expand its utility, enabling the development of stimuli-responsive systems that release drugs in response to specific conditions (pH, redox potential, or enzyme) within the tumor microenvironment. Additionally, pectin can be functionalized with different targeting ligands (antibodies or peptides) to enhance the selective delivery of chemotherapeutic agents to cancer cells while minimizing off-target effects [6]. The composition and structure of pectin offer a resilient and versatile foundation for the development of sophisticated drug delivery systems. The structural diversity, abundance of reactive functional groups, and adjustable degree of esterification render it a desirable material for targeted cancer therapy, presenting excellent prospects for the creation of unique and effective treatment regimens [30].

11.3 Functionalization and Modification of Pectin

The capacity to physically and chemically modify pectin makes it a versatile biological material that has led to the creation of sophisticated drug delivery systems that are specifically suited for cancer treatment [7]. Controlled and targeted drug administration is made possible by the functionalization of pectin, which improves its stability, biocompatibility, and therapeutic effectiveness. Modifying pectin for particular biological requirements has been achieved by several ways that take use of its availability of reactive groups, such as carboxyl and hydroxyl groups [31]. To improve medication loading, stability, and bioavailability, pectin is chemically modified to change its physicochemical characteristics. It is usual practice to functionalize the galacturonic acid backbone at the carboxyl groups [32]. One common method for making stable hydrogels and nanoparticles is ionic crosslinking using divalent cations like calcium or zinc. Encapsulating hydrophilic medicines and biomolecules is a specialty of this method, which allows for the development of a strong three-dimensional network *via* the "egg-box" mechanism [33–35]. Carboxyl group covalent alterations can make it possible to attach hydrophobic moieties, targeted ligands, or medicinal medicines [33]. For instance, pectin may be modified to better encapsulate sparsely soluble medicines and increase their bioavailability by conjugating it with hydrophobic groups like fatty acids or alkyl chains [36, 37].

Pectin's hydroxyl groups provide locations for grafting hydrophilic or hydrophobic polymers to produce hybrid composites with enhanced characteristics. For example, grafting polyethylene glycol (PEG) onto pectin molecules enhances the durability and circulation duration of pectin-based nanoparticles in the bloodstream, thereby improving medication delivery to tumor locations and so lowering early degradation [36]. Likewise, adding hydrophilic polymers—like poly(vinyl alcohol) (PVA)—improves the solubility and dispersity of pectin nanoparticles, therefore qualifying them for aqueous formulations [37]. These changes also improve pectin's stimuli-responsive properties, thus permitting exact medication release in response to certain triggers in the tumor microenvironment, such as acidic pH or raised redox potential [32]. Ligands may be conjugated to pectin to enhance the specificity of medication delivery systems. Pectin nanoparticles may selectively bind to overexpressed receptors on cancer cells by conjugating peptides, antibodies, or tiny compounds like folic acid, therefore reducing off-target effects [38]. Folic acid–modified pectin nanoparticles demonstrate superior absorption by cancer cells that overexpress folate receptors, resulting in increased therapeutic effectiveness and less systemic toxicity [39]. Furthermore, pectin functionalized with RGD peptides targets integrin receptors, often overexpressed in tumor vasculature, therefore facilitating efficient tumor targeting and drug distribution [40].

The advancement of hybrid systems that integrate pectin with other polymers or nanomaterials has broadened its uses in cancer treatment [41]. Hybrid nanoparticles that consist of pectin and chitosan utilize the synergistic characteristics of both biopolymers, leading to enhanced stability, increased drug encapsulation efficiency, and a responsive behavior to pH changes [42]. Pectin-based systems with inorganic nanomaterials like gold or iron oxide nanoparticles may be used for imaging and photothermal treatment. These hybrid technologies improve theranostics by diagnosing and treating simultaneously [43]. Microfluidics and spray drying have enabled large-scale manufacturing of functionalized pectin nanoparticles with exact size, shape, and drug loading efficiency [19]. Microfluidic methods rapidly combine pectin and crosslinking chemicals to create homogenous nanoparticles with consistent characteristics [44]. Spray-drying encapsulates thermosensitive medicines and bioactive molecules in pectin matrix, maintaining their stability and activity [45]. In summary, the functionalization and modification of pectin provide a flexible foundation for the development of sophisticated drug delivery systems in cancer treatment. Pectin-based nanoparticles may attain accurate, regulated, and targeted delivery of medicinal medicines by modifying their physicochemical characteristics and integrating targeting ligands or hybrid materials. These advances have substantial potential for enhancing the effectiveness and safety of cancer therapies, facilitating the practical use of pectin-based nanomedicine [46].

11.4 Applications in Targeted Cancer Therapy

Due to their promise, pectin-based nanoparticles are emerging as an effective option for targeted cancer therapy because of their versatility, biocompatibility, and functional tuneability [47]. These nanoparticles' capability of enhancing their efficacy includes the ability to target neoplastic tissues with little to no consequences on healthy tissues [48]. Their unique properties, including pH sensitivity, high drug loading capacity, and stability, provide an effective framework for addressing the limitations of pectin in formulating systems [7]. One of the most important exploits of these pectin nanoparticles is their use within the acidic tumor microenvironment [28].

The natural pH sensitivity of pectin allows the nanoparticles to degrade and release their payload at a gradual rate within the pH range of the tumors, while physically inactive healthy tissues are not touched [49]. In this regard, systems capable of using pH-sensitive materials for targeted systems in which the chemotherapeutic agents, e.g., doxorubicin, will be released only in the regions of tumors have been devised [50]. By controlling the regions that, e.g., doxorubicin, are released out of these systems, these systems are able to attain effective therapeutic results and minimal undesired side effects [6]. For encapsulating a variety of therapeutic agents, including both hydrophilic and hydrophobic medicines, pectin nanoparticles can provide flexible drug delivery platforms. Encapsulation increases solubility, shields the medications from breakdown in the circulation, and permits regulated and continuous release (Figure 11.3) [51]. Combination therapy targeting several cancer cell pathways are possible using functionalized pectin nanoparticles that co-deliver numerous medicines. Doxorubicin and curcumin in pectin-based nanoparticles have synergistic effects, increasing apoptosis and reducing drug resistance in cancer cells [46]. Targeting the tumor microenvironment is another important pectin nanoparticle use. Nanoparticles can modify the tumor microenvironment, enhancing cancer treatments [52]. Pectin nanoparticles cause oxidative stress and death in cancer cells by producing ROS [53]. Enzyme-responsive nanoparticles release their payload precisely when tumor-specific enzymes such as matrix metalloproteinases (MMPs) are present. These interactions with the tumor microenvironment boost therapeutic efficacy and reduce systemic toxicity [31, 54].

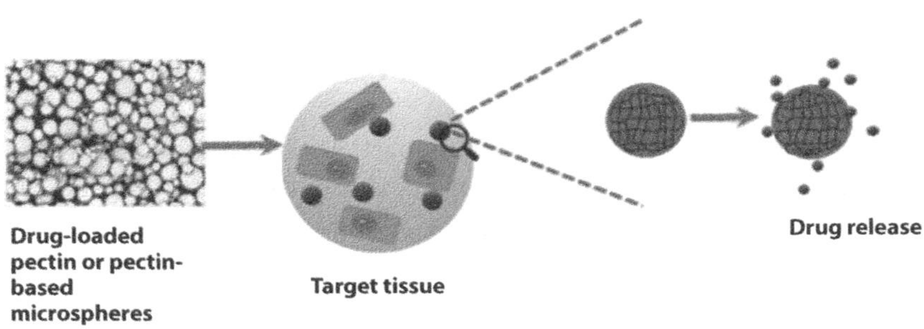

Figure 11.3 Schematic diagram of drug delivery approach using pectin or pectin-based microspheres with controlled release of the drug [31].

By functionalizing pectin nanoparticles with targeting ligands—such as monoclonal antibodies, RGD peptides, or folic acid—their selectivity for cancer cells has been much improved [46]. Folic acid–conjugated pectin nanoparticles, for example, especially target cancer cells overexpressed in folate receptors, hence optimizing medication delivery to the tumor and reducing exposure to healthy cells. In tumor vasculature, RGD peptide-functionalized nanoparticles also target integrin receptors, hence enhancing tumor targeting and lowering angiogenesis [55]. These receptor-mediated targeting techniques guarantee exact delivery of the therapeutic drugs to the tumor, thereby improving treatment effectiveness and lowering adverse effects [39]. Moreover, pectin-based nanoparticles have been used in multimodal treatments—that is, combinations of many therapeutic modalities for optimal outcomes [28]. Photodynamic treatment (PDT) has employed pectin nanoparticles loaded with photosensitizers, including porphyrins or pheophorbide-A, for example. These photosensitizers produce ROS upon light irradiation, therefore inducing localized tumor destruction [56]. By increasing DNA damage in cancer cells, pectin-coated nanoparticles with radiosensitizing chemicals, including platinum nanoparticles, have shown improved therapeutic efficacy in radiotherapy. By means of synergistic processes, the combination of photothermal treatment (PTT) and chemodynamic therapy (CDT) with chemotherapy utilizing pectin nanoparticles magnifies the anticancer effects [57, 58]. The expanding use of hybrid pectin systems in cancer treatment comes from their development. Hybrid systems get improved stability, drug encapsulation effectiveness, and multifunctionality by mixing pectin with other biopolymers, like chitosan or alginate, or using inorganic nanomaterials, including gold or iron oxide nanoparticles [4]. Combining therapy and imaging for real-time monitoring of treatment progress, these technologies also allow theranostics [59]. Also, new fabrication methods like 3D printing and microfluidics have made it possible to create drug delivery systems that target particular sites, such as 3D-printed tablets with pectin nanoparticles for colorectal cancer treatment [19, 60]. Pectin nanoparticles deliver therapeutic chemicals precisely, making them a powerful tool in targeted cancer treatment. They address drug resistance and systemic toxicity in cancer treatment because of their pH sensitivity, tumor microenvironment targeting, and multimodal therapeutic potential [61]. Pectin nanoparticles have the potential to revolutionize cancer nanomedicine and become widely used in clinical settings when new functionalization procedures and hybrid systems are developed [41, 62].

11.5 Mechanisms of Action in Cancer Cells

Pectin-based nanoparticles demonstrate diverse mechanisms of action against cancer cells, engaging multiple cellular pathways to inhibit tumor growth and promote the death of cancer cells [4]. These systems include disturbance of the cell cycle, induction of death by reactive oxygen species (ROS), and immune response modification [8, 51]. These mechanisms help pectin-based systems to be more effective in fighting cancer and to minimize harm to healthy cells [8]. Pectin nanoparticles mostly work by inducing programmed cell death, or death, which is one of the main processes causing their anticancer properties. Many times resistant to death, cancer cells may multiply wildly [63]. Pectin nanoparticles solve this problem by inducing the natural dying route mediated by the mitochondrial membrane [8]. A key element of this process is the formation of reactive oxygen species (ROS). Functionalized pectin nanoparticles—that is, those including photosensitizers or manganese ions—increase ROS generation in cancer cells, hence inducing oxidative stress. This oxidative stress damages DNA, proteins, and lipids, thus causing mitochondrial malfunction, cytochrome c release, and later caspase activation (Figure 11.4), the enzymes in charge of carrying out death [64]. Pectin nanoparticles reduce

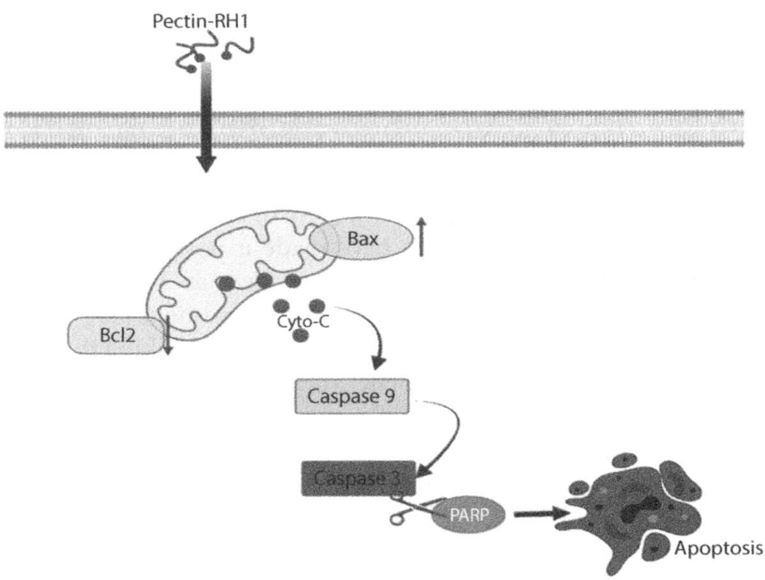

Figure 11.4 Pectin-induced caspase-3-dependent cell death [4].

toxicity to normal cells, which have higher antioxidant defenses, by selectively raising ROS levels in cancer cells [65].

Apart from causing death, pectin nanoparticles significantly disturb the cell cycle, a mechanism crucial for the growth of tumors [47]. Many chemotherapeutic drugs seek to stop cancer cell division by blocking the cell cycle at certain checkpoints [66]. By delivering medicines or functional moieties that interfere with important regulatory proteins engaged in the cell cycle, like cyclins and cyclin-dependent kinases (CDKs), pectin-based systems augment this impact [15, 67]. For example, pectin nanoparticles loaded with doxorubicin have been shown to cause cell cycle arrest in the G2/M phase, therefore stopping cancer cells from entering mitosis [68]. This disturbance causes growth inhibition and increases susceptibility to various treatment modalities like photodynamic therapy [66, 69]. Another important method by which pectin nanoparticles have anticancer action is the regulation of immunological responses [70]. Usually immunosuppressive, the tumor microenvironment lets cancer cells avoid immune monitoring [71]. By activating immune cells and boosting the anti-tumor immune response, pectin nanoparticles assist to offset this [72]. Pectin derivatives, for instance, have been shown to activate macrophages and dendritic cells, hence releasing pro-inflammatory cytokines that draw cytotoxic T lymphocytes to the tumor site [73]. Moreover, pectin-based systems may show tumor-associated antigens to immune cells thereby improving their capacity to identify and kill cancer cells [8]. Moreover, the immunogenic cell death caused by pectin nanoparticles, especially *via* ROS-mediated death, generates danger signals that boost the immune system and hence create a positive feedback loop to stop tumor development [8, 74–76].

Pectin nanoparticles' many and synergistic modes of action in cancer treatment include apoptosis induction *via* ROS production, cell cycle arrest, and immunological regulation [77]. Targeting the tumor microenvironment helps these multifarious activities not only boost the direct cytotoxic effects on cancer cells but also increase the general therapeutic efficiency of pectin-based systems [78]. Constant research of these processes will provide important information on how to maximize pectin nanoparticles for precision oncology.

11.6 Challenges and Limitations

Although pectin-based nanoparticles show great promise for targeted cancer treatment, various issues and restrictions have to be resolved if we are to enable their practical use [47]. The main concerns are the stability in physiological circumstances, manufacturing's scalability, and the natural complexity of tumor heterogeneity and medication resistance [79].

11.6.1 Stability Issues in Physiological Conditions

Ensuring pectin-based nanoparticles' stability under physiological settings is one of the main difficulties in their creation [79]. Naturally hydrophilic and prone to enzymatic breakdown, pectin could cause early drug release in systemic circulation [47, 80]. Maintaining the integrity of the nanoparticles and guaranteeing the regulated release of therapeutic medicines at the tumor site depend on this being seriously limited. Commonly utilized in the production of pectin nanoparticles [81], ionic crosslinking typically produces systems sensitive to ionic strength and pH changes in the circulation, therefore weakening their stability [82]. Strategies include covalent crosslinking, surface modification with hydrophobic polymers, or coating with protective materials like chitosan or polyethylene glycol (PEG), which have been investigated in order to solve these problems [83]. These methods might raise manufacturing complexity and expense even as they enhance stability. While these approaches improve stability, they may also increase production complexity and cost.

11.6.2 Scalability and Manufacturing Constraints

A major obstacle to commercial manufacturing of pectin-based nanoparticles still is scalability. Commonly utilized techniques for nanoparticle synthesis—such as ionic gelation or emulsion techniques—are appropriate for laboratory-scale production but difficult for commercial manufacture [84]. Large-scale manufacturing may be hampered by problems like batch-to-batch variability, limited repeatability, and yield inefficiencies. Further adding to the difficulty of the manufacturing process are the need for exact control over drug loading, size, and shape [83, 85]. By allowing high-throughput, repeatable synthesis with exact control over nanoparticle characteristics [86], emerging technologies as microfluidics and spray-drying provide interesting options. To reach cost-effectiveness, nevertheless, industrial use of these technologies calls for large investment and optimization [87].

11.6.3 Tumor Heterogeneity and Resistance

Tumor heterogeneity, both inter- and intra-tumoral, presents a substantial challenge in the effective application of pectin-based nanoparticles [47]. Tumors are highly diverse in terms of their genetic, cellular, and microenvironmental characteristics, which can significantly affect the uptake, distribution, and efficacy of nanoparticles [88]. Additionally, the presence of cancer stem cells, hypoxic regions, and variable expression of receptors across tumor cells can limit the effectiveness of targeted delivery systems [89]. Moreover, the development of multidrug resistance (MDR) mechanisms, such as overexpression of efflux pumps (e.g., P-glycoprotein) or enhanced DNA repair pathways, further reduces the efficacy of nanoparticle-based therapies [90]. To address these issues, pectin nanoparticles have been functionalized with dual-targeting ligands, incorporated with MDR inhibitors, or co-loaded with multiple therapeutic agents to tackle diverse tumor characteristics and resistance pathways [28, 91]. However, achieving consistent and effective outcomes across heterogeneous tumor populations remains a significant hurdle. Addressing these challenges is critical for advancing the clinical translation of pectin-based nanoparticles in cancer therapy. Innovative strategies to enhance nanoparticle stability, improve manufacturing scalability, and overcome tumor heterogeneity will be essential in optimizing these systems for real-world applications [92]. Collaborative efforts between researchers, clinicians, and industry stakeholders, coupled with advancements in technologies and computational modelling, will play a pivotal role in overcoming these limitations and unlocking the full potential of pectin-based nanomedicine in oncology [93, 94].

11.7 Future Perspectives

The future of pectin-based nanoparticles in cancer therapy is bright, driven by advancements in material science, biotechnology, and computational tools [95]. Emerging trends and innovations are addressing the current challenges, opening new avenues for more effective, precise, and personalized treatments. Below are key areas of development that highlight the promising future of pectin nanotechnology in cancer therapy [4].

11.7.1 Emerging Trends in Pectin Nanotechnology

Pectin nanotechnology is evolving to incorporate novel functionalities and expand its applications in cancer treatment. One significant trend is the development of stimuli-responsive nanoparticles that exploit the tumor microenvironment for controlled drug release [96, 97]. These systems respond to specific triggers, such as pH, redox potential, or enzymatic activity, ensuring the targeted delivery of drugs while sparing healthy tissues [98]. Additionally, the co-delivery of multiple therapeutic agents, such as chemotherapeutics, immune modulators, or gene-editing tools, is gaining traction [99, 100]. By combining these agents into a single nanoparticle, researchers aim to achieve synergistic effects that enhance treatment efficacy and overcome drug resistance [101]. Another emerging trend is the integration of imaging agents into pectin nanoparticles to create theranostic systems. These hybrid systems enable simultaneous cancer diagnosis and therapy, offering real-time monitoring of treatment progress and improving clinical decision-making [102]. The use of biodegradable and eco-friendly materials, such as pectin, aligns with the growing emphasis on sustainable and biocompatible solutions in nanomedicine [103].

11.7.2 Integration with Advanced Technologies

Advances in technology are revolutionizing the design and application of pectin-based nanoparticles, enhancing their functionality and scalability [96].

11.7.2.1 AI-Guided Design

Artificial intelligence (AI) and machine learning are becoming integral to the design of nanoparticles [104]. These technologies can analyze large datasets to predict optimal nanoparticle formulations, functionalization strategies, and drug release profiles [105]. AI-guided modelling can streamline the design process, reducing experimental costs and accelerating development timelines [106]. For instance, algorithms can identify the best combinations of functional groups, crosslinking agents, or targeting ligands to achieve desired therapeutic outcomes [107]. Additionally, AI can simulate nanoparticle interactions with the tumor microenvironment, providing insights into their distribution, uptake, and efficacy [108].

11.7.2.2 Hybrid Systems with Other Polymers

Combining pectin with other biopolymers or nanomaterials offers enhanced functionality and versatility [28]. Hybrid systems leverage the complementary properties of different materials, such as the stability of chitosan or the responsiveness of hyaluronic acid, to create multifunctional nanoparticles [31]. These systems can simultaneously address multiple therapeutic challenges, such as stability, drug loading, and targeting efficiency [79]. Moreover, the incorporation of inorganic materials like gold or iron oxide nanoparticles into pectin systems enables additional capabilities, such as photothermal therapy or magnetic targeting, expanding the therapeutic and diagnostic potential of these platforms [109, 110].

11.7.3 Toward Clinical Translation

While pectin-based nanoparticles have shown significant promise in preclinical studies, their clinical translation requires addressing several critical factors [8, 51]. Enhancing scalability and reproducibility in manufacturing is paramount. Techniques like microfluidics and 3D printing offer potential solutions, providing precise control over nanoparticle size, morphology, and drug loading at industrial scales [96, 111]. Regulatory approval processes also demand comprehensive data on the safety, efficacy, and pharmacokinetics of these nanoparticles, necessitating rigorous preclinical and clinical evaluations [112–114]. Another essential step toward clinical adoption is fostering collaboration among researchers, clinicians, and industry stakeholders. These partnerships can bridge the gap between laboratory research and real-world applications, ensuring that pectin-based systems are optimized for clinical needs [115, 116]. Furthermore, developing personalized formulations tailored to individual patient profiles is becoming increasingly feasible with advancements in precision medicine [117, 118]. By integrating pectin-based systems with patient-specific data, such as genetic or proteomic information, it will be possible to deliver more effective and targeted therapies [15, 31, 67].

The future of pectin nanotechnology in cancer therapy is marked by innovation and interdisciplinary collaboration. Emerging trends in stimuli-responsive systems, theranostics, and multimodal therapies are expanding the therapeutic potential of pectin-based nanoparticles [51, 96]. Integration with advanced technologies like AI and hybrid material systems further enhances their functionality and scalability [105, 106]. By addressing current challenges and advancing toward clinical translation, pectin nanoparticles are poised to become a cornerstone in the next generation of precision oncology, offering safer, more effective, and personalized cancer treatments [105, 106, 108, 110, 115].

11.8 Conclusion

Promising platform in the realm of cancer nanomedicine, pectin-based nanoparticles have special benefits like biocompatibility, biodegradability, and wide chemical functionalizing capability. For focused drug delivery systems, their natural characteristics—including pH sensitivity and strong drug-loading potential—make them perfect. Pectin nanoparticles solve important obstacles in cancer therapy including systemic toxicity, multidrug resistance, and tumor heterogeneity by allowing controlled release, receptor-mediated targeting, and multimodal therapeutic techniques. Pectin nanoparticles are flexible in that they may be customized for particular uses. Targeting ligands and functionalizing with other materials improves their stability, specificity, and therapeutic potency, hybridizing with other materials. Furthermore, extending their use are developments in stimuli-responsive systems, co-delivery platforms, and integration with imaging agents, thus facilitating concurrent diagnosis and treatment. These developments place pectin nanoparticles as a pillar of precision oncology as they may provide safer and more efficient therapies. Successful clinical translation depends on addressing issues such as stability in physiological circumstances, scalability in manufacturing, and tumor heterogeneity even if their great promise calls for attention. Promising methods to break through these limitations include emerging technologies such as 3D printing, microfluidic manufacturing, and AI-guided design. Preclinical research and clinical adoption will be bridged in great part by cooperative efforts among researchers, doctors, and industry players. Pectin-based nanoparticles, then, are a revolutionary development in cancer treatment. These technologies are ready to transform cancer therapy as research keeps improving their design and functioning and as material science and nanotechnology combine. Pectin-based nanoparticles have a bright future in the battle against cancer given their ability to provide tailored, exact, and less intrusive treatments.

AI disclosure statement: The author acknowledges the use of AI-based tools for minor language editing or grammatical correction. However, all intellectual contributions, analyses, and conclusions presented in this chapter are entirely the author's own.

References

1. Barrera-Chamorro, L., Fernandez-Prior, A., Rivero-Pino, F., Montserrat-de la Paz, S., A comprehensive review on the functionality and biological relevance of pectin and the use in the food industry. *Carbohydr. Polym.*, 348, 122794, 2025, https://doi.org/10.1016/J.CARBPOL.2024.122794.
2. Roy, S., Priyadarshi, R., Łopusiewicz, L., Biswas, D., Chandel, V., Rhim, J.W., Recent progress in pectin extraction, characterization, and pectin-based films for active food packaging applications: A review. *Int. J. Biol. Macromol.*, 239, 124248, 2023, https://doi.org/10.1016/J.IJBIOMAC.2023.124248.
3. Roman-Benn, A., Contador, C.A., Li, M.W., Lam, H.M., Ah-Hen, K., Ulloa, P.E., *et al.*, Pectin: An overview of sources, extraction and applications in food products, biomedical, pharmaceutical and environmental issues. *Food Chem. Adv.*, 2, 100192, 2023, https://doi.org/10.1016/J.FOCHA.2023.100192.
4. Picot-Allain, M.C.N. and Neergheen, V.S., Pectin a multifaceted biopolymer in the management of cancer: A review. *Heliyon*, 9, e22236, 2023, https://doi.org/10.1016/J.HELIYON.2023.E22236.
5. Yi, L., Cheng, L., Yang, Q., Shi, K., Han, F., Luo, W., *et al.*, Source, Extraction, Properties, and Multifunctional Applications of Pectin: A Short Review. *Polym.*, 16, 2883, 2024, https://doi.org/10.3390/POLYM16202883.
6. Hu, S., Zhao, R., Shen, Y., Lyu, B., Revolutionizing drug delivery: The power of stimulus-responsive nanoscale systems. *Chem. Eng. J.*, 496, 154265, 2024, https://doi.org/10.1016/J.CEJ.2024.154265.
7. Li, D., Li, J., Dong, H., Li, X., Zhang, J., Ramaswamy, S., *et al.*, Pectin in biomedical and drug delivery applications: A review. *Int. J. Biol. Macromol.*, 185, 49–65, 2021, https://doi.org/10.1016/J.IJBIOMAC.2021.06.088.
8. Emran, T.B., Islam, F., Mitra, S., Paul, S., Nath, N., Khan, Z., *et al.*, Pectin: A Bioactive Food Polysaccharide with Cancer Preventive Potential. *Molecules*, 27, 7405, 2022, https://doi.org/10.3390/MOLECULES27217405.
9. Salehi, F., Behboudi, H., Kavoosi, G., Ardestani, S.K., Oxidative DNA damage induced by ROS-modulating agents with the ability to target DNA: A comparison of the biological characteristics of citrus pectin and apple pectin. *Sci. Rep.*, 8, 1, 1–16, 2018, https://doi.org/10.1038/s41598-018-32308-2.
10. Chan, S.Y., Owh, C., Yan, Y., Lim, Q.R.T., Chee, P.L., Zhang, Y., *et al.*, Functionalization and structural evaluation of pectin, in: *Handb Nat Polym*, vol. 2 Funct Surf Modif Prop, pp. 123–54, 2024, https://doi.org/10.1016/B978-0-323-99856-7.00005-7.

11. Sun, L., Liu, H., Ye, Y., Lei, Y., Islam, R., Tan, S., *et al.*, Smart nanoparticles for cancer therapy. *Signal Transduct. Target. Ther.*, 8, 1, 1–28, 2023, https://doi.org/10.1038/s41392-023-01642-x.
12. Peng, X., Fang, J., Lou, C., Yang, L., Shan, S., Wang, Z., *et al.*, Engineered nanoparticles for precise targeted drug delivery and enhanced therapeutic efficacy in cancer immunotherapy. *Acta Pharm. Sin. B*, 14, 3432–56, 2024, https://doi.org/10.1016/J.APSB.2024.05.010.
13. Lara-Espinoza, C., Carvajal-Millán, E., Balandrán-Quintana, R., López-Franco, Y., Rascón-Chu, A., Pectin and Pectin-Based Composite Materials: Beyond Food Texture. *Mol. J. Synth. Chem. Nat. Prod. Chem.*, 23, 942, 2018, https://doi.org/10.3390/MOLECULES23040942.
14. Sahu, T., Ratre, Y.K., Chauhan, S., Bhaskar, L.V.K.S., Nair, M.P., Verma, H.K., Nanotechnology based drug delivery system: Current strategies and emerging therapeutic potential for medical science. *J. Drug Deliv. Sci. Technol.*, 63, 102487, 2021, https://doi.org/10.1016/J.JDDST.2021.102487.
15. Liu, L.S., Fishman, M.L., Kost, J., Hicks, K.B., Pectin-based systems for colon-specific drug delivery *via* oral route. *Biomaterials*, 24, 3333–43, 2003, https://doi.org/10.1016/S0142-9612(03)00213-8.
16. Overchuk, M., Weersink, R.A., Wilson, B.C., Zheng, G., Photodynamic and Photothermal Therapies: Synergy Opportunities for Nanomedicine. *ACS Nano*, 17, 7979–8003, 2023, https://doi.org/10.1021/ACSNANO.3C00891/ASSET/IMAGES/LARGE/NN3C00891_0007.JPEG.
17. Fang, L., Chen, Z., Dai, J., Pan, Y., Tu, Y., Meng, Q., *et al.*, Recent Advances in Strategies to Enhance Photodynamic and Photothermal Therapy Performance of Single-Component Organic Phototherapeutic Agents. *Adv. Sci.*, 12, 7, 2409157, 2025, https://doi.org/10.1002/ADVS.202409157.
18. Khan, M.K., Raza, M., Shahbaz, M., Farooq, U., Akram, M.U., Recent advancement in energy storage technologies and their applications. *J. Energy Storage*, 92, 112112, 2024, https://doi.org/10.1016/J.EST.2024.112112.
19. Liu, X., Sun, A., Brodský, J., Gablech, I., Lednický, T., Vopařilová, P., *et al.*, Microfluidics chips fabrication techniques comparison. *Sci. Rep.*, 14, 1, 1–13, 2024, https://doi.org/10.1038/s41598-024-80332-2.
20. Surolia, R. and Singh, A., Pectin—Structure, Specification, Production, Applications and various Emerging Sources: A Review, in: *World Sustain Ser*, pp. 267–82, 2024, Part F1813, https://doi.org/10.1007/978-3-031-46046-3_13.
21. Kameshwar, A.K.S. and Qin, W., Structural and functional properties of pectin and lignin–carbohydrate complexes de-esterases: A review. *Bioresour. Bioprocess.*, 5, 1–16, 2018, https://doi.org/10.1186/S40643-018-0230-8/FIGURES/5.
22. Khubber, S., Kazemi, M., Amiri Samani, S., Lorenzo, J.M., Simal-Gandara, J., Barba, F.J., Structural-functional Variability in Pectin and Effect of Innovative Extraction Methods: An Integrated Analysis for Tailored Applications. *Food Rev. Int.*, 39, 2352–77, 2023, https://doi.org/10.1080/87559129.2021.1952422.

23. Zdunek, A., Pieczywek, P.M., Cybulska, J., The primary, secondary, and structures of higher levels of pectin polysaccharides. *Compr. Rev. Food Sci. Food Saf.*, 20, 1101–17, 2021, https://doi.org/10.1111/1541-4337.12689.
24. Tang, C., Shi, Z., Wu, J., Zhu, T., Zeng, Q., Yuan, C., *et al.*, Effect of degree of esterification on the stability of high internal phase Pickering emulsions (HIPPEs) fabricated with pectin-whey protein isolate complexes. *Int. J. Food Sci. Technol.*, 59, 4154–65, 2024, https://doi.org/10.1111/IJFS.17175.
25. Abboud, K.Y., Iacomini, M., Simas, F.F., Cordeiro, L.M.C., High methoxyl pectin from the soluble dietary fiber of passion fruit peel forms weak gel without the requirement of sugar addition. *Carbohydr. Polym.*, 246, 116616, 2020, https://doi.org/10.1016/J.CARBPOL.2020.116616.
26. Cao, L., Lu, W., Mata, A., Nishinari, K., Fang, Y., Egg-box model-based gelation of alginate and pectin: A review. *Carbohydr. Polym.*, 242, 116389, 2020, https://doi.org/10.1016/J.CARBPOL.2020.116389.
27. Chandel, V., Biswas, D., Roy, S., Vaidya, D., Verma, A., Gupta, A., Current Advancements in Pectin: Extraction, Properties and Multifunctional Applications. *Foods*, 11, 2683, 2022, https://doi.org/10.3390/FOODS1117 2683.
28. Federico, O.D., Lizeth, L.E.C., Guadalupe, F.A.K., Zuleth, G.R.M., Gomez-Rodriguez Gabriel, H., Alfonso, S.V.J., *et al.*, Pectin nanoparticles: Fabrication and uses, in: *Polysacch Nanoparticles Prep Biomed Appl*, pp. 163–201, 2022, https://doi.org/10.1016/B978-0-12-822351-2.00022-X.
29. Gawkowska, D., Cybulska, J., Zdunek, A., Structure-Related Gelling of Pectins and Linking with Other Natural Compounds: A Review. *Polymers (Basel)*, 10, 7, 762, 2018, https://doi.org/10.3390/POLYM10070762.
30. Ridley, B.L., O'Neill, M.A., Mohnen, D., Pectins: structure, biosynthesis, and oligogalacturonide-related signaling. *Phytochemistry*, 57, 929–67, 2001, https://doi.org/10.1016/S0031-9422(01)00113-3.
31. Sultana, N., Biological Properties and Biomedical Applications of Pectin and Pectin-Based Composites: A Review. *Molecules*, 28, 7974, 2023, https://doi.org/10.3390/MOLECULES28247974.
32. Yue, Y., Wang, B., Xi, W., Liu, X., Tang, S., Tan, X., *et al.*, Modification methods, biological activities and applications of pectin: A review. *Int. J. Biol. Macromol.*, 253, 127523, 2023, https://doi.org/10.1016/J.IJBIOMAC.2023.127523.
33. Tan, J., Luo, Y., Guo, Y., Zhou, Y., Liao, X., Li, D., *et al.*, Development of alginate-based hydrogels: Crosslinking strategies and biomedical applications. *Int. J. Biol. Macromol.*, 239, 124275, 2023, https://doi.org/10.1016/J.IJBIOMAC.2023.124275.
34. Zhang, R., Qin, X., Kong, F., Chen, P., Pan, G., Improving cellular uptake of therapeutic entities through interaction with components of cell membrane. *Drug Deliv.*, 26, 328, 2019, https://doi.org/10.1080/10717544.2019.1582730.
35. Jiménez-Chillarón, J.C., Díaz, R., Ramón-Krauel, M., Omics Tools for the Genome-Wide Analysis of Methylation and Histone Modifications. *Compr.*

Anal. Chem., 63, 81–110, 2014, https://doi.org/10.1016/B978-0-444-62651-6.00004-0.

36. Said, N.S., Olawuyi, I.F., Lee, W.Y., Pectin Hydrogels: Gel-Forming Behaviors, Mechanisms, and Food Applications. *Gels*, 9, 732, 2023, https://doi.org/10.3390/GELS9090732.
37. Belmonte, G.K., Charles, G., Strumia, M.C., Weibel, D.E., Permanent hydrophilic modification of polypropylene and poly(vinyl alcohol) films by vacuum ultraviolet radiation. *Appl. Surf. Sci.*, 382, 93–100, 2016, https://doi.org/10.1016/J.APSUSC.2016.04.091.
38. Salahpour Anarjan, F., Active targeting drug delivery nanocarriers: Ligands. *Nano-Struct. Nano-Objects*, 19, 100370, 2019, https://doi.org/10.1016/J.NANOSO.2019.100370.
39. Yan, S., Na, J., Liu, X., Wu, P., Different Targeting Ligands-Mediated Drug Delivery Systems for Tumor Therapy. *Pharmaceutics*, 16, 248, 2024, https://doi.org/10.3390/PHARMACEUTICS16020248.
40. Thirumalai, A., Girigoswami, K., Pallavi, P., Harini, K., Gowtham, P., Girigoswami, A., Cancer therapy with iRGD as a tumor-penetrating peptide. *Bull. Cancer*, 110, 1288–300, 2023, https://doi.org/10.1016/J.BULCAN.2023.08.009.
41. Ferreira Soares, D.C., Domingues, S.C., Viana, D.B., Tebaldi, M.L., Polymer-hybrid nanoparticles: Current advances in biomedical applications. *Biomed. Pharmacother.*, 131, 110695, 2020, https://doi.org/10.1016/J.BIOPHA.2020.110695.
42. Rampino, A., Borgogna, M., Bellich, B., Blasi, P., Virgilio, F., Cesàro, A., Chitosan-pectin hybrid nanoparticles prepared by coating and blending techniques. *Eur. J. Pharm. Sci.*, 84, 37–45, 2016, https://doi.org/10.1016/J.EJPS.2016.01.004.
43. Sood, A., Arora, V., Shah, J., Kotnala, R.K., Jain, T.K., Multifunctional gold coated iron oxide core-shell nanoparticles stabilized using thiolated sodium alginate for biomedical applications. *Mater. Sci. Eng., C*, 80, 274–81, 2017, https://doi.org/10.1016/J.MSEC.2017.05.079.
44. Ogończyk, D., Siek, M., Garstecki, P., Microfluidic formulation of pectin microbeads for encapsulation and controlled release of nanoparticles. *Biomicrofluidics*, 5, 013405, 2011, https://doi.org/10.1063/1.3569944.
45. Akbarbaglu, Z., Peighambardoust, S.H., Sarabandi, K., Jafari, S.M., Spray drying encapsulation of bioactive compounds within protein-based carriers; different options and applications. *Food Chem.*, 359, 129965, 2021, https://doi.org/10.1016/J.FOODCHEM.2021.129965.
46. Chen, J., Mei, M.S., Xu, Y., Shi, S., Wang, S., Wang, H., Versatile functionalization of pectic conjugate: From design to biomedical applications. *Carbohydr. Polym.*, 306, 120605, 2023, https://doi.org/10.1016/J.CARBPOL.2023.120605.
47. Anjum, S., Hasan, N., Ilmi, R., Pectin-based nanoformulations for therapeutic applications, in: *Polym Nanosyst Theranostic Nanosyst*, vol. 1, pp. 405–39, 2023, https://doi.org/10.1016/B978-0-323-85656-0.00016-4.

48. Aparna, T.N., Kumar, R., Ali, S.R., Patel, D.J., Julekha, K., Begum, T., *et al.*, Silica Nanoparticles: A Promising Vehicle for Anti-Cancer Drugs Delivery. *AAPS PharmSciTech*, 26, 33, 2025, https://doi.org/10.1208/S12249-024-02982-9.
49. Elmizadeh, A., Goli, S.A.H., Mohammadifar, M.A., Characterization of pectin-zein nanoparticles encapsulating tanshinone: Antioxidant activity, controlled release properties, physicochemical stability to environmental stresses. *Food Chem.*, 460, 140613, 2024, https://doi.org/10.1016/J.FOODCHEM.2024.140613.
50. Le, Q.H., Neila, F., Smida, K., Li, Z., Abdelmalek, Z., Tlili, I., pH-responsive anticancer drug delivery systems: Insights into the enhanced adsorption and release of DOX drugs using graphene oxide as a nanocarrier. *Eng. Anal. Boundary Elem.*, 157, 157–65, 2023, https://doi.org/10.1016/J.ENGANABOUND.2023.09.008.
51. Shashidhara, V. and Alwarsamy, M., Pectin nanoforms—a multifaceted polysaccharide and a propitious nanocarrier for medical ailments. *Polym. Bull.*, 81, 4801–18, 2024, https://doi.org/10.1007/S00289-023-04972-6/TABLES/2.
52. Yang, M., Li, J., Gu, P., Fan, X., The application of nanoparticles in cancer immunotherapy: Targeting tumor microenvironment. *Bioact. Mater.*, 6, 1973–87, 2021, https://doi.org/10.1016/J.BIOACTMAT.2020.12.010.
53. Perillo, B., Di Donato, M., Pezone, A., Di Zazzo, E., Giovannelli, P., Galasso, G., *et al.*, ROS in cancer therapy: the bright side of the moon. *Exp. Mol. Med.*, 52, 2, 192–203, 2020, https://doi.org/10.1038/s12276-020-0384-2.
54. Li, M., Zhao, G., Su, W.K., Shuai, Q., Enzyme-Responsive Nanoparticles for Anti-tumor Drug Delivery. *Front. Chem.*, 8, 647, 2020, https://doi.org/10.3389/FCHEM.2020.00647.
55. Farran, B., Montenegro, R.C., Kasa, P., Pavitra, E., Huh, Y.S., Han, Y.K., *et al.*, Folate-conjugated nanovehicles: Strategies for cancer therapy. *Mater. Sci. Eng., C*, 107, 110341, 2020, https://doi.org/10.1016/J.MSEC.2019.110341.
56. Kou, J., Dou, D., Yang, L., Porphyrin photosensitizers in photodynamic therapy and its applications. *Oncotarget*, 8, 81591, 2017, https://doi.org/10.18632/ONCOTARGET.20189.
57. He, M., Chen, S., Yu, H., Fan, X., Wu, H., Wang, Y., *et al.*, Advances in nanoparticle-based radiotherapy for cancer treatment. *IScience*, 28, 111602, 2025, https://doi.org/10.1016/J.ISCI.2024.111602.
58. Shi, S., Zhong, H., Zhang, Y., Mei, Q., Targeted delivery of nano-radiosensitizers for tumor radiotherapy. *Coord. Chem. Rev.*, 518, 216101, 2024, https://doi.org/10.1016/J.CCR.2024.216101.
59. Zhang, W., Xu, P., Zhang, H., Pectin in cancer therapy: A review. *Trends Food Sci. Technol.*, 44, 258–71, 2015, https://doi.org/10.1016/J.TIFS.2015.04.001.
60. Su, R., Wang, F., McAlpine, M.C., 3D printed microfluidics: advances in strategies, integration, and applications. *Lab Chip*, 23, 1279–99, 2023, https://doi.org/10.1039/D2LC01177H.

61. Sun, Q., Yang, Z., Qi, X., Design and Application of Hybrid Polymer-Protein Systems in Cancer Therapy. *Polymers,* 15, 9, 2219, 2023, https://doi.org/10.3390/POLYM15092219.
62. Wieszczycka, K., Staszak, K., Woźniak-Budych, M.J., Litowczenko, J., Maciejewska, B.M., Jurga, S., Surface functionalization – The way for advanced applications of smart materials. *Coord. Chem. Rev.*, 436, 213846, 2021, https://doi.org/10.1016/J.CCR.2021.213846.
63. Yu, C.Y., Wang, Y.M., Li, N.M., Liu, G.S., Yang, S., Tang, G.T., *et al.*, *In vitro* and *in vivo* evaluation of pectin-based nanoparticles for hepatocellular carcinoma drug chemotherapy. *Mol. Pharm.*, 11, 638–44, 2014, https://doi.org/10.1021/MP400412C/ASSET/IMAGES/MEDIUM/MP-2013-00412C_0011.GIF.
64. Peng, Y., Li, X., Gu, P., Cheng, W., Zhang, R., Hu, K., Curcumin-loaded zein/pectin nanoparticles: Caco-2 cellular uptake and the effects on cell cycle arrest and apoptosis of human hepatoma cells (HepG2). *J. Drug Deliv. Sci. Technol.*, 74, 103497, 2022, https://doi.org/10.1016/J.JDDST.2022.103497.
65. Zhang, Q., Luo, Q., Liu, Z., Sun, M., Dong, X., Nano-ROS-generating approaches to cancer dynamic therapy: Lessons from nanoparticles. *Chem. Eng. J.*, 457, 141225, 2023, https://doi.org/10.1016/J.CEJ.2022.141225.
66. Alimbetov, D., Askarova, S., Umbayev, B., Davis, T., Kipling, D., Pharmacological Targeting of Cell Cycle, Apoptotic and Cell Adhesion Signaling Pathways Implicated in Chemoresistance of Cancer Cells. *Int. J. Mol. Sci.*, 19, 1690, 2018, https://doi.org/10.3390/IJMS19061690.
67. Mathew, A.A., Mohapathra, S., Panonnummal, R., Pectin-based drug delivery systems for biomedical applications, in: *Nat. Biopolym. Drug Deliv. Tissue Eng.*, pp. 301–46, 2023, https://doi.org/10.1016/B978-0-323-98827-8.00018-7.
68. Ouyang, J., Yang, M., Gong, T., Ou, J., Tan, Y., Zhang, Z., *et al.*, Doxorubicin-loading core-shell pectin nanocell: A novel nanovehicle for anticancer agent delivery with multidrug resistance reversal. *PLoS One*, 15, e0235090, 2020, https://doi.org/10.1371/JOURNAL.PONE.0235090.
69. Mills, C.C., Kolb, E.A., Sampson, V.B., Development of chemotherapy with cell cycle inhibitors for adult and pediatric cancer therapy. *Cancer Res.*, 78, 320, 2018, https://doi.org/10.1158/0008-5472.CAN-17-2782.
70. Strzelec, M., Detka, J., Mieszczak, P., Sobocińska, M.K., Majka, M., Immunomodulation—a general review of the current state-of-the-art and new therapeutic strategies for targeting the immune system. *Front. Immunol.*, 14, 1127704, 2023, https://doi.org/10.3389/FIMMU.2023.1127704.
71. Fiordoro, S., Rosano, C., Pechkova, E., Barocci, S., Izzotti, A., Epigenetic modulation of immune cells: Mechanisms and implications. *Adv. Biol. Regul.*, 94, 101043, 2024, https://doi.org/10.1016/J.JBIOR.2024.101043.
72. Moyano, D.F., Liu, Y., Peer, D., Rotello, V.M., Modulation of Immune Response using Engineered Nanoparticle Surfaces. *Small*, 12, 76, 2015, https://doi.org/10.1002/SMLL.201502273.

73. Blanco, P., Palucka, A.K., Pascual, V., Banchereau, J., Dendritic cells and cytokines in human inflammatory and autoimmune diseases. *Cytokine Growth Factor Rev.*, 19, 41, 2008, https://doi.org/10.1016/J.CYTOGFR.2007.10.004.
74. Moon, Y., Cho, H., Kim, K., Nano-Delivery of Immunogenic Cell Death Inducers and Immune Checkpoint Blockade Agents: Single-Nanostructure Strategies for Enhancing Immunotherapy. *Pharmaceutics*, 16, 795, 2024, https://doi.org/10.3390/PHARMACEUTICS16060795.
75. Duan, X., Chan, C., Lin, W., Nanoparticle-Mediated Immunogenic Cell Death Enables and Potentiates Cancer Immunotherapy. *Angew. Chem. Int. Ed. Engl.*, 58, 670–80, 2019, https://doi.org/10.1002/ANIE.201804882.
76. Sun, Y., Feng, X., Wan, C., Lovell, J.F., Jin, H., Ding, J., Role of nanoparticle-mediated immunogenic cell death in cancer immunotherapy. *Asian J. Pharm. Sci.*, 16, 129, 2020, https://doi.org/10.1016/J.AJPS.2020.05.004.
77. An, X., Yu, W., Liu, J., Tang, D., Yang, L., Chen, X., Oxidative cell death in cancer: mechanisms and therapeutic opportunities. *Cell Death Dis.*, 15, 8, 1–20, 2024, https://doi.org/10.1038/s41419-024-06939-5.
78. Nogueira, V. and Hay, N., Molecular pathways: reactive oxygen species homeostasis in cancer cells and implications for cancer therapy. *Clin. Cancer Res.*, 19, 4309–14, 2013, https://doi.org/10.1158/1078-0432.CCR-12-1424.
79. Zhou, S., Zhang, W., Han, X., Liu, J., Asemi, Z., The present state and future outlook of pectin-based nanoparticles in the stabilization of Pickering emulsions. *Crit. Rev. Food Sci. Nutr.*, 65, 13, 2562–86, 2025, https://doi.org/10.1080/10408398.2024.2351163.
80. Li, J., Peng, C., Mao, A., Zhong, M., Hu, Z., An overview of microbial enzymatic approaches for pectin degradation. *Int. J. Biol. Macromol.*, 254, 127804, 2024, https://doi.org/10.1016/J.IJBIOMAC.2023.127804.
81. Yetisgin, A.A., Cetinel, S., Zuvin, M., Kosar, A., Kutlu, O., Therapeutic Nanoparticles and Their Targeted Delivery Applications. *Molecules*, 25, 2193, 2020, https://doi.org/10.3390/MOLECULES25092193.
82. Arms, L., Smith, D.W., Flynn, J., Palmer, W., Martin, A., Woldu, A., *et al.*, Advantages and limitations of current techniques for analyzing the biodistribution of nanoparticles. *Front. Pharmacol.*, 9, 388902, 2018, https://doi.org/10.3389/FPHAR.2018.00802/BIBTEX.
83. Khan, I., Saeed, K., Khan, I., Nanoparticles: Properties, applications and toxicities. *Arab. J. Chem.*, 12, 908–31, 2019, https://doi.org/10.1016/J.ARABJC.2017.05.011.
84. Herdiana, Y., Wathoni, N., Shamsuddin, S., Muchtaridi, M., Scale-up polymeric-based nanoparticles drug delivery systems: Development and challenges. *OpenNano*, 7, 100048, 2022, https://doi.org/10.1016/J.ONANO.2022.100048.
85. Jenzsch, M., Gnoth, S., Kleinschmidt, M., Simutis, R., Lübbert, A., Improving the batch-to-batch reproducibility in microbial cultures during recombinant protein production by guiding the process along a predefined total biomass profile. *Bioprocess. Biosyst. Eng.*, 29, 315–21, 2006, https://doi.org/10.1007/S00449-006-0080-1/FIGURES/8.

86. Wu, L., Zhang, J., Watanabe, W., Physical and chemical stability of drug nanoparticles. *Adv. Drug Deliv. Rev.*, 63, 456–69, 2011, https://doi.org/10.1016/J.ADDR.2011.02.001.
87. Yu, Y., Mai, Y., Zheng, Y., Shi, L., Assessing and mitigating batch effects in large-scale omics studies. *Genome Biol.*, 25, 254, 2024, https://doi.org/10.1186/S13059-024-03401-9.
88. Marusyk, A. and Polyak, K., Tumor heterogeneity: causes and consequences. *Biochim. Biophys. Acta*, 1805, 105, 2009, https://doi.org/10.1016/J.BBCAN.2009.11.002.
89. Chen, Z., Han, F., Du, Y., Shi, H., Zhou, W., Hypoxic microenvironment in cancer: molecular mechanisms and therapeutic interventions. *Signal Transduct. Target. Ther.*, 8, 1, 1–23, 2023, https://doi.org/10.1038/s41392-023-01332-8.
90. Emami Nejad, A., Najafgholian, S., Rostami, A., Sistani, A., Shojaeifar, S., Esparvarinha, M., *et al.*, The role of hypoxia in the tumor microenvironment and development of cancer stem cell: a novel approach to developing treatment. *Cancer Cell Int.*, 21, 62, 2021, https://doi.org/10.1186/S12935-020-01719-5.
91. Zhang, F., Pei, X., Peng, X., Gou, D., Fan, X., Zheng, X., *et al.*, Dual crosslinking of folic acid-modified pectin nanoparticles for enhanced oral insulin delivery. *Biomater. Adv.*, 135, 212746, 2022, https://doi.org/10.1016/J.BIOADV.2022.212746.
92. Tong, F., Wang, Y., Gao, H., Progress and challenges in the translation of cancer nanomedicines. *Curr. Opin. Biotechnol.*, 85, 103045, 2024, https://doi.org/10.1016/J.COPBIO.2023.103045.
93. Younis, M.A., Tawfeek, H.M., Abdellatif, A.A.H., Abdel-Aleem, J.A., Harashima, H., Clinical translation of nanomedicines: Challenges, opportunities, and keys. *Adv. Drug Deliv. Rev.*, 181, 114083, 2022, https://doi.org/10.1016/J.ADDR.2021.114083.
94. Mundekkad, D. and Cho, W.C., Nanoparticles in Clinical Translation for Cancer Therapy. *Int. J. Mol. Sci.*, 23, 1685, 2022, https://doi.org/10.3390/IJMS23031685.
95. Wang, B., Hu, S., Teng, Y., Chen, J., Wang, H., Xu, Y., *et al.*, Current advance of nanotechnology in diagnosis and treatment for malignant tumors. *Signal Transduct. Target. Ther.*, 9, 1, 1–65, 2024, https://doi.org/10.1038/s41392-024-01889-y.
96. Huang, M., Sun, Y., Tan, C., Recent advances in emerging pectin-derived nanocarriers for controlled delivery of bioactive compounds. *Food Hydrocolloids*, 140, 108682, 2023, https://doi.org/10.1016/J.FOODHYD.2023.108682.
97. Ahmadi, S., Rabiee, N., Bagherzadeh, M., Elmi, F., Fatahi, Y., Farjadian, F., *et al.*, Stimulus-responsive sequential release systems for drug and gene delivery. *Nano Today*, 34, 100914, 2020, https://doi.org/10.1016/J.NANTOD.2020.100914.
98. Naser, I.H., Zaid, M., Ali, E., Jabar, H.I., Mustafa, A.N., Alubiady, M.H.S., *et al.*, Unveiling innovative therapeutic strategies and future trajectories on

stimuli-responsive drug delivery systems for targeted treatment of breast carcinoma. *Naunyn-Schmiedeberg's Arch. Pharmacol.*, 397, 6, 3747–70, 2023, https://doi.org/10.1007/S00210-023-02885-9.

99. Xu, W., Jia, A., Lei, Z., Wang, J., Jiang, H., Wang, S., *et al.*, Stimuli-responsive prodrugs with self-immolative linker for improved cancer therapy. *Eur. J. Med. Chem.*, 279, 116928, 2024, https://doi.org/10.1016/J.EJMECH.2024.116928.
100. Abdelhamid, M.S., Al-Hassan Wadan, S., Hager Saad, A., El-Dakroury, W.A., *et al.*, Nanoparticle innovations in targeted cancer therapy: advancements in antibody–drug conjugates. *Naunyn-Schmiedeberg's Arch. Pharmacol.*, 2025, 1–21, 2025, https://doi.org/10.1007/S00210-024-03764-7.
101. Yoo, H., Kim, Y., Kim, J., Cho, H., Kim, K., Overcoming Cancer Drug Resistance with Nanoparticle Strategies for Key Protein Inhibition. *Molecules*, 29, 3994, 2024, https://doi.org/10.3390/MOLECULES29173994.
102. Sun, R., Niu, Y., Li, M., Liu, Y., Wang, K., Gao, Z., *et al.*, Emerging trends in pectin functional processing and its fortification for synbiotics: A review. *Trends Food Sci. Technol.*, 134, 80–97, 2023, https://doi.org/10.1016/J.TIFS.2023.03.004.
103. Biswal, T., BadJena, S.K., Pradhan, D., Sustainable biomaterials and their applications: A short review. *Mater. Today Proc.*, 30, 274–82, 2020, https://doi.org/10.1016/J.MATPR.2020.01.437.
104. Olawade, D.B., Ige, A.O., Olaremu, A.G., Ijiwade, J.O., Adeola, A.O., The synergy of artificial intelligence and nanotechnology towards advancing innovation and sustainability - A mini-review. *Nano Trends*, 8, 100052, 2024, https://doi.org/10.1016/J.NWNANO.2024.100052.
105. Adir, O., Poley, M., Chen, G., Froim, S., Krinsky, N., Shklover, J., *et al.*, Integrating Artificial Intelligence and Nanotechnology for Precision Cancer Medicine. *Adv. Mater.*, 32, e1901989, 2019, https://doi.org/10.1002/ADMA.201901989.
106. Yang, L., Wang, H., Leng, D., Fang, S., Yang, Y., Du, Y., Machine learning applications in nanomaterials: Recent advances and future perspectives. *Chem. Eng. J.*, 500, 156687, 2024, https://doi.org/10.1016/J.CEJ.2024.156687.
107. Ertl, P., An algorithm to identify functional groups in organic molecules. *J. Cheminform.*, 9, 36, 2017, https://doi.org/10.1186/S13321-017-0225-Z.
108. Pratap Singh, R., Natarajan, A., Pandey, S., Kumar, D., Pratim Das, K., Nanoparticles and convergence of artificial intelligence for targeted drug delivery for cancer therapy: Current progress and challenges. *Front. Med. Technol.*, 4, 1067144, 2023, https://doi.org/10.3389/FMEDT.2022.1067144.
109. Unnikrishnan, G., Joy, A., Megha, M., Kolanthai, E., Senthilkumar, M., Exploration of inorganic nanoparticles for revolutionary drug delivery applications: a critical review. *Discov. Nano*, 18, 1, 1–44, 2023, https://doi.org/10.1186/S11671-023-03943-0.

110. Mitchell, M.J., Billingsley, M.M., Haley, R.M., Wechsler, M.E., Peppas, N.A., Langer, R., Engineering precision nanoparticles for drug delivery. *Nat. Rev. Drug Discov.*, 20, 2, 101–24, 2020, https://doi.org/10.1038/s41573-020-0090-8.
111. Rosales, T.K.O. and Fabi, J.P., Pectin-based nanoencapsulation strategy to improve the bioavailability of bioactive compounds. *Int. J. Biol. Macromol.*, 229, 11–21, 2023, https://doi.org/10.1016/J.IJBIOMAC.2022.12.292.
112. Halamoda-Kenzaoui, B., Holzwarth, U., Roebben, G., Bogni, A., Bremer-Hoffmann, S., Mapping of the available standards against the regulatory needs for nanomedicines. *Wiley Interdiscip. Rev. Nanomed. Nanobiotechnol.*, 11, e1531, 2018, https://doi.org/10.1002/WNAN.1531.
113. Gupta, D.K., Tiwari, A., Yadav, Y., Soni, P., Joshi, M., Ensuring safety and efficacy in combination products: regulatory challenges and best practices. *Front. Med. Technol.*, 6, 1377443, 2024, https://doi.org/10.3389/FMEDT.2024.1377443.
114. Ali, F., Neha, K., Parveen, S., Current regulatory landscape of nanomaterials and nanomedicines: A global perspective. *J. Drug Deliv. Sci. Technol.*, 80, 104118, 2023, https://doi.org/10.1016/J.JDDST.2022.104118.
115. Castonguay, L.G. and Muran, J.C., Fostering collaboration between researchers and clinicians through building practice-oriented research: an introduction. *Psychother. Res.*, 25, 1–5, 2015, https://doi.org/10.1080/10503307.2014.966348.
116. Shepherd, M., Endacott, R., Quinn, H., Bridging the gap between research and clinical care: strategies to increase staff awareness and engagement in clinical research. *J. Res. Nurs.*, 27, 168, 2022, https://doi.org/10.1177/17449871211034545.
117. Ho, D., Quake, S.R., McCabe, E.R.B., Chng, W.J., Chow, E.K., Ding, X., *et al.*, Enabling technologies for personalized and precision medicine. *Trends Biotechnol.*, 38, 497, 2020, https://doi.org/10.1016/J.TIBTECH.2019.12.021.
118. Mathur, S. and Sutton, J., Personalized medicine could transform healthcare. *Biomed. Rep.*, 7, 3, 2017, https://doi.org/10.3892/BR.2017.922.

12

Alginate Nanoparticles: Advances in Cancer Therapy

Andleeb Amin[1] and Showkat Ali Ganie[2]*

[1]*Department of Chemistry, School of Chemical Engineering and Physical Sciences, Lovely Professional University, Phagwara, Punjab, India*
[2]*Department of Chemistry and Earth Sciences, College of Arts and Sciences, Qatar University, Doha, Qatar*

Abstract

Alginate-based nanoparticles have emerged as a versatile platform in cancer therapy, addressing critical challenges such as poor drug solubility, systemic toxicity, and multidrug resistance. Derived from natural sources, alginate offers exceptional biocompatibility, biodegradability, and functional versatility, enabling the development of nanoparticles tailored for precise drug delivery and controlled release. Advanced fabrication techniques, such as ionic gelation and microfluidics, have facilitated the creation of alginate nanoparticles with enhanced stability and targeting capabilities. These nanoparticles are utilized in multimodal therapies, including chemo-photothermal-radiotherapy, and stimuli-responsive systems that release therapeutic agents in response to tumor-specific triggers like pH and redox potential. Despite challenges such as scalability and tumor heterogeneity, innovations like hybrid systems and AI-guided design are paving the way for clinical translation. Alginate nanoparticles represent a promising advancement in precision oncology, offering safer and more effective therapeutic options for cancer treatment.

***Keywords*:** Alginate nanoparticles, cancer therapy, drug delivery systems, stimuli-responsive nanocarriers, multimodal cancer treatment, precision oncology

**Corresponding author*: alishowkat443@gmail.com

Luqman Jameel Rather, Showkat Ali Ganie and Mohammed A. Assiri (eds.) Polysaccharide Biomaterials in Cancer Research and Therapy: From Lab to Life, (365–392) © 2026 Scrivener Publishing LLC

12.1 Introduction

Alginate, a naturally occurring polysaccharide derived from brown seaweed, has garnered significant attention in the field of nanomedicine for its unique properties and versatile applications. Composed of mannuronic acid (M) and guluronic acid (G) units, alginate exhibits excellent biocompatibility, biodegradability, and the ability to form hydrogels through ionic crosslinking [1]. These characteristics make it an ideal candidate for the development of nanoparticles designed to address critical challenges in cancer therapy. In cancer treatment, the use of nanoparticles has revolutionized drug delivery by enabling precise targeting, controlled release, and reduced systemic toxicity. Alginate-based nanoparticles stand out due to their ability to encapsulate a wide variety of therapeutic agents, including hydrophilic and hydrophobic drugs, nucleic acids, and peptides [2]. Additionally, their tunable properties allow for modifications that enhance drug stability and delivery efficiency. For example, ionic gelation, a simple and eco-friendly fabrication technique, enables the production of alginate nanoparticles with minimal use of harsh chemicals, ensuring compatibility with sensitive therapeutic agents.

Alginate nanoparticles offer significant advantages in overcoming the limitations of conventional cancer therapies. Their ability to respond to tumor-specific stimuli, such as pH and enzyme activity, ensures the localized release of drugs in the tumor microenvironment, minimizing damage to healthy tissues. Furthermore, alginate nanoparticles can be functionalized with targeting ligands, such as antibodies or peptides, to selectively bind to cancer cells, enhancing the therapeutic index of encapsulated agents [3]. These features make them highly effective in tackling multidrug resistance and improving treatment outcomes. Recent advancements in alginate nanoparticle technology have expanded their scope of application, from delivering chemotherapeutics and gene therapies to acting as carriers for combination treatments. Their role in modulating the tumor microenvironment, improving drug permeability, and enhancing immune response has opened new avenues in cancer nanomedicine. Moreover, the integration of alginate nanoparticles with advanced technologies, such as stimuli-responsive systems and hybrid materials, is paving the way for the next generation of cancer therapies. The alginate nanoparticles represent a powerful tool in the fight against cancer, offering a combination of biocompatibility, versatility, and therapeutic efficacy [4]. As research continues to refine their design and functionality, alginate-based systems are poised to play a pivotal role in advancing precision medicine and improving patient outcomes in cancer therapy.

12.2 Structure and Chemistry of Alginate

Alginate is a naturally occurring anionic polysaccharide primarily extracted from the cell walls of brown seaweed. Its unique structure and chemical properties make it an attractive material for biomedical applications, particularly in the development of nanoparticles for cancer therapy. Chemically, alginate is composed of two monomeric units: β-D-mannuronic acid (M) and α-L-guluronic acid (G), linked through 1→4 glycosidic bonds. These units are arranged in homopolymeric (MM or GG) and heteropolymeric (MG) blocks along the alginate chain. The ratio and sequence of these blocks vary depending on the source of the alginate, significantly influencing its physical and chemical properties [5]. For instance, alginate with a high G content forms stronger hydrogels due to the tight packing of GG blocks, whereas alginate with higher M content exhibits more flexibility.

A defining feature of alginate is its ability to undergo ionic gelation in the presence of divalent cations such as calcium (Ca^{2+}) or barium (Ba^{2+}). This property enables the formation of crosslinked hydrogels and nanoparticles without the need for harsh chemical reagents. The "egg-box" model explains the gelation process, where divalent cations bind selectively to G blocks, forming a three-dimensional network. This crosslinking mechanism provides alginate nanoparticles with excellent mechanical stability and tunable properties, such as swelling and degradation rates, which are essential for controlled drug delivery [6]. The chemical versatility of alginate lies in its abundance of hydroxyl and carboxyl functional groups. These groups facilitate various chemical modifications to enhance the functionality of alginate for specific applications:

- **Conjugation of targeting ligands**: Functional groups can be used to attach molecules such as folic acid, antibodies, or peptides, enabling selective targeting of cancer cells.
- **Hydrophobic modifications**: By attaching hydrophobic moieties, alginate can encapsulate hydrophobic drugs, improving their solubility and stability.
- **Stimuli-responsive functionalization**: Alginate can be modified to respond to pH, temperature, or enzymatic activity, enabling precise drug release in the tumor microenvironment.

Alginate's biocompatibility and biodegradability further enhance its appeal as a biomaterial for cancer therapy [6]. It degrades naturally into harmless monosaccharides through hydrolysis or enzymatic activity, making it safe for use *in vivo*. Its biocompatibility ensures minimal immunogenic response, reducing the risk of adverse effects in clinical applications. In conclusion, the structure and chemistry of alginate provide a versatile foundation for designing nanoparticles tailored to specific therapeutic needs. Its ability to form stable crosslinked networks, combined with chemical modifiability and biocompatibility, makes alginate an indispensable material in the field of cancer nanomedicine [7]. These properties not only enable efficient drug delivery but also open opportunities for developing advanced multifunctional therapeutic systems.

12.3 Synthesis of Alginate Nanoparticles

The synthesis of alginate nanoparticles is a critical step in leveraging alginate's properties for biomedical applications, particularly in cancer therapy [8]. Several techniques have been developed to fabricate alginate nanoparticles, each with unique advantages and applications. These methods focus on achieving desired nanoparticle size, stability, and drug encapsulation efficiency while maintaining the biocompatibility of the alginate material.

12.3.1 Ionic Gelation

Ionic gelation is one of the most widely used methods for synthesizing alginate nanoparticles due to its simplicity, mild conditions, and eco-friendliness [9]. This technique involves the crosslinking of alginate molecules with divalent cations, such as calcium (Ca^{2+}), under aqueous conditions.

- **Process**: A solution of sodium alginate is mixed with a solution containing divalent cations. The cations bind to the guluronic acid (G) residues in alginate, forming crosslinked nanoparticles through the "egg-box" model.
- **Applications**: This method is particularly effective for encapsulating hydrophilic drugs or sensitive biological molecules such as proteins and peptides.
- **Advantages**: It avoids the use of organic solvents and harsh chemicals, ensuring compatibility with sensitive therapeutic agents.

12.3.2 Emulsion Techniques

Emulsion-based methods are used to create alginate nanoparticles by forming a dispersed phase of alginate in an immiscible organic phase [10].

- **Water-in-oil (W/O) emulsion**: Alginate is dispersed in an organic solvent, and crosslinking is induced by adding calcium chloride or other cationic crosslinkers. The emulsion droplets act as templates, and the size of the nanoparticles is controlled by varying the emulsion conditions.
- **Advantages**: This method is ideal for encapsulating both hydrophilic and hydrophobic drugs, as the dispersed phase can be tailored to accommodate various payloads.
- **Limitations**: The use of organic solvents can pose challenges for biocompatibility and scalability.

12.3.3 Nanoprecipitation

Nanoprecipitation is a solvent displacement method where alginate is dissolved in a solvent that is miscible with water but does not dissolve alginate [11].

- **Process**: Alginate is precipitated by adding a non-solvent phase, typically under stirring, which results in the formation of nanoparticles.
- **Applications**: This technique is useful for fabricating alginate nanoparticles with high drug loading efficiency and controlled particle size.
- **Advantages**: It is a straightforward and reproducible process suitable for large-scale production.

12.3.4 Spray Drying

Spray drying is a scalable method used to produce alginate nanoparticles by atomizing alginate solutions into a hot air chamber [12].

- **Process**: Alginate and crosslinking agents are fed into a spray dryer, where rapid solvent evaporation forms dry nanoparticles.
- **Applications**: It is widely used for encapsulating drugs that require long-term stability and for creating inhalable nanoparticles for lung cancer therapy.

- **Advantages**: This method offers excellent control over particle size and morphology, making it suitable for industrial-scale production.

12.3.5 Microfluidics

Microfluidic techniques involve the controlled mixing of alginate and crosslinking solutions in microchannels to form nanoparticles with high precision [13].

- **Process**: Alginate is introduced into microfluidic devices, where it interacts with calcium ions in a controlled manner to produce uniform nanoparticles.
- **Applications**: Microfluidics is ideal for producing monodisperse nanoparticles for advanced applications, such as drug delivery systems tailored to specific therapeutic needs.
- **Advantages**: This method provides precise control over nanoparticle size and structure, enhancing reproducibility and scalability.

12.3.6 Polyelectrolyte Complexation

Polyelectrolyte complexation involves the interaction of alginate with positively charged polymers, such as chitosan, to form nanoparticles [14].

- **Process**: Alginate and chitosan solutions are mixed under mild conditions, leading to the formation of nanoparticles through electrostatic interactions.
- **Applications**: This method is particularly useful for creating multi-functional nanoparticles with enhanced stability and drug release profiles.
- **Advantages**: It allows for the incorporation of multiple functional agents, making it versatile for diverse therapeutic applications.

The choice of synthesis method for alginate nanoparticles depends on the intended application, desired particle size, and type of therapeutic agent to be encapsulated. Ionic gelation and emulsion techniques are widely used for their simplicity and versatility, while advanced methods like microfluidics and spray drying are gaining popularity for their scalability and precision [15]. By optimizing these synthesis techniques, alginate nanoparticles can be tailored to meet the complex demands of cancer therapy, ensuring efficient drug delivery and improved patient outcomes.

12.4 Application in Cancer Therapy

Alginate-based nanoparticles have emerged as a versatile and effective tool in modern cancer therapy, addressing limitations in conventional treatments such as systemic toxicity, poor drug solubility, and multi-drug resistance [2]. This section outlines the innovative strategies and mechanisms employed by alginate nanoparticles in the delivery of therapeutic agents, highlighting their multifunctionality, biocompatibility, and targeted delivery capabilities. The synthesis and characterization of SnO_2–sodium alginate–polyethylene glycol crocin nanoparticles were accomplished, focusing on their structural, optical, and potential applications in anticancer and antimicrobial fields [16]. This novel methodology shows potential in tackling the issues of antibiotic resistance, cancer therapy, and the advancement of more efficient and accurate medicinal remedies. The nanoparticle cytotoxicity was assessed on HeLa cells using MTT assay. The administration of nanoparticles exhibited a potential increase in cellular apoptosis in HeLa cells, as evidenced by the results of the MTT assay. The effects of the nanoparticles on endogenous reactive oxygen species generation in HeLa cells were tested, and the results showed that the nanoparticles increased reactive oxygen species production. This leads to the occurrence of apoptotic cell death and nuclear damage, which is distinguished by the depolarization of the mitochondrial membrane and a reduction in the level of matrix metalloproteinase [17]. Tumor environment dual-response nanoparticles were prepared by using a facial assembly of alginate oligosaccharides, halloysite, and doxorubicin to overcome the tumor penetration, poor stability, and uncontrolled drug release of the nanoparticle-based drug delivery. Following the modification of halloysite with hydrophilic alginate oligosaccharides, it is expected that the EPR effect will result in the halloysite exhibiting effective accumulation and circulation within the tumor. Enzymes that are found in the microenvironment of the tumor can degrade the alginate oligosaccharides that are pH-responsive and lysozyme-degradable, which are wrapping the surface of the halloysite and allow these particles to be released. The cytotoxicity of the nanoparticles was assessed in lung cancer cell model A549 cells and normal cell model L132 cells by using MTT assay, which reveals that the cancer cell death induction occurs through reactive oxygen species and mitochondrial membrane potential [18]. Sodium alginate SnO_2 nanoparticles were prepared through a one pot green approach using Amomum subulatum as a reducing agent. The WST-1 assay was used to explore anticancer and toxicity study on breast cancer MDAMB-231, MCF-7, and fibroblast cells. The sodium alginate SnO_2 nanoparticles treated with both breast cancer cells exhibit lower IC_{50} values and lower colony count as compared to SnO_2 nanoparticles. These nanoparticles exhibit reduced particle sizes and increased surface defects, namely oxygen vacancies. Consequently, upon interaction with cancer cells, these nanoparticles induce a heightened production of reactive oxygen species, which have the ability to oxidize and degrade macromolecules. This leads to substantial oxidative stress, which has the potential to degrade cancer cells. These nanoparticles produce Sn ions, which can engage with macromolecules and induce death

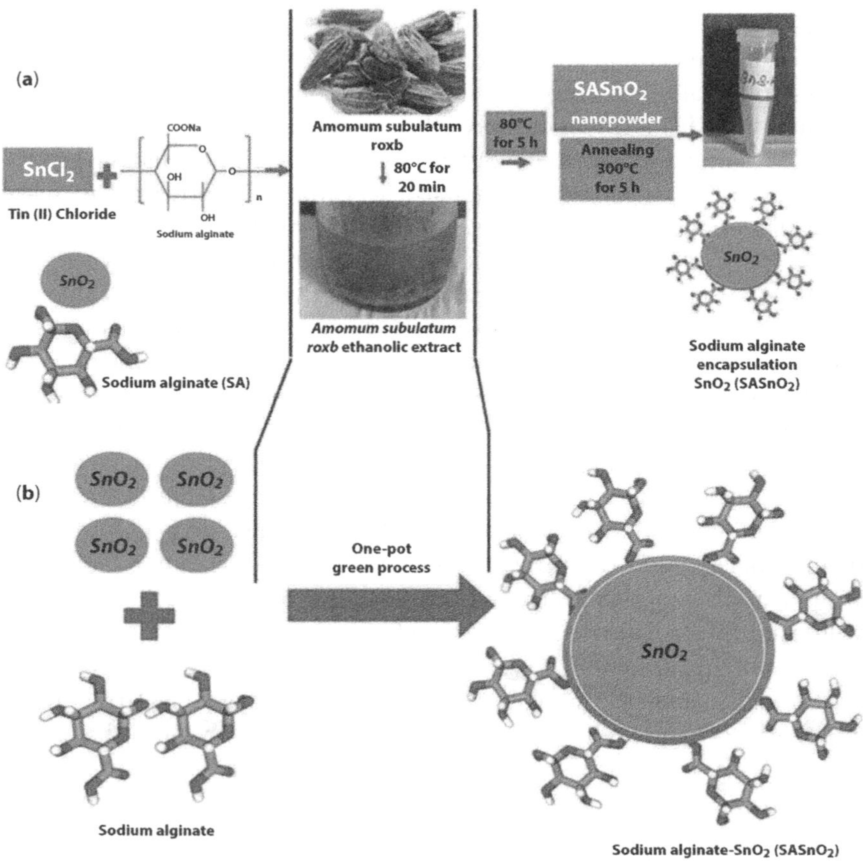

Figure 12.1 Synthesis of alginate nanoparticles using different methods [19].

to cancer cells. The mitochondrial electron transport pathway produces reactive oxygen species, the most common kind of free radicals, when cell is under oxidative stress, which leads to increased DNA damage in cancer cells [19] (Figure 12.1).

Luminescent nanoparticles based on alginate and curcumin were designed, synthesized, and tested for anticancer applications. The fluorescent polymer nanoparticles based on alginate were first produced *via* a multicomponent Ugi reaction. Three cell lines (L929 cells, MC3T3-E1 cells, and SV-HUC-1 cells) were used in the cell counting kit-8 (CCK-8) experiment to study the cell toxicity of these nanoparticles. The cytotoxicity studies show that there was essentially no change in the cell viability values after incubating three cell lines with varying concentrations of these nanoparticles. In particular, the nanoparticles continued to display remarkable cell viability and even a propensity to stimulate cell growth at the higher doses. These nanoparticles were endowed with fluorescent property through the introduction of aggregation-induced emission active material, resulting in clear excitation-dependent fluorescence. The emission, which encompasses a range of colors from blue to red, demonstrated exceptional capabilities in multicolor imaging. The synthesized nanoparticles exhibited consistent micelle characteristics, rendering them suitable for drug administration within microenvironments [20] (Figure 12.2).

An ideal formulation of niosome-based carrier that is coated with alginate for the transport of herbal extract Gingerol was developed for the treatment of cancer cells and infections caused by intracellular pathogens. The cytotoxicity of the nanoparticles was studied against the normal HFF cell lines and breast cancer cell lines MDA-MB-231 through MTT assay. The slow release of Gingerol in normal pH from nanoparticles causes less

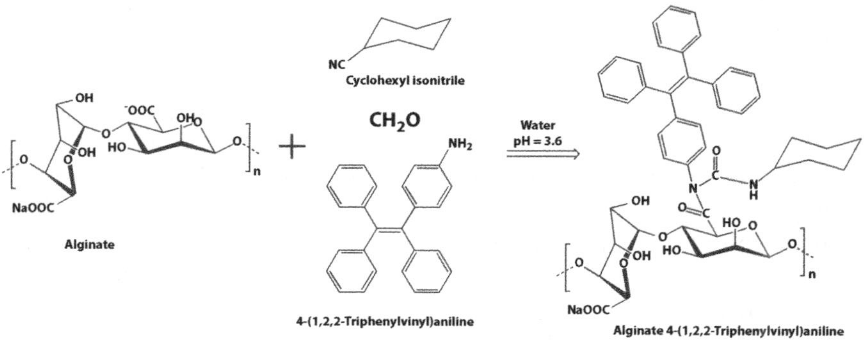

Figure 12.2 The synthetic scheme of alginate triphenyl vinyl aniline [20].

toxicity toward the normal cell line. The cytotoxicity of the nanoparticles was greater in cancer cell lines due to the protective nature of the niosome structure, which hindered the breakdown of drugs and enhanced their uptake by cells. The elevated cytotoxicity seen in modified niosome nanoparticles incorporating alginate can be attributed to the enhanced engagement between nanocarriers and cancer cells facilitated by the presence of alginate on the surface of niosome vesicles. This interaction subsequently results in an accelerated release rate of the drug within the cancer cells [21]. A microfluidic technology was employed to prepare hybrid nanoparticles consisting of carboplatin-loaded alginate and poly(amidoamine). Subsequently, epidermal growth factor was conjugated onto the surface of these nanoparticles to facilitate receptor-targeted delivery. The interaction between epidermal growth factor and the surface of nanoparticles, along with the overexpression of the epidermal growth factor receptor on the surface of non-small cell lung cancer cells, has the potential to trigger receptor-mediated endocytosis. This process can result in enhanced cellular uptake of nanoparticles and a subsequent decrease in cancer cell proliferation. Therefore, the process of epidermal growth factor conjugation was accomplished using carbodiimide chemistry subsequent to the microfluidic synthesis of nanoparticles. Subsequently, the therapeutic efficacy of epidermal growth factor nanoparticles was assessed in both 2D *in vitro* culture and 3D spheroid culture, and their correlation with antitumorigenic activities *in vivo* was examined. The incorporation of epidermal growth factor as a ligand onto the surfaces of nanoparticles leads to increased cytotoxicity in both 2D and 3D tumor cells, in comparison to unconjugated nanoparticles and free carboplatin. The quantitative analysis of tumor tissue revealed that the fluorescence intensity, as assessed by *in vivo* imaging, was significantly reduced when treated with these nanoparticles. This suggests that the tumor size was less compared to the other groups. It is likely that these nanoparticles entered tumor tissues through the epidermal growth factor action and had an antitumor effect. The histological data from the biochemical analysis revealed that the tumor tissues in the groups treated with epidermal growth factor nanoparticles had a greater degree of suppression in comparison to the other groups, resulting in reductions in tumor sizes. At the conclusion of the 21st day, the group that received epidermal growth factor nanoparticles exhibited full eradication of tumor tissue in the mice [22].

An alginate nanogel with multi-stimulus responsiveness was formulated to react to variations in pH and redox potential inside the tumor microenvironment. The nanogels were designed by reacting oxidized alginate with 4-mercapto phenylboronic acid and pheophorbide-A, a hydrophobic photosensitizer, for conjugation with adipic acid dihydrazide. Additionally, doxorubicin, a cytotoxic drug, was included into the nanogel matrix to facilitate the administration of chemotherapy. The alginate nanogel demonstrated the pH-dependent release of both pheophorbide-A and doxorubicin, while also decreasing the redox potential, which improved photodynamic therapy by promoting the generation of reactive oxygen species [23]. A highly effective nanocomposite was synthesized by combining sodium alginate with polyethylene glycol. This nanocomposite was then filled with tin oxide nanoparticles, which were created through the utilization of carvacrol, a phenolic monoterpene that is found in the essential oil of plants belonging to the Lamiaceae family. The cytotoxic effect of the nanocomposite on carcinoma cells was evaluated by subjecting the nanocomposite to KYSE-150–7 cells, which are squamous carcinoma cells of the esophagus. In KYSE-150–7 cells, the nanocomposite dramatically increases the rate of cell death, as revealed by MTT assay experiment. The nanocomposite treatment results rise in the formation of reactive oxygen species as well as an increase in the potential of the mitochondrial membrane, which ultimately led to the death of the cells. In addition to causing a considerable reduction in the levels of glutathione and superoxide dismutase, the nanocomposite also caused a rise in the levels of thiobarbituric acid reactive compounds, which is an indicative of cell damage [24].

A nanocomposite was formulated by combining α-Fe_2O_3 sodium alginate eugenol to examine their synergism in *in vivo* hepatotoxicity models and on liver cancer cells. MTT assay was used to determine the cytotoxicity of the nanocomposite against Hep3B cells. The impact of the nanocomposite on the cell growth of Hep3B cells through MTT assay revealed that the exposure of the nanocomposite reduced the cell growth in a dose-dependent manner. The impact of nanoparticles on the levels of reactive oxygen species in Hep3B cells was investigated using DCFH-DA staining. The results indicated that control cells did not exhibit any fluorescence. However, when cells were exposed to nanocomposites prior to being combined with DCFH-DA, a significant increase in fluorescence was observed. The results demonstrated a heightened fluorescence spike compared to the control cells, indicating that the nanocomposite exposure results in an augmentation of reactive oxygen species accumulation. These results indicate that nanocomposites enhance the buildup of endogenous reactive oxygen species in tumor cells. The nanocomposites were able to reduce mitochondrial membrane potential, induced DNA alterations, significantly lengthened comet tails in the Hep3B cells, and damaged the DNA of liver cancer cells. The histopathological examination of zebrafish liver tissue after a 7-day exposure to these nanocomposites revealed no significant alterations. This suggests that nanocomposites exhibit a non-toxic character across several dosages [25].

The synthesis, characterization, and implementation of alginate coated platinum nanoparticles were carried out to enhance the efficacy of X-ray therapy in breast cancer by acting as a radiosensitizer. A simple and eco-friendly method was developed to obtain these nanoparticles in aqueous solution. Alginate solution was supplemented with platinum salt, which underwent reduction by sodium borohydride through its interaction with negative functional groups and subsequent entrapment within the unoccupied spaces of the alginate. After the formation of platinum nanoparticles, the process of dialysis was employed to achieve the purification of the nanoparticles and eliminate any unreacted ions. The alginate polymer is of significant importance in enhancing the aqueous solubility, physical stability, and biocompatibility platinum nanoparticles. The cytotoxicity of these nanoparticles was studied against mouse breast carcinoma cell line (4 T1 cell line) through MTT assay, which showed that the cytotoxicity was dependent on the concentration of the nanoparticles. At a concentration of 50 μg/mL, the cell viability was 86%. However, as the concentration increased to 400 μg/mL, the cell viability decreased to 57%. At equivalent concentrations, the vitality of normal cells was shown to be approximately 91% and 72%, respectively. The radiosensitizing effect of these nanoparticles was evaluated by exposing the cancerous cells to X-rays in conjunction with the nanoparticles. The combination of irradiation and nanoparticle therapy had a positive effect on the reduction of cell viability. There was a considerable decrease in the number of viable cells that were present after the cells were exposed to X-rays. The radiosensitizing action of the nanoparticles following X-ray irradiation was responsible for the considerable increase in cytotoxicity that was obtained by increasing the concentration of the nanoparticles [26].

To create a regulated release of etoposide while simultaneously improving its hydrophilicity, a pH-responsive alginate-based nanogel was synthesized. This was accomplished by grafting alginate with 2-hydroxypropyl methacrylamide using a microwave-supported approach. MTT assay was performed on fibroblast and H1299 cells, respectively, in order to evaluate the biocompatibility of the drug-free nanogels as well as the anticancer activity of the etoposide-loaded nanogels. When the sample concentration was increased, the proportion of viable cells treated with copolymer and drug-free nanogels maintained approximately 90%, in comparison to the control group. In general, there was a modest decrease in cell viability observed in the nanogels when compared to the copolymer. The MTT assay demonstrated a significant anticancer effect of etoposide-loaded nanogels in a dose-dependent manner. The nanogels showed a maximum cytotoxicity of 70.86% at a concentration of 160 μg/mL in comparison to free etoposide, which exhibited a cytotoxicity of 62.30% under the same conditions. This indicates that the nanogel formulation has a higher anticancer activity against the growth of H1299 cells. The synergistic effects were seen as a result of the trapping of etoposide by the nanogels. The nanogels exhibit exceptional stability and dispersity, which, in conjunction with their high etoposide release in the culture medium, is likely to have enhanced cellular absorption in comparison to free etoposide [27] (Figure 12.3).

Alginate nanoparticles containing S-nitroso-mercaptosuccinic acid and/or silver nanoparticles were prepared, characterized, and evaluated for their anticancer and antibacterial activity. Nanoparticles of alginate were generated using ionotropic gelation with calcium ions, and these nanoparticles were then utilized to integrate either silver nanoparticles or NO donor nanoparticles. The cytotoxic effects of the nanoparticles at different concentrations were evaluated against fibroblast-like cells of African green monkey cell line (Vero cells) through an MTT assay. After conducting an MTT assay, it was found that alginate nanoparticles did not exhibit cytotoxicity at any of the concentrations that were examined. On the other hand, nanoparticles that included the nitric oxide donor or silver nanoparticles exhibited a toxicity that was dependent on the quantity of the nanoparticles. The combination of S-nitroso-mercaptosuccinic acid with silver nanoparticles enhanced the cytotoxicity of the nanoparticles. The fact that nitric oxide has been shown to be cytotoxic at high doses in

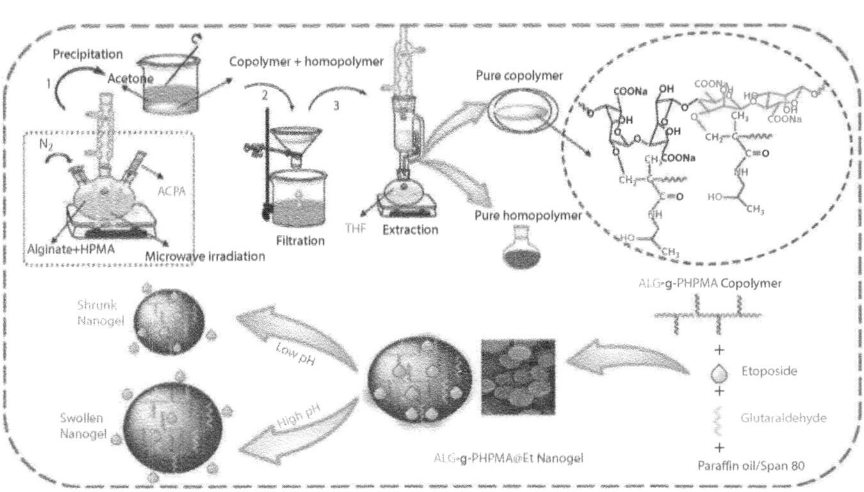

Figure 12.3 Schematic diagram of the nanogel synthesis and pH-responsive release [26].

the past indicates that such type of nanoparticles has the potential to be used in anticancer applications [28].

Sodium alginate, a naturally occurring anionic polysaccharide, was used to stabilize the reduction of silver ions into silver nanoparticles during the synthesis of silver nanoparticles that were built over alginate modified magnetite nanoparticles. The cytotoxicity and anti-lung cancer properties of the synthesized nanocomposite were assessed using the MTT assay on common lung cancer cell lines NCI-H1975, NCI-H1563, and NCI-H1299. The synthesized nanocomposite exhibited a significant decrease in cell viability and showed a dose-dependent increase in anti-lung cancer activity against the NCI-H1975, NCI-H1563, and NCI-H1299 cell lines. Notably, no cytotoxicity was observed on the normal cell line, specifically the human umbilical vein endothelial cells (HUVECs) [29] (Figure 12.4).

Alginate-coated silver sulfide nanoparticles were synthesized, characterized, and evaluated for their cytotoxicity against HFF-2, MCF-7, and 4 T1 cell lines for radio enhancement ability evaluation and biocompatibility. The viability of cultivated HFF-2 cells can be observed to decrease as the concentration of nanoparticles increases. Nevertheless, nanoparticles lacking an alginate coating exhibit an adverse impact on viable cells. An increase in the concentration of nanoparticles results in a considerable rise in cytotoxicity, which can be related to the radiosensitizing impact of the nanoparticles when they are exposed to X-rays. The presence of these nanoparticles increases the susceptibility of cancer cells to radiotherapy, highlighting the crucial role of reactive oxygen species producing nanomaterials in improving the effectiveness of radiotherapy and making cancer cells more responsive to radiation [30]. In an effort to reduce drug dosages and address the issue of multidrug resistance, a novel formulation of

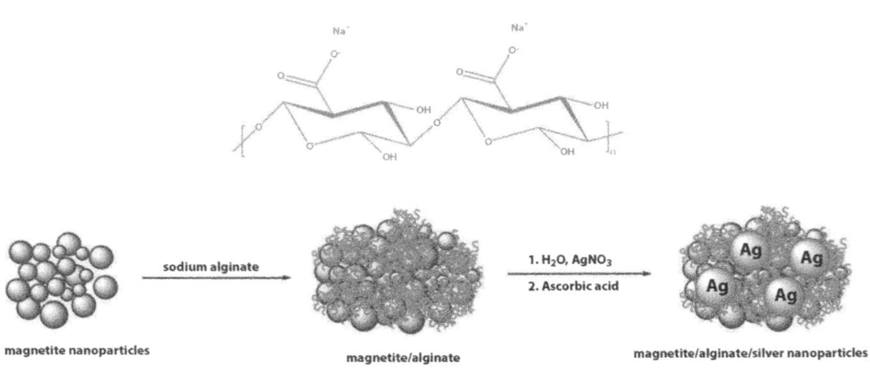

Figure 12.4 Schematic preparation of magnetite/alginate/silver nanocomposite.

alginate-coated niosome-based nanocarriers was developed for the simultaneous administration of doxorubicin and cisplatin in the treatment of breast and ovarian malignancies. The cytotoxicity of the nanocarriers was investigated by MTT assay against MCF-7, A2780, and HFF cells. The IC50 value of the alginate nanocarrier was significantly lower compared to both the alginate-free formulations and the free drugs, as demonstrated by the MTT experiment. Alginate-based nanocarriers were shown to significantly enhance the rate of apoptosis induction and cell cycle arrest in MCF-7 and A2780 cancer cells, as evidenced by cellular and molecular studies. Moreover, the activity of Caspase 3/7 exhibited an increase subsequent to the administration of alginate coated niosomes in comparison to both uncoated niosomes and the drug-free condition. The combined effects of cisplatin and doxorubicin in these nanocarriers in inhibiting cell proliferation were observed in MCF-7 and A2780 cancer cells, suggesting the potential synergistic efficacy of combination chemotherapy in the treatment of ovarian and breast cancers. Also, *in vivo* research can provide further insight into the possible applications of these nanocarriers as a therapeutic agent for cancer treatment [31].

A versatile nanocomplex that combines photothermal therapy, chemotherapy, and radiotherapy was created using alginate hydrogel and co-loaded with gold nanoparticles and cisplatin. When compared to free cisplatin, the nanocomplex significantly increased tumor growth suppression and significantly increased drug delivery efficiency. When exposed to a 532-nm laser, the tumor treated with nanocomplex exhibited an enhanced rate of heating, showing the nanocomplex's capacity for photothermal conversion. The rate of tumor growth was significantly slowed down by thermo-chemotherapy, thermo-radiotherapy, and chemoradiation therapy employing this nanocomplex, but radiotherapy alone only slightly inhibited tumor growth. The nanocomplex may facilitate a trimodal thermo-chemo-radiotherapy upon 532-nm laser and 6-MV X-ray, which resulted in total tumor shrinkage with no sign of relapse throughout the 90-day follow-up period. The study's findings showed that cisplatin and gold nanoparticles added to an alginate hydrogel network can successfully combine radiation, chemotherapy, and photothermal therapy to produce a locally synergistic cancer treatment [32]. 3D-printed tablets with good drug content uniformity and selective release of oxaliplatin in the colonic environment were prepared from Eudragit L100-55 filament that contained oxaliplatin loaded alginate nanoparticles. The tablets exhibited a high level of uniformity in the drug content and demonstrated selective release of oxaliplatin within the colonic environment. An assessment was conducted to compare the antitumor efficacy of 3D-printed tablets containing nanoparticles with the administration of oxaliplatin solution intravenously and orally in CT-26 tumor-bearing mice. Additionally, compressed tablets containing oxaliplatin nanoparticles, prepared using the direct compression method with the same formulation, were also evaluated. The 3D-printed tablets containing these nanoparticles exhibited a noteworthy and similar antitumor effect to intravenous oxaliplatin solution ($p < 0.05$), while also demonstrating a superior safety profile. However, compressed tablets did not exhibit any significant antitumor effect, likely due to non-selective drug release in the stomach and upper intestine environments. This work emphasizes the potential of integrating nanotechnology and 3D printing to develop drug delivery systems specifically designed for the colon. These systems are intended to deliver chemotherapeutic drugs that exhibit favorable antitumor activity, tumor targetability, and safety profile, making them suitable for the treatment of colorectal cancer [33].

A biohybrid drug carrier consisting of sodium alginate and colloidal silica nanoparticles loaded with doxorubicin was prepared through the process of evaporation-induced self-assembly through the application of the spray-drying technique. The cytotoxicity of empty carriers and doxorubicin-loaded carriers was assessed through MTT assay in mouse lymphocytes and A549 cells, respectively. The impact of free doxorubicin on cell viability was found to be statistically insignificant at all tested doses. In contrast to free doxorubicin, the entrapment of doxorubicin in nanoparticles resulted in a notable decrease in cell viability at a concentration of 500 nM. This finding indicates that the utilization of entrapped doxorubicin within nanoparticles exhibits enhanced efficacy against cancer cells, even when administered at lower dosages (Figure 12.5) [34]. The perfect synergistic chemotherapy/chemodynamic therapy nanoplatform was prepared using doxorubicin-loaded nanogels comprising alginate and manganese ions through a microfluidic technique. The doxorubicin, which was encapsulated within the nanogels, was promptly liberated because of the pH-sensitive characteristics of alginate. This not only induces direct apoptosis of cancer cells but also significantly elevates the concentration of endogenous hydrogen peroxide. The increased concentration of hydrogen peroxide might be transformed into an adequate quantity of hydroxide (·OH) by these nanogels, which then initiate a Fenton-like reaction for the purpose of chemodynamic therapy of tumors, ultimately leading to synergistic chemodynamic therapy and chemotherapy combinations. These nanogels have the potential to stimulate a strong immunological response against cancer. This could be attributed to the fact that both chemotherapy caused by doxorubicin and chemodynamic therapy mediated by manganese ions can trigger the death of tumor cells through immunogenic mechanisms (Figure 12.6) [35].

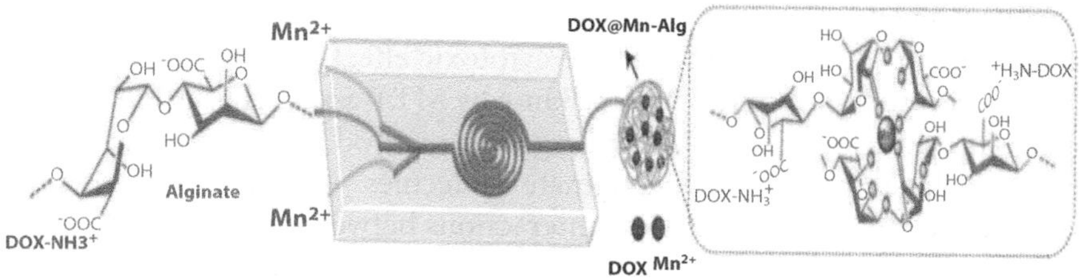

Figure 12.5 Schematic diagram of microfluidic chip to construct doxorubicin manganese alginate nanogel [34].

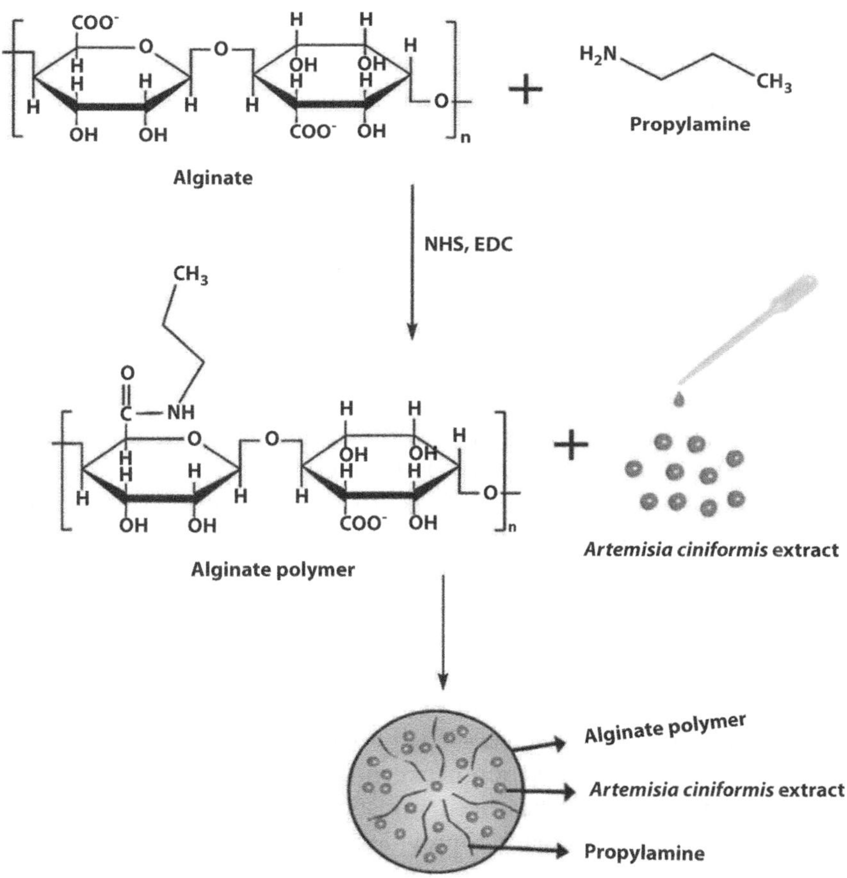

Figure 12.6 Alginate nanogel encapsulated *artemisia ciniformis* extract [35].

The alginate nanocarrier encapsulating Artemisia ciniformis extract was prepared and evaluated for the cytotoxic effects on the cell death and apoptosis induction in the AGS cell line by MTT assay. The alginate nanogel was synthesized *via* a self-aggregation method, wherein propylamine was employed to modify the alginate molecules. Alginate nanogels were synthesized by forming covalent interactions between the carboxyl groups of alginates and the amine groups of propylamine. The conversion of the hydrophilic alginate molecule into an amphipathic molecule was achieved through this process. The alginate carboxylic groups were activated using the EDC and NHS. The hydrophobic component was loaded with the plant extract. Consequently, the incorporation of a propylamine group into alginate resulted in the encapsulation of hydrophobic substances within the alginate polymer [36]. The MTT assay indicates that the cytotoxicity effects were enhanced, and the proliferative activity of the cells was reduced as a result of increasing the concentration of alginate nanogel encapsulating *A. ciniformis* and extending the treatment duration. Following an extension of the treatment duration utilizing the free extract and nanogel containing *A. ciniformis*, there was an observed augmentation in cellular apoptosis. The apoptotic response of AGS cells was shown to be less apparent when treated with nanogel alone, in comparison to the combination of extract and nanogel encapsulating *A. ciniformis*. The assessment of apoptosis in AGS cells by flow cytometry revealed that the nanogel containing the extract exhibited greater efficacy in inducing apoptosis compared to both the free extract and the nanogel alone [37].

Iron oxide–sodium alginate–thymoquinone nanocomposites were synthesized and evaluated for their cytotoxic and apoptotic potential on MDA-MB-231 cells by MTT assays, FACS-based cell cycle studies, annexin-V-PI staining, ELISA, and qRT-PCR. The cytotoxicity of nanocomposites leads to a decrease in cell growth in MDA-MB-231 cells. The FACS study revealed that the nanocomposite exhibited nuclear damage, formation of reactive oxygen species, and increased levels of annexin-V. Consequently, this led to cell cycle arrest specifically in the S phase. In the presence of PI3K-Akt-mTOR inhibitors, the nanocomposite in MDA-MB-231 cells was seen to decrease the activity of PI3K-Akt-mTOR regulatory pathways. This indicates that these regulatory pathways play a role in apoptotic cell death. The molecular interaction between thymoquinone and PI3K-Akt-mTOR receptor proteins has been investigated using *in silico* docking experiments. These investigations provide evidence that the nanocomposite effectively inhibits PI3K-Akt-mTOR signaling in MDA-MB-231 cells. Based on the findings of this work, it can be inferred that the nanocomposite exhibits inhibitory effects on the PI3K-Akt-mTOR pathway in breast cancer cell lines, hence inducing apoptotic cell death [38]. An injectable nanocomposite hydrogel that responds to pH and near-infrared light was prepared for the treatment of melanoma and the promotion of skin regeneration from biomimetic polydopamine-Fe(III)-doxorubicin and sodium alginate graft dopamine nanoparticles. The nanocomposite hydrogel can accurately transport doxorubicin to the tumor site, minimizing its loss and off-target damage. Additionally, it can convert light into heat energy when exposed to near-infrared irradiation, effectively killing cancer cells. This nanocomposite hydrogel can convert excessive endogenous hydrogen peroxide into oxygen, hence mitigating tumor hypoxia. The hydrogel shown efficacy in inhibiting the proliferation and migration of tumor cells using a combination of photothermal, chemotherapeutic, and nanozyme synergetic therapy, as evidenced by both *in vivo* and *in vitro* studies [39]. The anticancer drug paclitaxel was encapsulated more efficiently in plasmonic magnetic nanocomposites prepared from hydrophobically modified thiolated sodium alginate, amine-terminated poly butyl methacrylate, which was synthesized using free radical polymerization and iron oxide nanoparticles encased in a gold shell. The cytotoxicity of paclitaxel, paclitaxel loaded nanocomposite, and blank nanocomposite were evaluated against PLC/PRF/5 cells using MTT assay. Plasmonic magnetic nanocomposites exhibited essentially minimal toxicity to PLC/PRF/5 cells, and the cells retained around 90% of their vitality across all doses. Paclitaxel and paclitaxel-loaded plasmonic magnetic nanocomposites demonstrated a dose-dependent reduction in cell viability, with an IC-50 value of around 40 nM for paclitaxel and 35 nM for nanocomposites, respectively [40–44].

12.5 Challenges and Future Directions

Alginate-based nanoparticles hold immense potential in cancer therapy; however, several challenges must be addressed to fully realize their clinical applications. These challenges include issues related to stability, drug loading efficiency, scalability, and the complexity of tumor microenvironments. At the same time, emerging innovations offer promising solutions that pave the way for the future of alginate nanoparticles in cancer therapeutics. One significant challenge is the stability of alginate nanoparticles during storage and in physiological environments. Alginate's natural hydrophilicity and susceptibility to enzymatic degradation can lead to premature drug release or loss of functionality. While modifications such as cross-linking with calcium ions or coating with stabilizing agents improve stability, these approaches can affect the biocompatibility and release profile of the nanoparticles [45]. Future advancements in formulation strategies, including covalent crosslinking or the incorporation of hybrid materials, are expected to enhance the robustness of alginate-based systems.

Another hurdle is optimizing drug loading efficiency without compromising the structural integrity of the nanoparticles. Although alginate's carboxyl and hydroxyl groups provide ample opportunities for drug binding, the encapsulation of hydrophobic drugs remains a challenge. Strategies like chemical functionalization with hydrophobic moieties or combining alginate with amphiphilic polymers have shown promise in addressing this limitation. Further research into multi-drug encapsulation and synergistic drug delivery systems will be crucial for enhancing the versatility of alginate nanoparticles. The scalability of alginate nanoparticle production is another critical issue. Techniques like ionic gelation and emulsion methods are widely used at the laboratory scale but face challenges when translated to industrial production. Factors such as batch-to-batch variability, process reproducibility, and cost-effectiveness need to be addressed. Emerging technologies, such as spray drying, microfluidics, and 3D printing, offer scalable and reproducible solutions that can streamline large-scale manufacturing.

In addition, overcoming the complexity of tumor microenvironments remains a significant challenge. Tumors are heterogeneous, with varying pH, enzyme activity, and oxygen levels, which complicates the design of universally effective nanoparticles. Stimuli-responsive nanoparticles that release their payloads in response to specific tumor conditions (e.g., pH or redox potential) are a promising solution. However, achieving precise control over these mechanisms requires further refinement. Despite these challenges, the future of alginate nanoparticles in cancer therapy is bright. The integration of advanced technologies, such as artificial intelligence (AI) and machine learning, offers new opportunities for optimizing nanoparticle design and predicting therapeutic outcomes. AI-guided algorithms can identify optimal formulations, functionalization strategies, and release profiles, reducing the time and cost of experimental trials. Hybrid systems that combine alginate with other biopolymers, such as chitosan or hyaluronic acid, are emerging as a powerful approach to enhance the functionality of nanoparticles. These systems can simultaneously improve stability, targeting capabilities, and drug loading efficiency, making them highly versatile in addressing various therapeutic needs.

Moreover, the use of 3D printing technology for designing personalized drug delivery systems integrated with alginate nanoparticles holds immense potential. By tailoring nanoparticle formulations to the specific needs of individual patients, precision medicine can achieve higher efficacy and reduced side effects. Finally, clinical translation remains the ultimate goal. While preclinical studies have demonstrated the potential of alginate nanoparticles, large-scale clinical trials are necessary to establish their safety, efficacy, and regulatory compliance. Collaborative efforts among researchers, clinicians, and industry stakeholders will be essential to bridge the gap between laboratory research and real-world applications. In conclusion, while challenges remain in the development and application of alginate nanoparticles, ongoing innovations and interdisciplinary efforts are paving the way for their successful integration into clinical cancer therapy. By addressing current limitations and leveraging emerging technologies, alginate nanoparticles have the potential to revolutionize the field of oncology and improve patient outcomes on a global scale.

12.6 Conclusion

Alginate-based nanoparticles have emerged as a transformative tool in cancer therapy, offering solutions to some of the most persistent challenges in oncology. Their unique properties, including biocompatibility, biodegradability, and chemical versatility, enable precise drug delivery, enhanced therapeutic efficacy, and reduced systemic toxicity [45–49]. Through advancements in synthesis methods, functionalization techniques, and targeted delivery strategies, these nanoparticles have demonstrated remarkable potential in overcoming limitations associated with conventional treatments. The wide range of applications discussed, from reactive oxygen species (ROS) generation to stimuli-responsive drug release and combination therapies, highlights the versatility of alginate nanoparticles. They not only improve the delivery of chemotherapeutics but also facilitate multimodal therapies such as photothermal therapy, radiotherapy, and immunotherapy. This adaptability positions them as a cornerstone in the development of personalized and precision medicine [50–53].

Despite their advantages, challenges such as stability during storage, scalability for industrial production, and optimization of drug loading efficiency remain significant barriers. Moreover, the complexity of tumor microenvironments necessitates further refinement in the design of stimuli-responsive and hybrid systems. However, these challenges are being addressed through innovations in fabrication techniques, such as 3D printing and microfluidics, and the integration of AI for design optimization. The future prospects for alginate nanoparticles are promising. Advances in hybrid systems, combining alginate with other biopolymers or inorganic materials, are expected to enhance their functionality and broaden their applications [54–58]. Furthermore, efforts to translate preclinical successes into clinical practice will pave the way for their widespread adoption, bringing the benefits of this technology to patients worldwide. In conclusion, alginate nanoparticles represent a paradigm shift in cancer nanomedicine, bridging the gap between advanced drug delivery systems and real-world therapeutic needs [59]. As research continues to address current challenges and push the boundaries of innovation, alginate nanoparticles are poised to revolutionize cancer therapy, offering hope for more effective, targeted, and less invasive treatments in the fight against cancer.

AI disclosure statement: The author acknowledges the use of AI-based tools for minor language editing or grammatical correction. However, all intellectual contributions, analyses, and conclusions presented in this chapter are entirely the author's own.

References

1. Zia, K.M., Zia, F., Zuber, M., Rehman, S., Ahmad, M.N., Alginate based polyurethanes: A review of recent advances and perspective. *Int. J. Biol. Macromol.*, *79*, 377–387, 2015.
2. Konwarh, R., Singh, A.P., Varadarajan, V., Cho, W.C., Harnessing alginate-based nanocomposites as nucleic acid/gene delivery platforms to address diverse biomedical issues: A progressive review. *Carbohydr. Polym. Technol. Appl.*, 7, 100404, 2024.
3. Jahan, S.T., Sadat, S.M., Walliser, M., Haddadi, A., Targeted therapeutic nanoparticles: an immense promise to fight against cancer. *J. Drug Deliv.*, *2017*, 1, 9090325, 2017.
4. Dodero, A., Alberti, S., Gaggero, G., Ferretti, M., Botter, R., Vicini, S., Castellano, M., An up-to-date review on alginate nanoparticles and nanofibers for biomedical and pharmaceutical applications. *Adv. Mater. Interfaces*, *8*, 22, 2100809, 2021.
5. Boucelkha, A., Petit, E., Elboutachfaiti, R., Molinié, R., Amari, S., Yahaoui, R.Z., Production of guluronate oligosaccharide of alginate from brown algae Stypocaulon scoparium using an alginate lyase. *J. Appl. Phycol.*, *29*, 509–519, 2017.
6. Teng, K., An, Q., Chen, Y., Zhang, Y., Zhao, Y., Recent development of alginate-based materials and their versatile functions in biomedicine, flexible electronics, and environmental uses. *ACS Biomater. Sci. Eng.*, *7*, 4, 1302–1337, 2021.

7. Afshari, H., Maleki, M., Hakimian, M., Tanha, R.A., Salouti, M., Immunogenicity evaluating of the SLNs-alginate conjugate against Pseudomonas aeruginosa. *J. Immunol. Methods*, *488*, 112938, 2021.
8. Hasany, M., Talebian, S., Sadat, S., Ranjbar, N., Mehrali, M., Wallace, G.G., Mehrali, M., Synthesis, properties, and biomedical applications of alginate methacrylate (ALMA)-based hydrogels: Current advances and challenges. *Appl. Mater. Today*, *24*, 101150, 2021.
9. Budnicka, M., Sobiech, M., Kolmas, J., Luliński, P., Frontiers in ion imprinting of alkali-and alkaline-earth metal ions–Recent advancements and application to environmental, food and biomedical analysis. *TrAC, Trends Anal. Chem.*, *156*, 116711, November 2022.
10. Li, D., Wei, Z., Xue, C., Alginate-based delivery systems for food bioactive ingredients: An overview of recent advances and future trends. *Compr. Rev. Food Sci.*, *20*, 6, 5345–5369, 2021.
11. Lopes, M., Abrahim, B., Veiga, F., Seiça, R., Cabral, L.M., Arnaud, P., Ribeiro, A.J., Preparation methods and applications behind alginate-based particles. *Expert Opin. Drug Deliv.*, *14*, 6, 769–782, 2017.
12. Sosnik, A. and Seremeta, K.P., Advantages and challenges of the spray-drying technology for the production of pure drug particles and drug-loaded polymeric carriers. *Adv. Colloid Interface Sci.*, *223*, 40–54, 2015.
13. Luo, X., Su, P., Zhang, W., Raston, C.L., Microfluidic devices in fabricating nano or micromaterials for biomedical applications. *Adv. Mater. Technol.*, *4*, 12, 1900488, 2019.
14. Sarmento, B., Ribeiro, A.J., Veiga, F., Ferreira, D.C., Neufeld, R.J., Insulin-loaded nanoparticles are prepared by alginate ionotropic pre-gelation followed by chitosan polyelectrolyte complexation. *J. Nanosci. Nanotechnol.*, *7*, 8, 2833–2841, 2007.
15. Roy, A.A., Mutalik, S., Dhas, N., Unleashing the power of polymeric nanoparticles—Creative triumph against antibiotic resistance: A review. *Int. J. Biol. Macromol.*, 278, 134977, October 2024.
16. Chen, H., Govindasamy, C., Oh, D.H., Chelliah, R., Ramamoorthy, A., Rengarajan, T., Thangavelu, I., Synthesis of SnO2-Sodium alginate-polyethylene glycol-crocin nanocomposite for enhanced antimicrobial and anticancer activity. *J. Drug Deliv. Sci. Technol.*, *93*, 105449, 2024.
17. Hu, A., Alarfaj, A.A., Hirad, A.H., Veeraraghavan, V.P., Surapaneni, K.M., Hussein-Al-Ali, S.H., Elayappan, P.K., Chitosan-sodium alginate-polyethylene glycol-crocin nanocomposite treatment inhibits esophageal cancer KYSE-150 cell growth *via* inducing apoptotic cell death. *Arab. J. Chem.*, *15*, 6, 103844, 2022.
18. Huang, P., Chen, Z., Li, T., Ying, K., Xie, L., Ruan, B., Fabrication of facile assembly shrinkable double-responsive nanoparticles: Investigation of anticancer activity in lung cancer cells and apoptosis induction. *Process Biochem.*, 137, 175–186, 2024.

19. Karthikeyan, C., Varaprasad, K., Kim, S., Jangid, A.K., Lee, W., Hameed, A.S.H., Kim, K., Size-dependent cellular uptake of sodium alginate passivated tin dioxide nanoparticles in triple-negative breast cancer cells. *J. Ind. Eng. Chem.*, 123, 2023, 476–487, 2023.
20. Lin, F., Liu, H., Zhou, Q., Zhang, S., Zhou, Y., Feng, Y., Li, J., Amphiphilic alginate-based fluorescent polymer nanoparticles: Fabrication and multifunctional applications. *Int. J. Biol. Macromol.*, 258, 128957, 2024.
21. Ilhan-Ayisigi, E., Saglam-Metiner, P., Sanci, E., Bakan, B., Yildirim, Y., Buhur, A., Yesil-Celiktas, O., Receptor mediated targeting of EGF-conjugated alginate-PAMAM nanoparticles to lung adenocarcinoma: 2D/3D *in vitro* and *in vivo* evaluation. *Int. J. Biol. Macromol.*, 261, 129758, 2024.
22. Pillarisetti, S., Vijayan, V., Rangasamy, J., Bardhan, R., Uthaman, S., Park, I.K., A multistimuli responsive alginate nanogel for anticancer chemo-photodynamic therapy. *J. Ind. Eng. Chem.*, 123, 361–370, 2023.
23. Jiang, G., Mohideen, A.P., Seshadri, V.D., Rengarajan, T., Biosynthesized tin oxide-sodium alginate-polyethylene glycol-carvacrol nanocomposite shows anticancer activity on esophagus squamous carcinoma cells. *Process Biochem.*, 121, 403–412, 2022.
24. Elderdery, A.Y., Alzerwi, N.A., Alzahrani, B., Alsrhani, A., Alsultan, A., Rayzah, M., Mok, P.L., Nanocomposites of iron oxide, sodium alginate, and eugenol induce apoptosis *via* PI3K/Akt/mTOR signaling in Hep3 cells and *in vivo* hepatotoxicity in the zebrafish model. *Int. J. Biol. Macromol.*, 256, 127490, 20242024.
25. Rashidzadeh, H., Seidi, F., Ghaffarlou, M., Salehiabar, M., Charmi, J., Yaray, K., Ertas, Y.N., Preparation of alginate coated Pt nanoparticle for radiosensitization of breast cancer tumor. *Int. J. Biol. Macromol.*, 233, 123273, 20232023.
26. Geyik, G., Güncüm, E., Işıklan, N., Design and development of pH-responsive alginate-based nanogel carriers for etoposide delivery. *Int. J. Biol. Macromol.*, 250, 126242, 2023.
27. Urzedo, A.L., Gonçalves, M.C., Nascimento, M.H.M., Lombello, C.B., Nakazato, G., Seabra., A.B., Multifunctional alginate nanoparticles containing nitric oxide donor and silver nanoparticles for biomedical applications. *Mater. Sci. Eng., C*, 112, 110933, 2020.
28. Huang, J., Guo, J., Zhu, J., Zou, X., Supported silver nanoparticles over alginate-modified magnetic nanoparticles: Synthesis, characterization and treat the human lung carcinoma. *J. Saudi Chem. Soc.*, 26, 101393, 2022.
29. Mousazadeh, N., Seidi, F., Ghaffarlou, M., Rashidzadeh, H., Hosseinmirzaei, A., Mozafari, F., Nosrati, H., Silver sulfide coated alginate radioenhancer for enhanced X-ray radiation therapy of breast cancer. *Int. J. Biol. Macromol.*, 234, 23636, 2023.
30. Sharafshadeh, M.S., Tafvizi, F., Khodarahmi, P., Ehtesham, S., Preparation and physicochemical properties of cisplatin and doxorubicin encapsulated

by niosome alginate nanocarrier for cancer therapy. *Int. J. Biol. Macromol.*, 235, 123686, 2023.

31. Mirrahimi, M., Beik, J., Mirrahimi, M., Alamzadeh, Z., Teymouri, S., Mahabadi, V.P., Moustakis, C., Triple combination of heat, drug and radiation using alginate hydrogel co-loaded with gold nanoparticles and cisplatin for locally synergistic cancer therapy. *Int. J. Biol. Macromol.*, 158, 617–626, 2020.
32. Mirdamadian, S.Z., Varshosaz, J., Minaiyan, M., Taheri, A., 3D printed tablets containing oxaliplatin loaded alginate nanoparticles for colon cancer targeted delivery. An *in vitro/in vivo* study. *Int. J. Biol. Macromol.*, 205, 90–109, 2022.
33. Mishra, A., Pandey, V.K., Shankar, B.S., Melo, J.S., Spray drying as an efficient route for synthesis of silica nanoparticles-sodium alginate biohybrid drug carrier of doxorubicin. *Colloids Surf. B Biointerfaces*, 197, 111445, 2021.
34. Su, M., Zhu, Y., Chen, J., Zhang, B., Sun, C., Chen, M., Yang, X., Microfluidic synthesis of manganese-alginate nanogels with self-supplying H_2O_2 capability for synergistic chemo/chemodynamic therapy and boosting anticancer immunity. *Chem. Eng. J.*, 435, 134926, 2022.
35. Rahimivand, M., Tafvizi, F., Noorbazargan, H., Synthesis and characterization of alginate nanocarrier encapsulating Artemisia ciniformis extract and evaluation of the cytotoxicity and apoptosis induction in AGS cell line. *Int. J. Biol. Macromol.*, 158, 338–357, 2020.
36. Bourbour, M., Khayam, N., Noorbazargan, H., Yaraki, M.T., Lalami, Z.A., Akbarzadeh, I., Tan, Y.N., Evaluation of anti-cancer and anti-metastatic effects of folate-PEGylated niosomes for co-delivery of letrozole and ascorbic acid on breast cancer cells. *Mol. Syst. Des. Eng.*, 7, 9, 1102–1118, 2022.
37. Alzahrani, B., Elderdery, A.Y., Alsrhani, A., Alzerwi, N.A., Althobiti, M.M., Elkhalifa, A.M., Mok, P.L., Sodium alginate encapsulated iron oxide decorated with thymoquinone nanocomposite induces apoptosis in human breast cancer cells *via* PI3K-Akt-mTOR pathway. *Int. J. Biol. Macromol.*, 244, 125054, 2023.
38. Li, P., Li, Y., Fu, R., Duan, Z., Zhu, C., Fan, D., NIR-and pH-responsive injectable nanocomposite alginate-graft-dopamine hydrogel for melanoma suppression and wound repair. *Carbohydr. Polym.*, 314, 120899, 2023.
39. Arora, V., Sood, A., Kumari, S., Kumaran, S.S., Jain, T.K., Hydrophobically modified sodium alginate conjugated plasmonic magnetic nanocomposites for drug delivery & magnetic resonance imaging. *Mater. Today Commun.*, 25, 101470, 2020.
40. da Silva, P.B., Oliveira, R.J.A., Araújo, M., Caires, H.R., Bidarra, S.J., Barrias, C.C., An integrative alginate-based 3D *in vitro* model to explore epithelial-stromal cell dynamics in the breast tumor microenvironment. *Carbohydr. Polym.*, 342, 122363, 15 October 2024.

41. Emam, A.N., Girgis, E., Khalil, W.K., Mohamed, M.B., Toxicity of plasmonic nanomaterials and their hybrid nanocomposites, in: *Advances in Molecular Toxicology*, vol. 8, pp. 173–202, 2014.
42. Reddy, L.H., Arias, J.L., Nicolas, J., Couvreur, P., Magnetic nanoparticles: design and characterization, toxicity and biocompatibility, pharmaceutical and biomedical applications. *Chem. Rev.*, *112*, 11, 5818–5878, 2012.
43. Sotiriou, G.A., Hirt, A.M., Lozach, P.Y., Teleki, A., Krumeich, F., Pratsinis, S.E., Hybrid, silica-coated, Janus-like plasmonic-magnetic nanoparticles. *Chem. Mater.*, *23*, 7, 1985–1992, 2011.
44. Balestri, A., Cardellini, J., Berti, D., Gold and silver nanoparticles as tools to combat multidrug-resistant pathogens. *Curr. Opin. Colloid Interface Sci.*, *66*, 101710, 2023.
45. Xu, Z., Chen, L., Duan, X., Li, X., Ren, H., Microparticles based on alginate/chitosan/casein three-dimensional system for oral insulin delivery. *Polym. Adv. Technol.*, *32*, 11, 4352–4361, 2021.
46. Motwani, S.K., Chopra, S., Talegaonkar, S., Kohli, K., Ahmad, F.J., Khar, R.K., Chitosan–sodium alginate nanoparticles as submicroscopic reservoirs for ocular delivery: Formulation, optimisation and *in vitro* characterisation. *Eur. J. Pharm. Biopharm.*, *68*, 3, 513–525, 2008.
47. Kolawole, O.M., Ifeanafor, A.R., Ifade, W.A., Akinleye, M.O., Patrojanasophon, P., Silva, B.O., Osuntoki, A.A., Formulation and evaluation of paclitaxel-loaded boronated chitosan/alginate nanoparticles as a mucoadhesive system for localized cervical cancer drug delivery. *J. Drug Deliv. Sci. Technol.*, *87*, 104810, 2023.
48. Zhan, Y., Qin, S., Zeng, Y., Xu, Q., McClements, D.J., Hu, K., Pickering emulsions stabilized by egg white protein-alginate nanoparticles: Freeze-thaw stability after heating. *Food Hydrocoll.*, *150*, 109675, 2024.
49. Fatima, M., Almalki, W.H., Khan, T., Sahebkar, A., Kesharwani, P., Harnessing the Power of Stimuli-Responsive Nanoparticles as an Effective Therapeutic Drug Delivery System. *Adv. Mater.*, 36, 2312939, 2024.
50. Majumder, J. and Minko, T., Multifunctional and stimuli-responsive nanocarriers for targeted therapeutic delivery. *Expert Opin. Drug Deliv.*, *18*, 2, 205–227, 2021.
51. Ashrafizadeh, M., Saebfar, H., Gholami, M.H., Hushmandi, K., Zabolian, A., Bikarannejad, P., Mostafavi, E., Doxorubicin-loaded graphene oxide nanocomposites in cancer medicine: stimuli-responsive carriers, co-delivery and suppressing resistance. *Expert Opin. Drug Deliv.*, *19*, 4, 355–382, 2022.
52. Shi, Z., Liu, J., Tian, L., Li, J., Gao, Y., Xing, Y., Liang, C., Insights into stimuli-responsive diselenide bonds utilized in drug delivery systems for cancer therapy. *Biomed. Pharmacother.*, *155*, 113707, 2022.
53. Cook, A.B. and Decuzzi, P., Harnessing endogenous stimuli for responsive materials in theranostics. *ACS Nano*, *15*, 2, 2068–2098, 2021.
54. Maity, C. and Das, N., Alginate-based smart materials and their application: Recent advances and perspectives. *Top. Curr. Chem.*, *380*, 1, 3, 2022.

55. Pinto, L., Bonifacio, M.A., De Giglio, E., Santovito, E., Cometa, S., Bevilacqua, A., Baruzzi, F., Biopolymer hybrid materials: Development, characterization, and food packaging applications. *Food Packag. Shelf Life*, *28*, 100676, 2021.
56. Alshangiti, D.M., El-Damhougy, T.K., Zaher, A., Madani, M., Revolutionizing biomedicine: Advancements, applications, and prospects of nanocomposite macromolecular carbohydrate-based hydrogel biomaterials: A review. *RSC Adv.*, *13*, 50, 35251–35291, 2023.
57. Khan, A., Alamry, K.A., Asiri, A.M., Multifunctional biopolymers-based composite materials for biomedical applications: a systematic review. *ChemistrySelect*, *6*, 2, 154–176, 2021.
58. Zia, F., *et al.*, Alginate-based hybrid nanocomposite materials, in: *Algae Based Polymers, Blends, and Composites*, pp. 603–648, Elsevier, Radarweg, Amsterdam, Netherlands, The Boulevard, Langford Lane, Kidlington, Oxford, United Kingdom, Cambridge, United States, 2017.
59. Alvarez, M.M., Aizenberg, J., Analoui, M., Andrews, A.M., Bisker, G., Boyden, E.S., Khademhosseini, A., Emerging trends in micro-and nanoscale technologies in medicine: From basic discoveries to translation. *ACS Nano*, *11*, 6, 5195–5214, 2017.

Index

Printed and bound by CPI Group (UK) Ltd, Croydon, CR0 4YY

17/09/2026

14964265-0005